Current Trends in Otorhinolaryngology and Head and Neck Pathology

Current Trends in Otorhinolaryngology and Head and Neck Pathology

Editors

Adriana Neagos
Daniela Vrinceanu
Codrut Sarafoleanu
Mahmut Tayyar Kalcioglu

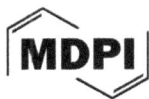 Basel • Beijing • Wuhan • Barcelona • Belgrade • Novi Sad • Cluj • Manchester

Editors

Adriana Neagos
ENT Department, George
Emil Palade University of
Medicine, Pharmacy, Science
and Technology of Targu
Mures
Tirgu Mures, Romania

Daniela Vrinceanu
ENT Department, Carol
Davila University of
Medicine and Pharmacy
Bucharest, Romania

Codrut Sarafoleanu
ENT Department, Carol
Davila University of
Medicine and Pharmacy
Bucharest, Romania

Mahmut Tayyar Kalcioglu
Chief of the Department of
ORL & HNS, Istanbul
Medeniyet University
Istanbul, Turkey

Editorial Office
MDPI
St. Alban-Anlage 66
4052 Basel, Switzerland

This is a reprint of articles from the Special Issue published online in the open access journal *Medicina* (ISSN 1648-9144) (available at: https://www.mdpi.com/journal/medicina/special_issues/489JPD1HN5).

For citation purposes, cite each article independently as indicated on the article page online and as indicated below:

Lastname, A.A.; Lastname, B.B. Article Title. *Journal Name* **Year**, *Volume Number*, Page Range.

ISBN 978-3-0365-9264-0 (Hbk)
ISBN 978-3-0365-9265-7 (PDF)
doi.org/10.3390/books978-3-0365-9265-7

© 2023 by the authors. Articles in this book are Open Access and distributed under the Creative Commons Attribution (CC BY) license. The book as a whole is distributed by MDPI under the terms and conditions of the Creative Commons Attribution-NonCommercial-NoDerivs (CC BY-NC-ND) license.

Contents

About the Editors ix

Preface xi

Daniela Vrinceanu, Codrut Sarafoleanu, Mahmut Tayyar Kalcioglu and Adriana Neagos
Multidisciplinarity and Transdisciplinarity as Current Trends in Otorhinolaryngology and Head and Neck Pathology
Reprinted from: *Medicina* 2022, 58, 1661, doi:10.3390/medicina58111661 1

Daniela Vrinceanu, Mihai Dumitru, Matei Popa-Cherecheanu, Andreea Nicoleta Marinescu, Oana-Maria Patrascu and Florin Bobirca
Extracranial Facial Nerve Schwannoma—Histological Surprise or Therapeutic Planning?
Reprinted from: *Medicina* 2023, 59, 1167, doi:10.3390/medicina59061167 3

Michał Gontarz, Jolanta Orłowska-Heitzman, Krzysztof Gąsiorowski, Jakub Bargiel, Tomasz Marecik, Paweł Szczurowski and et al.
Myoepithelial Carcinoma Arising in a Salivary Duct Cyst of the Parotid Gland: Case Presentation
Reprinted from: *Medicina* 2023, 59, 184, doi:10.3390/medicina59020184 23

Dimitrinka Kisova, Tihomir Dikov, Vesela Ivanova, Hristo Stoyanov and Greta Yordanova
Mixed Eccrine Cutaneous Tumor with Folliculo–Sebaceous Differentiation: Case Report and Literature Review
Reprinted from: *Medicina* 2023, 59, 1465, doi:10.3390/medicina59081465 29

Cosmin Ioan Faur, Mădălina Anca Moldovan, Mădălina Văleanu, Horațiu Rotar, Laura Filip and Rareș Călin Roman
The Prevalence and Treatment Costs of Non-Melanoma Skin Cancer in Cluj-Napoca Maxillofacial Center
Reprinted from: *Medicina* 2023, 59, 220, doi:10.3390/medicina59020220 39

Balica Nicolae Constantin, Trandafir Cornelia Marina, Stefanescu Horatiu Eugen, Enatescu Ileana and Gluhovschi Adrian
Tongue Base Ectopic Thyroid Tissue—Is It a Rare Encounter?
Reprinted from: *Medicina* 2023, 59, 313, doi:10.3390/medicina59020313 53

Constantin Stan, Laszlo Peter Ujvary, Cristina Maria Blebea, Doinița Vesa, Mihai Ionuț Tănase, Mara Tănase and et al.
Sheep's Head as an Anatomic Model for Basic Training in Endoscopic Sinus Surgery
Reprinted from: *Medicina* 2023, 59, 1792, doi:10.3390/medicina59101792 61

Irina-Gabriela Ionita, Viorel Zainea, Catalina Voiosu, Cristian Dragos Stefanescu, Cristina Aura Panea, Adrian Vasile Dumitru and et al.
Management of Capillary Hemangioma of the Sphenoid Sinus
Reprinted from: *Medicina* 2023, 59, 858, doi:10.3390/medicina59050858 71

Do Hyun Kim, Jun-Beom Park, Sung Won Kim, Gulnaz Stybayeva and Se Hwan Hwang
Effect of Infraorbital and/or Infratrochlear Nerve Blocks on Postoperative Care in Patients with Septorhinoplasty: A Meta-Analysis
Reprinted from: *Medicina* 2023, 59, 1659, doi:10.3390/medicina59091659 83

Ana Maria Vlad, Cristian Dragos Stefanescu, Iemima Stefan, Viorel Zainea and
Razvan Hainarosie
Comparative Efficacy of Velopharyngeal Surgery Techniques for Obstructive Sleep Apnea: A Systematic Review
Reprinted from: *Medicina* 2023, *59*, 1147, doi:10.3390/medicina59061147 97

Trandafir Cornelia Marina, Balica Nicolae Constantin, Baderca Flavia, Sarau Oana Silvana,
Poenaru Marioara and Cristian Andrei Sarau
Olfactory Neuroblastoma—A Challenging Fine Line between Metastasis and Hematology
Reprinted from: *Medicina* 2023, *59*, 731, doi:10.3390/medicina59040731 113

Ana Maria Vlad, Cristian Dragos Stefanescu, Catalina Voiosu and Razvan Hainarosie
The Role of Inverted Papilloma Surgical Removal for Sleep Apnea Treatment Success—A Case Report
Reprinted from: *Medicina* 2023, *59*, 444, doi:10.3390/medicina59030444 123

Veronica Epure, Razvan Hainarosie and Dan Cristian Gheorghe
Efficacy of Continuous Suctioning in Adenoidectomy Haemostasis—Clinical Study
Reprinted from: *Medicina* 2023, *59*, 1534, doi:10.3390/medicina59091534 133

Mihai Dumitru, Daniela Vrinceanu, Bogdan Banica, Romica Cergan,
Iulian-Alexandru Taciuc, Felicia Manole and Matei Popa-Cherecheanu
Management of Aesthetic and Functional Deficits in Frontal Bone Trauma
Reprinted from: *Medicina* 2022, *58*, 1756, doi:10.3390/ medicina58121756 145

Florentina Severin, Andrei-Mihail Rosu, Mirela Tiglis, Laura-Elisabeta Checherita,
Gina Stegaru, Mihail Dan Cobzeanu, Razvan Hainarosie and et al.
Multidisciplinary Therapeutic Management in Complex Cervical Trauma
Reprinted from: *Medicina* 2023, *59*, 596, doi:10.3390/medicina59030596 155

Andrei-Mihail Roșu, Florentina Severin, Oana Cristina Roșu, Bogdan Mihail Cobzeanu,
Stefan Gherasimescu, Florin Petrică Sava and et al.
Patterns and Characteristics of Midface Fractures in North-Eastern Romania
Reprinted from: *Medicina* 2023, *59*, 510, doi:10.3390/medicina59030510 169

Cornelia M. Trandafir, Nicolae Constantin Balica, Delia I. Horhat, Ion C. Mot,
Cristian A. Sarau and Marioara Poenaru
Granulomatosis with Polyangiitis (GPA)—A Multidisciplinary Approach of a Case Report
Reprinted from: *Medicina* 2022, *58*, 1837, doi:10.3390/medicina58121837 181

Adeline Josephine Cumpata, Dragos Peptanariu, Ana-Lacramioara Lungoci,
Luminita Labusca, Mariana Pinteala and Luminita Radulescu
Towards Regenerative Audiology: Immune Modulation of Adipose-Derived Mesenchymal Cells Preconditioned with Citric Acid-Coated Antioxidant-Functionalized Magnetic Nanoparticles
Reprinted from: *Medicina* 2023, *59*, 587, doi:10.3390/medicina59030587 191

Violeta Necula, Alma Aurelia Maniu, László-Péter Ujváry, Maximilian-George Dindelegan,
Mara Tănase, Mihai Tănase and et al.
Vertigo Associated with Otosclerosis and Stapes Surgery—A Narrative Review
Reprinted from: *Medicina* 2023, *59*, 1485, doi:10.3390/medicina59081485 209

Leo De Raeve, Marinela-Carmen Cumpăt, Aimée van Loo, Isabel Monteiro Costa,
Maria Assunção Matos, João Canossa Dias and et al.
Quality Standard for Rehabilitation of Young Deaf Children Receiving Cochlear Implants
Reprinted from: *Medicina* 2023, *59*, 1354, doi:10.3390/medicina59071354 221

Iemima Stefan, Cristian Dragos Stefanescu, Ana Maria Vlad, Viorel Zainea and Răzvan Hainarosie
Postoperative Outcomes of Endoscopic versus Microscopic Myringoplasty in Patients with Chronic Otitis Media—A Systematic Review
Reprinted from: *Medicina* **2023**, *59*, 1074, doi:10.3390/medicina59061074 . . . . **235**

Dan Cristian Gheorghe, Veronica Epure, Doru Oprea and Adina Zamfir-Chiru-Anton
Persistent Stapedial Artery, Oval Window Atresia and Congenital Stapes Agenesis—Case Report
Reprinted from: *Medicina* **2023**, *59*, 461, doi:10.3390/medicina59030461 . . . . **247**

About the Editors

Adriana Neagos

Is an Associate Professor of ENT and HNS Surgery, Head of the ENT Department in Targu Mures, Romania. She has a continous ENT practice since 1997. Doctor Neagos is one of the ENT Specialists focusing on Ear Surgery. Also leads one of the most complex private Sleep Clinics in Romania. She has an interest in ENT pathology, imaging modalities, sleep apnea and quality of life, allergic reactions, implants in ENT and head and neck pathology, cochlear implants, ear surgery, artificial intelligence, and translation of interdisciplinary management into current practice. Currently Associate Professor Neagos defended her habilitation thesis enabling her to train future young PhD students.

Daniela Vrinceanu

Is an Associate Professor of ENT and HNS Surgery, Head of the ENT Department at Bucharest University Emergency Hospital. The beginning of her academic career from 1998 till 2006 as assitant professor in the Physiology Department at Carol Davila University of Medicine and Pharmacy, Bucharest, Romania. Since 2004 Doctor Vrinceau developed the ENT Department from Bucharest University Emergency Hospital. Doctor Vrinceanu defended her PhD thesis in 2007. Since 2022 is responsible for resident training. Doctor Vrinceanu wrote 4 books and more than 30 articles with impact factor. Doctor Vrinceanu is an active reviewer for more than 5 journals indexed in international databases. Moreover she organised more than 7 interdisciplinary conference with an interest in oncology—head and neck surgery, artificial intelligence, interdisciplinary management into current practice, rhinology, and allergy.

Codrut Sarafoleanu

Is Professor of ENT and HNS Surgery, Head of ENT Department at Saint Mary Clinical Hospital in Bucharest. He is a member of the Senate of the University since 2008. Also held the position of Underdean of the Faculty of Dental Medicine between 2008-2016. Till present he is General Secretary of Romanian Rhinologic Society and Founding Member since 2010. Member of the General Comitte of the European Rhinologic Society and ENT Societas Latina. Moreover he is Editor in Chief at the Journal of Romanian Rhinologic Society. Organiser of more than 10 international ENT conferences and more than 15 hands-on endoscopic sinus surgery courses. Professor Sarafoleanu is also Associated Professor at the University of Medicine N. Testimitianu from Chisinau. He is leading PhD research since 2010 with an interest in imaging, allergy, rhinology and skull base, treatment of ENT pathology, interdisciplinary management into current practice, implants in ENT and head and neck pathology, and sleep medicine.

Mahmut Tayyar Kalcioglu

Is a Professor of ENT and HNS Surgery, Chief of the Department of ORL & HNS, Istanbul Medeniyet University, Istanbul, Turkey. Professor Kalcioglu published more than 4 books on ENT subjects and more than 50 articles indexed in international databases with impact factor. Moreover he was involved in more than 15 research grants. Currently is editor at more than 9 medical journals with an interest in ENT pathology treatment, imaging ENT, sleep aprea, allergy, implants in ENT and head and neck pathology, artificial intelligence, cochlear implant, and ear surgery. Profesor Kalcioglu is board member of European Union of Medical Specialists ORL Board since 2016. Proof to the high level of research is the H-index of 19 with almost 1000 citations in Web of Science.

Preface

This Special Issue, entitled "Current Trends in Otorhinolaryngology and Head and Neck Pathology", aimed to illustrate, from an interdisciplinary point of view, complex aspects of ENT practice. There are 22 interesting materials that cover almost all fields of activity of otorhinolaryngologists: head and neck tumors, cranio-facial and cervical trauma, rhinology, and ear pathology. The topics of the materials range from surgical approaches in multidisciplinary teams to experimental techniques in ENT pathology and very rare clinical cases. The authors are renowned specialists from different countries all over the world. The conclusion of this Special Issue is that complex cases can be solved only in trained interdisciplinary teams, and this is the future of ENT practice. We welcome suggestions on behalf of our readers.

Adriana Neagos, Daniela Vrinceanu, Codrut Sarafoleanu, and Mahmut Tayyar Kalcioglu
Editors

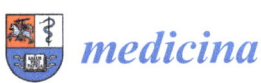

Editorial

Multidisciplinarity and Transdisciplinarity as Current Trends in Otorhinolaryngology and Head and Neck Pathology

Daniela Vrinceanu [1,*], Codrut Sarafoleanu [1], Mahmut Tayyar Kalcioglu [2] and Adriana Neagos [3,*]

1 ENT Department, Carol Davila University of Medicine and Pharmacy, 020021 Bucharest, Romania
2 Department of ORL & HNS, Istanbul Medeniyet University, 34720 Istanbul, Turkey
3 ENT Department, George Emil Palade University of Medicine, Pharmacy, Science and Technology of Targu Mures, 540142 Targu Mures, Romania
* Correspondence: vrinceanudana@yahoo.com (D.V.); neagos.adriana@gmail.com (A.N.)

The specialty of otorhinolaryngology and cervicofacial surgery has experienced accelerated development in recent decades through the development of the techniques and technologies involved. Thus, from the classic image of the ENT specialist who operated on tonsils and adenoids during in-office procedures in the late 1970s, we have reached a type of ENT specialist and surgeon who tackles difficult and complex fields and pathologies, continuously exceeding the predefined limits of the specialty. A significant challenge for otolaryngologists was the COVID-19 pandemic and the infection with the SARS-CoV-2 virus; in this context, our specialty is at the entrance gate of the virus, generating new clinical pictures but also developmental directions for topical nasal vaccines, assuming and continuing collaboration with infectious disease specialists [1]. Endoscopic rhinosinusal surgery and neuro-navigation systems have progressively pushed the limits of endonasal surgery, especially for sinonasal tumors and transnasal surgery, which involves the skull base approach and working with a neurosurgeon [2]. Obstructive sleep apnea syndrome (OSA) involves teams with a pulmonologist, maxillofacial surgeon, and ENT surgeon, with results that lead to an increase in the quality of life of our patients [3].

Associated with classically approached head and neck pathology, several chapters of pathology are considered "no man's land" and addressed by several surgical specialties. An example is the infratemporal fossa approach, frequently shared between the neurosurgeon, the maxillofacial surgeon, and the ENT surgeon. Another example is cervicofacial vascular malformations, a delicate chapter often burdened with disappointments and limitations shared between the vascular surgeon, maxillofacial surgeon, ENT surgeon, and plastic surgeon. Craniofacial and cervical trauma involves, due to the loco-regional anatomical and functional adjacencies, a multidisciplinary approach because it involves an ENT surgeon, maxillofacial surgeon, ophthalmologist, neurosurgeon, plastic surgeon, vascular surgeon, thoracic surgeon, and anesthesiologist. Thyroid surgery has to be completed together with an endocrinologist and sometimes with a thoracic surgeon [4].

Of course, the most complex field that constantly transcends boundaries is represented by head and neck oncology. Head and neck oncological surgery with tumor ablative time and reconstructive time to limit aesthetic and functional deficits requires joint-trained teams involving all types of surgeons already mentioned, along with an anesthetist, imager, and pathologist [5]. Adjuvant or neoadjuvant therapy involves tumor boarding with an oncologist, radiotherapist, speech therapist, and psychologist, and the list is permanently open [6].

In solving complex cases, a single surgical specialty is seldom enough. It is necessary to develop a multidisciplinary perspective, which involves bringing together several skills in diagnosing and treating a patient. However, multidisciplinarity goes beyond gathering consultations from several specialties in a given case, an undoubtedly important aspect from a medico-legal point of view, but also finding an optimal therapeutic solution. Modern

Citation: Vrinceanu, D.; Sarafoleanu, C.; Kalcioglu, M.T.; Neagos, A. Multidisciplinarity and Transdisciplinarity as Current Trends in Otorhinolaryngology and Head and Neck Pathology. *Medicina* **2022**, *58*, 1661. https://doi.org/10.3390/medicina58111661

Received: 31 October 2022
Accepted: 15 November 2022
Published: 16 November 2022

Publisher's Note: MDPI stays neutral with regard to jurisdictional claims in published maps and institutional affiliations.

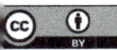

Copyright: © 2022 by the authors. Licensee MDPI, Basel, Switzerland. This article is an open access article distributed under the terms and conditions of the Creative Commons Attribution (CC BY) license (https://creativecommons.org/licenses/by/4.0/).

pathology requires transdisciplinary case-solving, which represents the integration of skills introduced by mixed teams of different specialists that address head and neck pathology without going beyond the legal limits of medical practice that define malpraxis [7]. The multidisciplinary teams acquire training over time, according to the solution of the cases, learning from each other from successes and cases with a less favorable evolution. In essence, multidisciplinarity also includes the ability to see the patient through the eyes of a colleague from another specialty; to intraoperative mobility with successive operating times; to sequenced treatment stages with the essential aim of identifying the optimal therapeutic solution, often individualized for each patient, because certainly many minds think better than one.

We proposed that the multidisciplinary and transdisciplinary approach to head and neck pathology be the theme of this Special Issue entitled "Current trends in Otorhinolaryngology and Head and Neck pathology". We invite specialists in this pathology to cross the borders between specialties, submit research articles to share clinical and surgical experience, generate discussions that lead to progress, and enrich our daily practice.

Author Contributions: Conceptualization, D.V., C.S., M.T.K. and A.N.; methodology, D.V., C.S., M.T.K. and A.N.; software, D.V., C.S., M.T.K. and A.N.; validation, D.V., C.S., M.T.K. and A.N.; formal analysis, D.V., C.S., M.T.K. and A.N.; investigation, D.V., C.S., M.T.K. and A.N.; resources, D.V., C.S., M.T.K. and A.N.; data curation, D.V., C.S., M.T.K. and A.N.; writing—original draft preparation, D.V., C.S., M.T.K. and A.N.; writing—review and editing, D.V., C.S., M.T.K. and A.N.; visualization, D.V., C.S., M.T.K. and A.N.; supervision, D.V., C.S., M.T.K. and A.N.; project administration, D.V., C.S., M.T.K. and A.N.; funding acquisition, D.V., C.S., M.T.K. and A.N. All authors have read and agreed to the published version of the manuscript.

Funding: This research received no external funding.

Institutional Review Board Statement: Not applicable.

Informed Consent Statement: Not applicable.

Data Availability Statement: Not applicable.

Conflicts of Interest: The authors declare no conflict of interest.

References

1. El-Anwar, M.W.; Elzayat, S.; Fouad, Y.A. ENT manifestation in COVID-19 patients. *Auris Nasus Larynx* **2020**, *47*, 559–564. [CrossRef] [PubMed]
2. Vrinceanu, D.; Dumitru, M.; Patrascu, O.M.; Costache, A.; Papacocea, T.; Cergan, R. Current diagnosis and treatment of rhinosinusal aspergilloma (Review). *Exp. Med.* **2021**, *22*, 1264. [CrossRef] [PubMed]
3. Neagos, A.; Vrinceanu, D.; Dumitru, M.; Costache, A.; Cergan, R. Demographic, anthropometric, and metabolic characteristics of obstructive sleep apnea patients from Romania before the COVID-19 pandemic. *Exp. Med.* **2021**, *22*, 1487. [CrossRef] [PubMed]
4. Díez, J.J.; Galofré, J.C. Thyroid cancer patients' view of clinician professionalism and multidisciplinary approach to their management. *J. Multidiscip. Healthc.* **2021**, *14*, 1053–1061. [CrossRef] [PubMed]
5. Winters, D.A.; Soukup, T.; Sevdalis, N.; Green, J.S.; Lamb, B.W. The cancer multidisciplinary team meeting: In need of change? History, challenges and future perspectives. *BJU Int.* **2021**, *128*, 271–279. [CrossRef] [PubMed]
6. Chang, Y.L.; Lin, C.Y.; Kang, C.J.; Liao, C.T.; Chung, C.F.; Yen, T.C.; Peng, H.L.; Chen, S.C. Association between multidisciplinary team care and the completion of treatment for oral squamous cell carcinoma: A cohort population-based study. *Eur. J. Cancer Care* **2021**, *30*, e13367. [CrossRef] [PubMed]
7. Choi, B.C.; Pak, A.W. Multidisciplinarity, interdisciplinarity and transdisciplinarity in health research, services, education and policy: 1. Definitions, objectives, and evidence of effectiveness. *Clin. Investig. Med.* **2006**, *29*, 351–364.

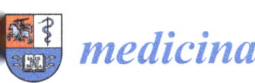

Review

Extracranial Facial Nerve Schwannoma—Histological Surprise or Therapeutic Planning?

Daniela Vrinceanu [1], Mihai Dumitru [1,*], Matei Popa-Cherecheanu [2,*], Andreea Nicoleta Marinescu [3], Oana-Maria Patrascu [4] and Florin Bobirca [5]

1. ENT Department, Carol Davila University of Medicine and Pharmacy, 050472 Bucharest, Romania; vrinceanudana@yahoo.com
2. Department of Cardiovascular Surgery, "Prof. Dr. Agrippa Ionescu" Emergency Clinical Hospital, 011356 Bucharest, Romania
3. Radiology Department, Carol Davila University of Medicine and Pharmacy, 020021 Bucharest, Romania; andreea_marinescu2003@yahoo.com
4. Department of Pathology, Carol Davila University of Medicine and Pharmacy, 050096 Bucharest, Romania; oanamaria.patrascu@gamil.com
5. Department of Surgery, Carol Davila University of Medicine and Pharmacy, 011437 Bucharest, Romania; florin.bobirca@umfcd.ro
* Correspondence: orldumitrumihai@yahoo.com (M.D.); matei.cherecheanu@gmail.com (M.P.-C.)

Abstract: Schwannomas (neurilemomas) are benign, slow-growing, encapsulated, white, yellow, or pink tumors originating in Schwann cells in the sheaths of cranial nerves or myelinated peripheral nerves. Facial nerve schwannomas (FNS) can form anywhere along the course of the nerve, from the pontocerebellar angle to the terminal branches of the facial nerve. In this article, we propose a review of the specialized literature regarding the diagnostic and therapeutic management of schwannomas of the extracranial segment of the facial nerve, also presenting our experience in this type of rare neurogenic tumor. The clinical exam reveals pretragial swelling or retromandibular swelling, the extrinsic compression of the lateral oropharyngeal wall like a parapharyngeal tumor. The function of the facial nerve is generally preserved due to the eccentric growth of the tumor pushing on the nerve fibers, and the incidence of peripheral facial paralysis in FNSs is described in 20–27% of cases. Magnetic Resonance Imaging (MRI) examination is the gold standard and describes a mass with iso signal to muscle on T1 and hyper signal to muscle on T2 and a characteristic "darts sign." The most practical differential diagnoses are pleomorphic adenoma of the parotid gland and glossopharyngeal schwannoma. The surgical approach to FNSs requires an experienced surgeon, and radical ablation by extracapsular dissection with preservation of the facial nerve is the gold standard for the cure. The patient's informed consent is important regarding the diagnosis of schwannoma and the possibility of facial nerve resection with reconstruction. Frozen section intraoperative examination is necessary to rule out malignancy or when sectioning of the facial nerve fibers is necessary. Alternative therapeutic strategies are imaging monitoring or stereotactic radiosurgery. The main factors which are considered during the management are the extension of the tumor, the presence or not of facial palsy, the experience of the surgeon, and the patient's options.

Keywords: schwannoma; facial nerve; extracranial; facial palsy; surgery; histology

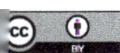

1. Introduction

Schwannomas (neurilemomas) were first described by Virchow in 1908. They are benign, slow-growing, encapsulated, white, yellow, or pink tumors originating in Schwann cells in the sheaths of cranial nerves or myelinated peripheral nerves. Their capsule continues directly with the epinerve. Occasionally, they may show calcifications or cystic degeneration [1].

One in four schwannomas originates in the nerve structures of the head and neck. When located in the head and neck, most schwannomas involve the facial nerve. Facial nerve schwannomas (FNS) can form anywhere along the course of the nerve, from the pontocerebellar angle to the terminal branches of the facial nerve. They are rare tumors, representing less than 1% of schwannomas. Many are located in the intratemporal region, and only 9% involve the extratemporal segment [2].

Of all FNS, approximately 9% occur in the intraparotid segment. Intraparotid FNSs represent 0.2–1.5% of all facial nerve tumors. Caughey et al., in a 38-year retrospective study of FNS involving the parotid gland, found 3722 patients with schwannoma, of whom 29 were FNS and only eight involved the parotid segment of the facial nerve [3].

Since it is a rare type of tumor, it is relatively difficult to standardize diagnostic and therapeutic management. In this article, we propose a review of the specialized literature regarding the diagnostic and therapeutic management of schwannomas of the extracranial segment of the facial nerve. Also, we present our experience with this type of rare neurogenic tumor. Articles in the English language about the management of FNS have been selected and critically reviewed. When we searched for facial nerve schwannoma, we found 3179 results. When we added the extracranial segment, there were 51 results, and when we used intraparotid facial nerve schwannoma, we found 84 results.

2. Anatomical Reminder

It is important to remember that three distinct segments of the extracranial portion of the facial nerve are described: retro parotid segment, intraparotid segment, and extra parotid segment. The retroparotid segment is the shortest (10–12 mm), but it is the most important from a surgical point of view because it is discovered at this level [4]. It exits the skull through the stylomastoid foramen with an antero-infero-external trajectory. It crosses the external face of the styloid apophysis and the styloid diaphragm between the posterior belly of the digastric (external) and the stylohyoid muscle (internal), finally reaching the parotid gland (Figure 1). The intraparotid segment is approximately 2 cm long and projects to the skin on a line that joins the earlobe to the wing of the nose. This segment has an anterior and external course, becoming shallower at the ramification [5]. It crosses the external carotid artery, passing laterally. Afterward, it encounters the external jugular vein—near the posterior margin of the mandible. There, it classically divides into two terminal branches—the temporofacial branch and the cervicofacial branch (Figure 2). Davis et al. were the first to describe the branching variability of the facial nerve plexus and propose a classification [6]. Last year Poutoglidis et al. published a systematic review of the branching patterns of the facial nerve, concluding that type III is the most common branching pattern instead of type I according to the Davis classification [7]. The complexity of these branching patterns creates a difficult field for the surgeon to orient and dissect the facial nerve inside the parotid gland. Recently immunohistochemistry studies showed that the fibers traveling inside the postparotid terminal cranial nerve VII branch connections are not exclusively motor, and this could explain synkinesis after surgery [8]. The branching pattern of the facial nerve is of extreme importance also in the newer techniques for facial reanimation surgery using the nerve fibers supplying the zygomaticus major muscle [9]. One of the rarest branching patterns is that of double main trunks FN, not mentioned in the Davis classification system [10].

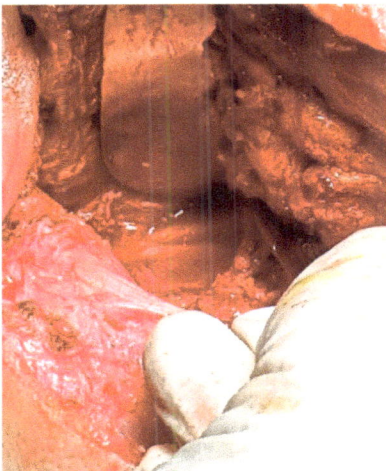

Figure 1. Intraoperative view of the right facial nerve trunk on the external face of the right styloid process, after ablation of a facial nerve schwannoma in the retro parotid segment of the nerve, with preservation of the nerve trunk.

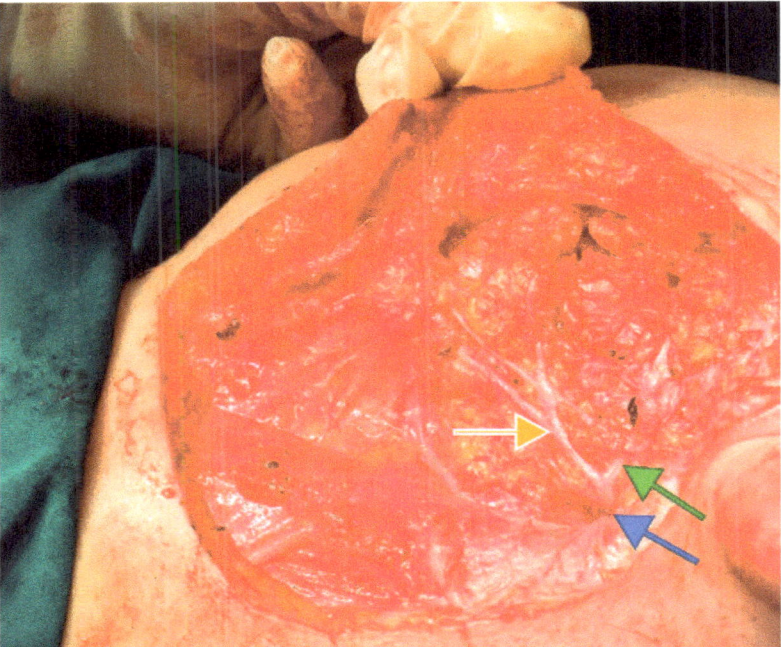

Figure 2. The trunks and branches of the facial nerve, after superficial parotidectomy. Shown here are the trunk of the facial nerve (blue arrow), which bifurcates into the temporal-facial branch (green arrow), and the cervicofacial branch (yellow arrow).

The pharyngeal extension of the parotid gland can extend into the parapharyngeal space and displace the pharyngeal wall when a tumor develops at this level [11]. Schwannomas of the extracranial segment of the facial nerve can extend into the infratemporal fossa. The infratemporal fossa represents an irregular, retro maxillary space, bordered as follows: superiorly by the greater wing of the sphenoid (medial) and by the squama temporal (lateral); medial to the lateral surface of the lateral blade of the pterygoid process; anterior to the posterior wall of the maxillary sinus; inferior has direct communication with the neck and is partially closed by the medial pterygoid muscle [12]. The parapharyngeal space and infratemporal fossa can be occupied by schwannomas developed from the extracranial portion of the facial nerve, especially from the retroparotid portion or the deep parotid lobe [13].

3. The Clinical Picture of Extracranial FNSs

The clinical picture of the extracranial segment of FNS is uncharacteristic, and only 20% of patients show symptoms because the tumor has slow growth and a late clinical onset [14]. The clinical picture can be represented by a painless preauricular swelling or by a tumor of the deep parotid lobe with a clinical picture like that of a parapharyngeal tumor (Figure 3). In this context, through the development of the tumor in the parapharyngeal space or the infratemporal fossa through the compression of the Eustachian tube, we can clinically encounter a picture of chronic serous otitis [15]. In the variant of FNS that develops at the level of the stylomastoid foramen concerning the trunk of the facial nerve, it is possible to deform the lower wall of the bony external auditory canal (tympanic bone) with canalicular stenosis and hearing loss (Figure 4). Also, the tumor can become, after a certain period of evolution, palpable as retroangulomandibular swelling (Figure 5). Although it is a tumor that develops from the facial nerve sheath, the function of the facial nerve is generally preserved due to the eccentric growth of the tumor pushing on the nerve fibers and, secondarily, the ability of the parotid gland to accommodate the growth of the tumor. The incidence of peripheral facial paralysis in FNS is described in the literature as between 20–27% of cases [16].

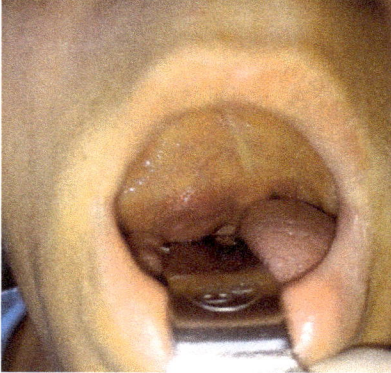

Figure 3. Right parotid deep lobe schwannoma, with clinical presentation of right parapharyngeal tumor, with bulging at the level of the right oropharynx and pushing the right palatine tonsil downward and anteriorly.

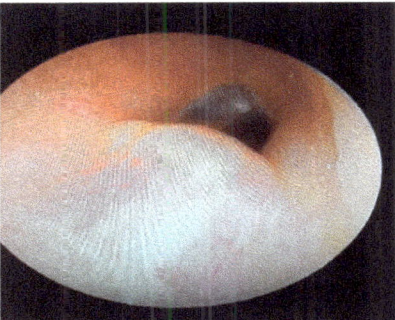

Figure 4 Otic endoscopy view of the right ear in a patient with a right deep parotid lobe tumor pushing and deforming the inferior wall of the right external auditory canal with secondary canal stenosis.

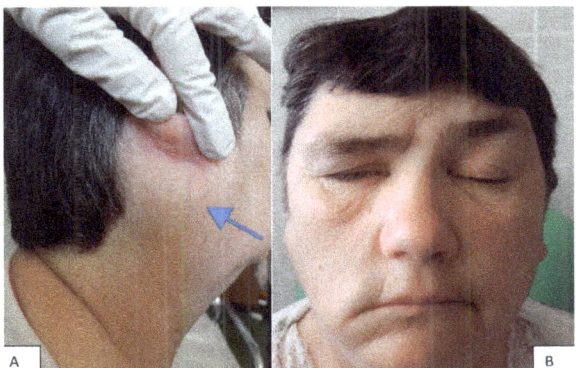

Figure 5. (**A**). Clinical appearance for right deep parotid lobe tumor, with right retroangulomandibular swelling (arrow). (**B**). Right peripheral facial paresis, more than 6 months old.

4. Imagery in Extracranial FNSs

Imaging is essential for therapeutic planning. Contrast-enhanced cervical CT scan shows an inhomogeneous, well-circumscribed lesion and may reveal compression bone lysis lesions (Figures 6 and 7). Detailed information can be provided by the CT scan of the temporal bone, which can highlight FNS development at the level of the stylomastoid foramen with secondary changes induced in the mastoid portion of the facial nerve (Figure 8). MRI examination is the gold standard in the formulation of high suspicion of schwannoma even before performing any fine needle aspiration cytology (FNAC) maneuver or any surgical exploration [17]. MRI examination describes a mass with iso signal to muscle on T1 and hyper signal to muscle on T2 [18]. The "darts sign" is characteristic, with a weak central signal and high peripheral signal in T2, being suggestive of benign or malignant neurogenic tumors (Figures 9 and 10). Carotid angiography [19] can be useful in large tumors, having an exploratory purpose, and in selected cases, with voluminous tumors, it can also have a therapeutic purpose through preoperative selective embolization (Figures 11 and 12).

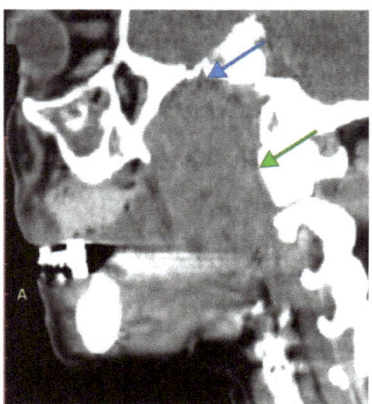

Figure 6. Cervical CT view in the sagittal plane showing an extensive facial nerve schwannoma in the right infratemporal fossa, retro maxillary, with the upper pole in contact with the base of the skull (blue arrow) and the posterior pole in the prevertebral plane (green arrow).

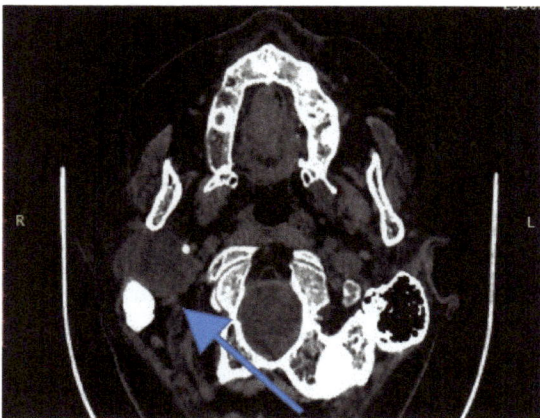

Figure 7. Contrast-enhanced cervical CT view showing deep lobe tumor of the right parotid gland, with extension into the right infratemporal fossa widening the distance between the styloid process and the mastoid process of the temporal bone (arrow).

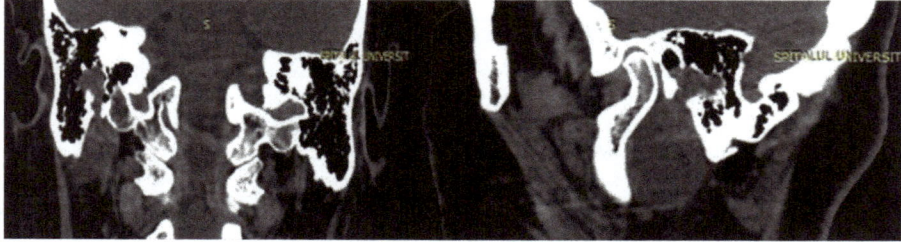

Figure 8. Temporal bone CT showing facial nerve schwannoma developed at the level of the stylomastoid foramen with minimal extension into the mastoid segment of the facial nerve (coronal and sagittal sections).

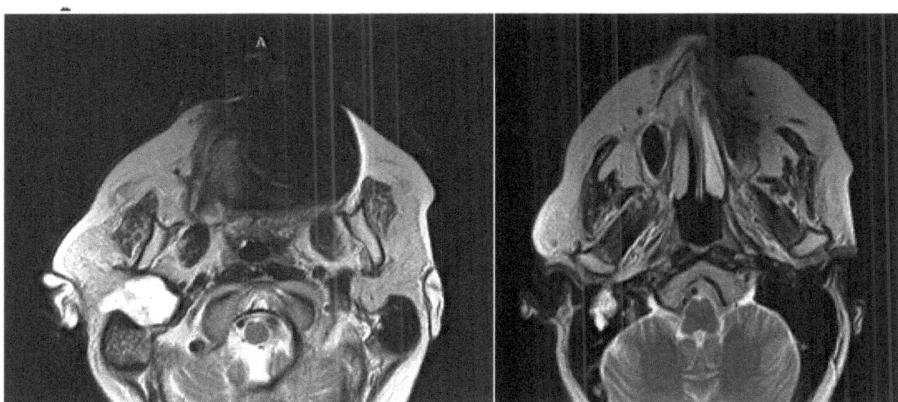

Figure 9. Cervical MRI depicting a deep lobe tumor of the right parotid gland with schwannoma histology after surgery, with extension in the right infratemporal fossa towards the stylomastoid foramen (axial sections).

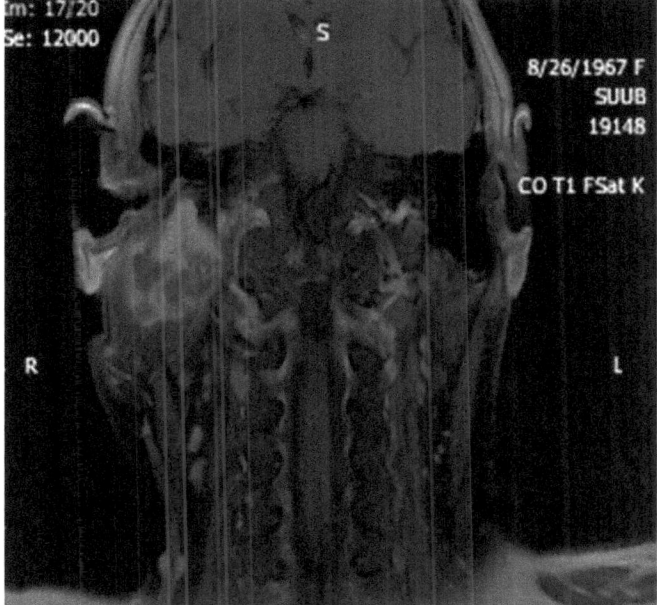

Figure 10. MRI appearance of a nonhomogeneous tumor developed at the level of the right stylomastoid foramen, with an appearance suggestive of a schwannoma of the right facial nerve (coronal section).

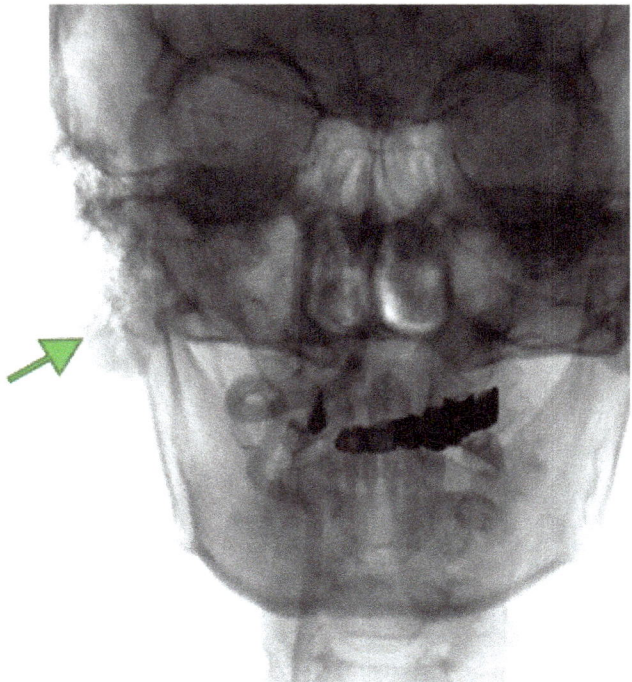

Figure 11. Right carotid angiography, with tumoral blush (green arrow) at the level of a facial nerve schwannoma of the right deep parotid lobe, with the normal angiographic appearance of the carotid system, in the image showing a normal route of the right occipital artery that is in contact with lower tumor pole.

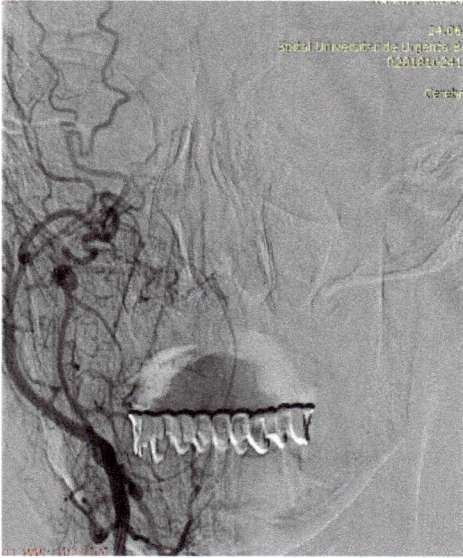

Figure 12. Right carotid angiography with tumor blush in a patient with voluminous facial nerve schwannoma extending into the right infratemporal fossa.

Ultrasound examination is insufficient for diagnosis, as well as for preparation for surgery, but it can be useful in raising the suspicion of a tumor of the deep parotid lobe and in the dimensional monitoring of an already detected tumor [20]. FNAC, which is a common procedure to treat tumoral pathology of the parotid gland, does not bring the same benefit in FNS, even performed under ultrasound guidance, being burdened by the risk of damaging the facial nerve threads and inconclusive results which, in any case, do not change the need for surgical exploration and obtaining a significant sample for histological diagnosis [21]. Of course, under the conditions of an experienced surgeon-pathologist team, FNAC can bring significant diagnostic benefits. Essentially, in the absence of histology, preoperative diagnosis is practically impossible if there is only a high suspicion of schwannoma following the MRI examination and especially if there is also clinical peripheral facial palsy.

5. Histology

Histology is the only one that provides the diagnosis with certainty, the result being, sometimes, surprising for a tumor of the deep parotid lobe. On macroscopic examination, FNSs appear as a well-defined cystic mass with a smooth surface and a variety of colors (yellowish, pinkish, grayish-white, reddish) and, in some cases, lobulated (Figures 13 and 14). From a histological point of view, two types of areas are described in FNS: Antoni A areas are hypercellular areas with elongated, fusiform cells, with nuclei aligned in the palisade and Verocay bodies (acellular zones, located between the nuclear palisades) and Antoni B areas are hypocellular, with cellular pleiomorphism, without a palisade aspect for the nuclei [22]. Both types of areas are found in different proportions in FNS (Figures 15 and 16). Nerve fibers (axons of the facial nerve) are not part of the tumor, recalling that the tumor develops from the sheath of Schwann and pushes the axons to one side (Figures 17 and 18). The histological paraffin examination should be completed with immunohistochemistry for the S100 marker—necessary to establish the neural origin, and for SMA (Smooth Muscle Actin)—to exclude a leiomyoma [23].

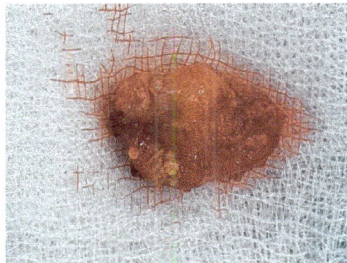

Figure 13. Macroscopic appearance of facial nerve schwannoma: cystic appearance with a thin wall and yellowish friable intraluminal material.

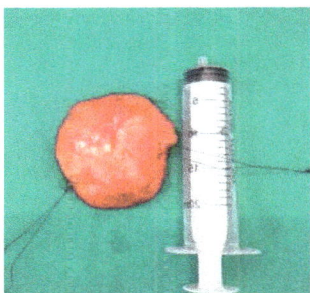

Figure 14. Macroscopic appearance of nodular facial nerve schwannoma.

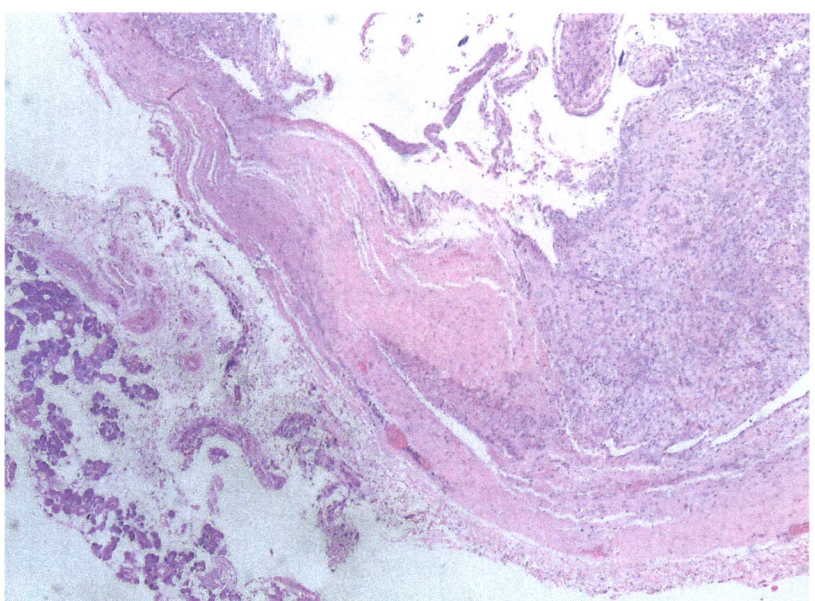

Figure 15. On the left side of the image, there is a glandular tissue of the parotid gland, and on the right side, there is a spindle-cell proliferation with a thick fibrous capsule and a hyalin stroma, HE, 40×.

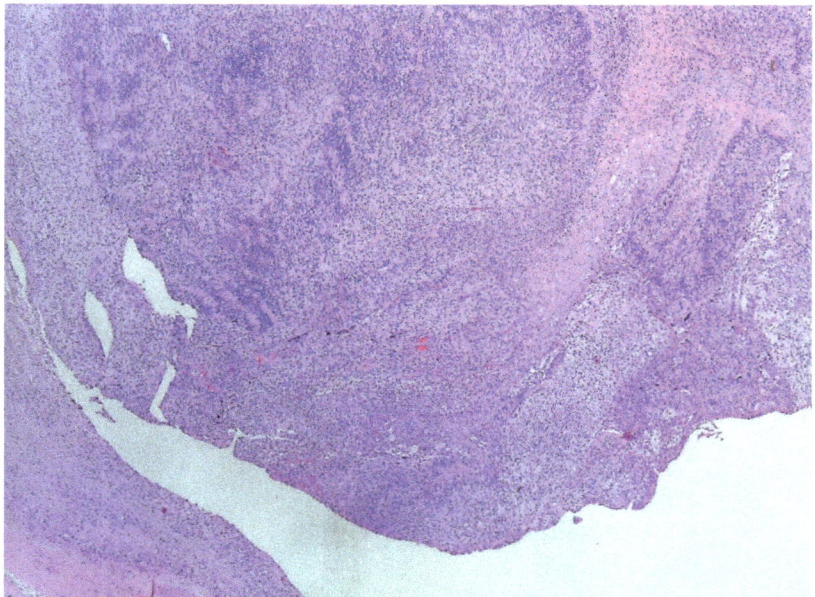

Figure 16. Encapsulated nodular proliferation with spindle cell originating in Schwann cell and cells with clear cytoplasm admixed a fibro-hyalin stroma, HE, 40×.

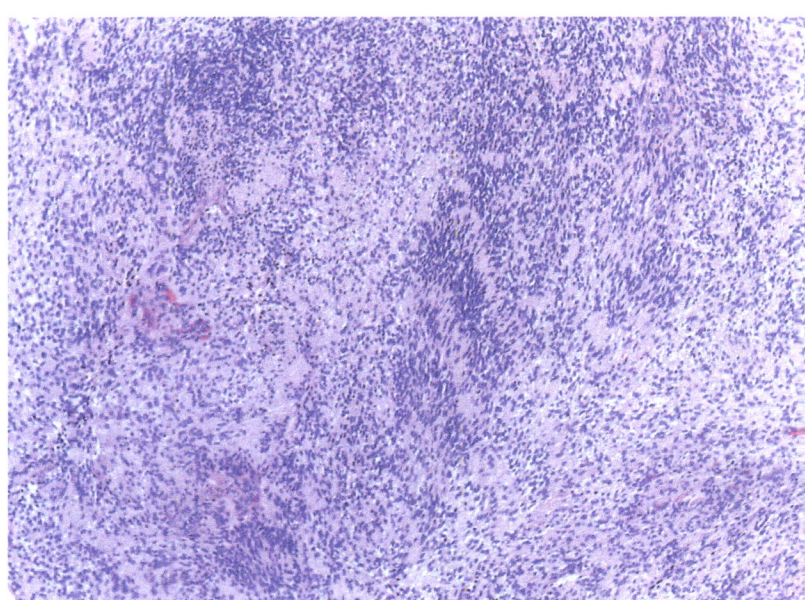

Figure 17. Details of the spindle cell proliferation pattern, with hypercellular Antoni A areas with Verocay bodies (where the nuclei of the cells are arranged in a palisaded architecture); a hyalinized blood vessel can also be seen, HE, 100×.

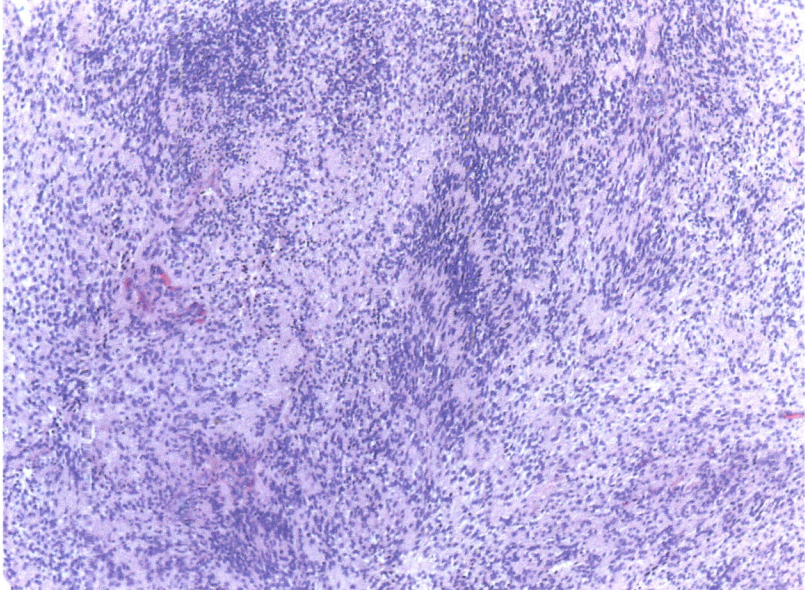

Figure 18. Details of the myxoid area (Antoni B area) and blood vessels with thick hyalinized walls, HE 100×.

6. Differential Diagnosis of the Extracranial FNS

The differential diagnosis must be made, most often, with a pleomorphic adenoma of the parotid gland that is difficult to differentiate from imaging studies such as CT and MRI [24]. FNAC does not provide conclusive results, so a definite diagnosis is possible only after surgical ablation and histological and immunohistochemical examinations. Schwannoma-like pleomorphic adenoma, a rare histopathological variant of pleiomorphic adenoma, is also described [25]. Leiomyoma is another variant of histological diagnosis [26]. For FNS located at the level of the deep parotid lobe, the differential diagnosis of schwannoma of the glossopharyngeal nerve can also be considered [27]. Other differential diagnoses that can be considered include the fluctuating parotid cyst, the lymphoepithelial cyst in HIV-positive patients, and autoimmune diseases that usually cause bilateral lesions and frequently have systemic manifestations [28]. Neurofibromatosis can associate neurofibromas along the facial nerve, but they are usually accompanied by facial paralysis associated with other neurological deficits depending on the location of the neurofibromas, burden, and the risk of recurrence after ablation [29].

7. Therapeutic Strategies in the Management of FNS Extracranial Segment

The gold standard treatment of FNS of the parotid segment consists of the surgical excision of the tumor with preservation of the facial nerve. Because these tumors are most often without preoperative peripheral facial palsy, there is a very high moral and medico-legal liability for the surgeon, and it is a fine line between choosing conservatory treatment versus surgical ablation, given the risk of intraoperative damage to the facial nerve [30]. It is possible that in certain selected cases where the imaging arguments are strong in favor of the diagnosis of schwannoma and there is no clinical peripheral facial palsy, the conservative attitude of imaging monitoring of the tumor for a short time may be considered. But, considering that the diagnosis of certainty cannot be formulated by histological examination, and the increase in the size of the tumor also increases the surgical risks, the wisest attitude seems to be informed consent of the patient regarding the operative risks, with the presentation of the possibility of intraoperative reconstruction of a damaged facial nerve [31]. As a consequence, choosing surgery depends on the location and extension of the tumor, the preoperative function of the facial nerve, the experience of the surgeon, and the results obtained previously regarding the reconstruction of the nerve, but also on the patient's preferences. Large tumors with extension into the mastoid cavity and with preoperative facial paralysis are indications for surgical intervention. An approach to the infratemporal fossa, parapharyngeal space, or parotid gland may be considered [32].

The current approach is an arciform submandibular cervical approach or a modified Redon approach (Figures 19 and 20). Tumor ablation by extracapsular dissection with preservation of the facial nerve is ideal. Superficial or total parotidectomy with preservation of the facial nerve can also be considered. In tumors involving the medial aspect of the deep lobe, parotidectomy is usually not necessary (Figures 21–23). Frozen sections examination must be done intraoperatively to rule out malignancy, especially if sectioning of the facial nerve fibers is required.

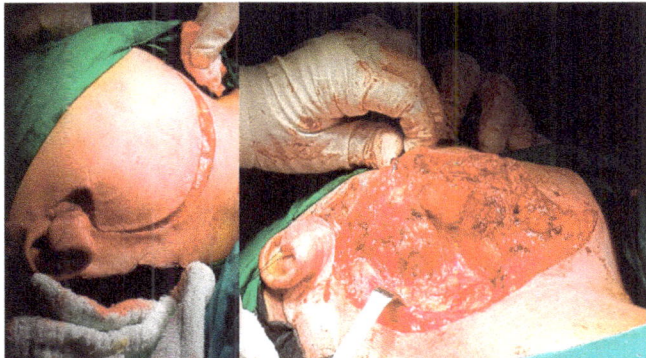

Figure 19. Modified Redon-type cervical parotid approach for deep parotid lobe tumor with the histological result of schwannoma.

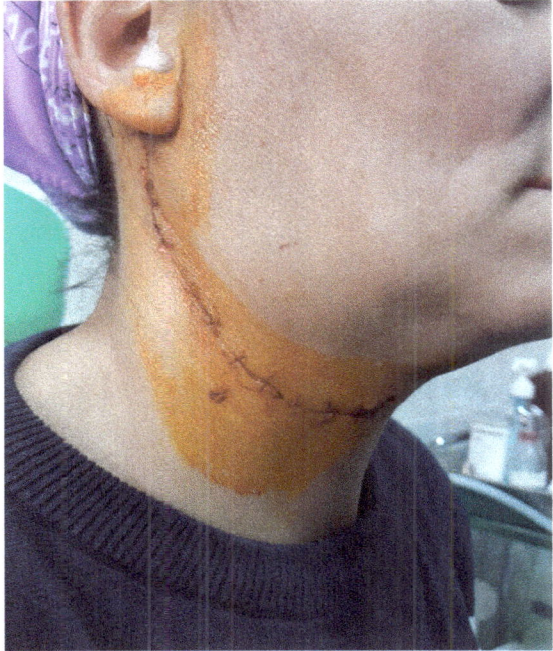

Figure 20. Submandibular arciform approach for right facial nerve schwannoma, from the tip of the mastoid to under the chin, with the steepest point near the hyoid bone in a patient without preoperative peripheral facial palsy.

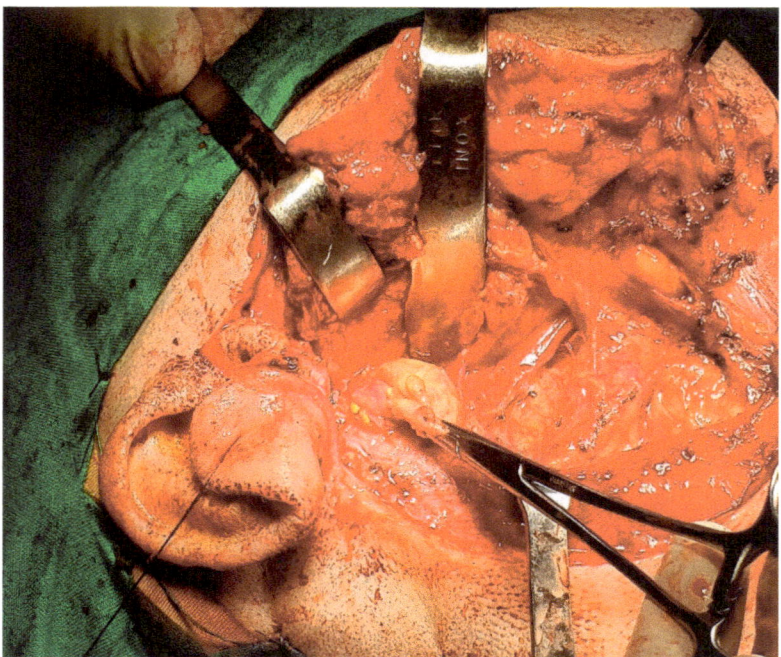

Figure 21. Intraoperative appearance of schwannoma of the facial nerve developed from the retro parotid segment of the facial nerve, with the characteristic yellowish appearance. The right parotid gland is under the retractors.

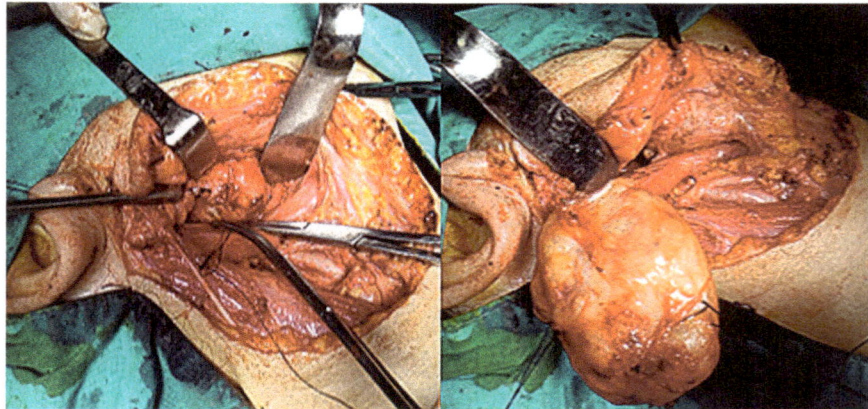

Figure 22. Intraoperative appearance of schwannoma of the facial nerve, of the right deep parotid lobe, with right parapharyngeal evolution, operated using the right submandibular arciform approach—the tumor was removed by extracapsular dissection with preservation of the facial nerve.

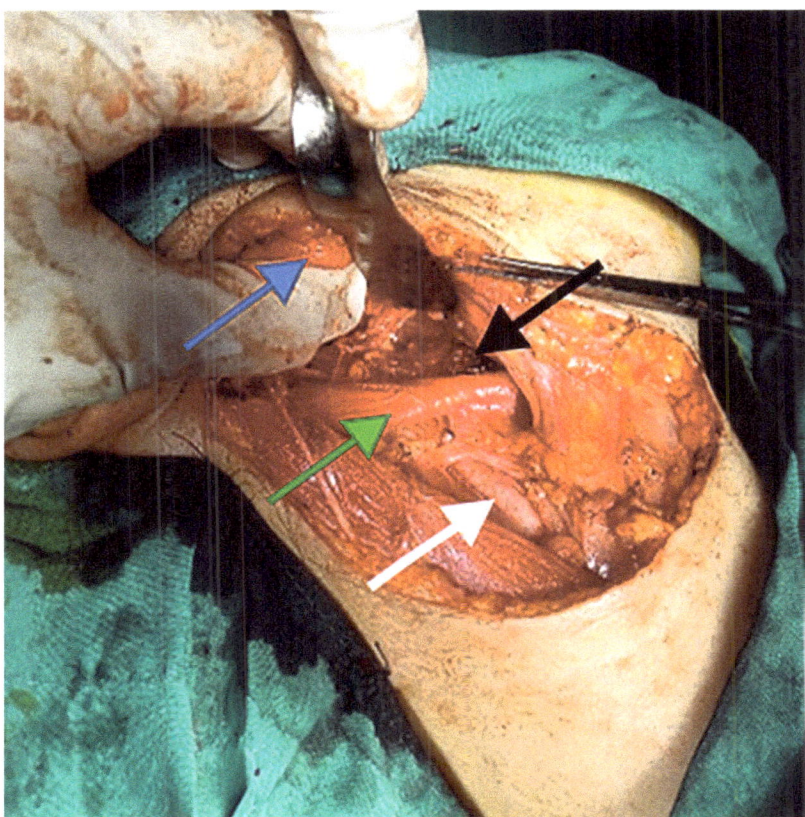

Figure 23. Intraoperative appearance after ablation of a bulky schwannoma of the right deep parotid lobe, with the parotid gland digitally retracted (blue arrow), the posterior belly of the digastric (green arrow), the common carotid artery at the bifurcation (white arrow) and the right parapharyngeal space (black arrow).

Marchioni D. et al. classify intraparotid FNSs [33] according to the relationship with the facial nerve path into four types of SNF: type A, in which the tumor can be resected without sacrificing the facial nerve; this type of tumor rarely produces preoperative facial paralysis; type B, in which the tumor can be resected, but with a partial sacrifice of peripheral branches or distal divisions; immediate reconstruction, using either a nerve graft or direct neurorrhaphy, is required, and the prognosis is dependent on the affected branch rather than the type of reconstruction; type C, in which resection of the tumor requires the sacrifice of the trunk of the facial nerve; and type D, in which tumor resection requires the sacrifice of the facial nerve trunk and at least one of the temporofacial or cervicofacial branches.

Half of the intraparotid segment FNSs are described in the literature as originating in the trunk of the facial nerve, making it virtually impossible to discover the trunk. Peripheral facial paralysis is reported in intraparotid NSF in which only biopsy or even resection was performed with apparent preservation of the nerve due to the individual sensitivity of the facial nerve to dissection and the particularities of nerve microvascularization [34]. Therefore, even in the conditions of preservation of the facial nerve, after tumor ablation, a reversible peripheral facial paresis is possible under cortisone treatment and group B vitamin therapy (Figure 24). Facial gymnastics initiated immediately postoperatively is essential for motor recovery as quickly as possible [35]. In the case of FNSs with preoperative peripheral facial paresis, the recovery of the facial motor deficit, in the conditions of preservation of the facial nerve, is very unlikely; even in these cases, it is worth starting facial gymnastics immediately postoperatively and chronic treatment with neurotrophic drugs for 60 days (Figure 25).

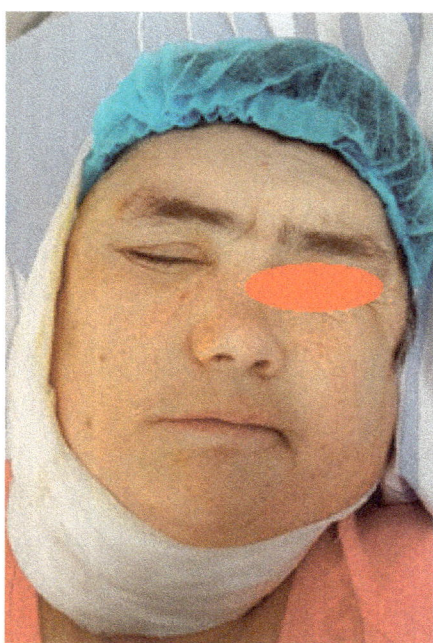

Figure 24. Immediate postoperative appearance of a patient with preoperative right peripheral facial weakness, in whom the facial nerve was preserved, with possible right palpebral occlusion.

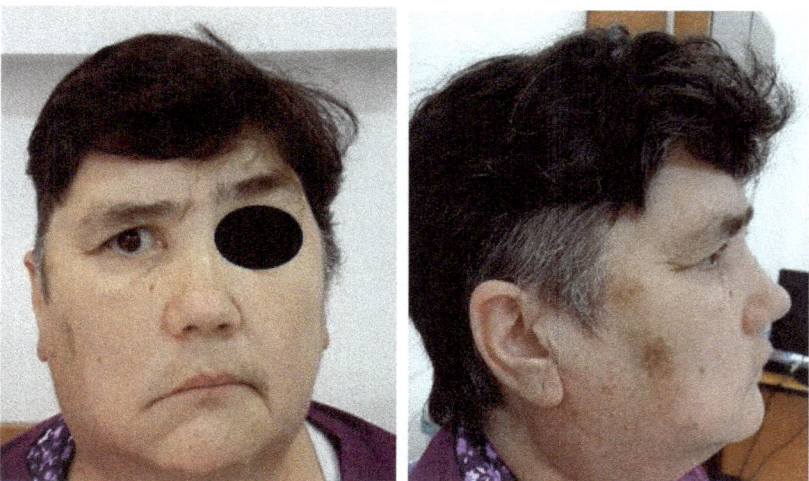

Figure 25. Postoperative appearance at 30 days in a patient with schwannoma of the right facial nerve, parotid segment, with preoperative right peripheral facial paresis older than 6 months, where the right facial nerve was preserved, but in which motor recovery was only partially achieved due to the age of the compressed nerve fibers.

A therapeutic alternative worth considering in the case of extracranial FNS is stereotactic hyper-fractionated radiosurgery which can be chosen as a therapeutic option when the surgical planning offers few chances of preserving the facial nerve when there is already peripheral facial paralysis, and we still aim to preserve the motor function of the facial nerve [36]. The literature also mentions subtotal excision, with annual radiological follow-up, in cases where dissection of the nerve tumor is difficult, but—in our experience—this therapeutic option only prolongs or postpones the moment of a definitive, radical decision and greatly increases the risks of facial nerve sacrifice in revision surgery.

8. Discussions

Because extracranial FNS is a rare neurogenic tumor, however, there is no firm consensus regarding the management of the different types of extracranial FNSs. The therapeutic strategy in extracranial FNSs is done keeping account of the location and extension of the tumor, the preoperative function of the facial nerve, the experience of the surgeon regarding cervical surgery, and the reconstruction of the facial nerve, but also the patient's options [37]. However, the surgical procedures are extensive and pose a great risk to the overall prognosis of the patient, given the possible associated pathologies such as cardiovascular disease, bleeding disorders, or allergic reactions [38]. In current practice, the surgeon approaching a tumor which can be an extracranial FNS has to keep in mind a type of protocol based on these factors. In the type A or B of FNSs (after Marchioni Classification), or in case of a pre-operative facial nerve palsy House-Brackmann (HB) grade IV or worse, the surgery with ablation and, if it is necessary, the reconstruction of the nerve could be the reasonable strategy [39]. In the case of pre-operative facial nerve palsy HB grade III or better and type C or D of FNSs (after Marchioni classification), the biopsy is to exclude a malignant variant and conservative management with imaging monitoring every 12 months [40].

9. Conclusions

Schwannomas of the extracranial segment, particularly of the parotid segment of the facial nerve, are rare tumors that require careful diagnostic and therapeutic management. MRI and CT Scan imaging is essential, often providing complementary information and formulating a diagnosis of high suspicion for schwannoma and allowing planning for surgery. The surgical approach to FNSs requires an experienced surgeon, and radical ablation by extracapsular dissection with preservation of the facial nerve is the gold standard. The patient's informed consent is important regarding the diagnosis of schwannoma and the possibility of facial nerve resection with reconstruction. Extemporaneous histological examination is mandatory to rule out malignancy or when sectioning of the facial nerve fibers is necessary. The histological examination, which can sometimes be a surprise, must be completed with immunohistochemistry to confirm the diagnosis of schwannoma. Alternative therapeutic strategies are imaging monitoring or stereotactic radiosurgery. The main factors which are influencing the management are the extension of the tumor, the presence or not of facial palsy, the experience of the surgeon, and the patient's options.

Author Contributions: Conceptualization, D.V. and M.D.; methodology, D.V.; software, M.D.. validation, D.V., M.D. and M.P.-C.; formal analysis, M.P.-C.; investigation, A.N.M.; resources, O.-M.P.; data curation, O.-M.P.; writing—original draft preparation, D.V.; writing—review and editing, M.D.; visualization, A.N.M.; supervision, F.B.; project administration, F.B.; funding acquisition, F.B. All authors have read and agreed to the published version of the manuscript.

Funding: This research received no external funding.

Institutional Review Board Statement: Not applicable.

Informed Consent Statement: Informed consent was obtained from all subjects involved in the study.

Data Availability Statement: All data are available from the corresponding authors on request.

Acknowledgments: The authors thank Cristina Veronica Andreescu from the Medical English Department at Carol Davila University of Medicine and Pharmacy, Bucharest, Romania. She kindly agreed to proofread the manuscript.

Conflicts of Interest: The authors declare no conflict of interest.

References

1. Haider, M.Y.; Rahim, M.; Bashar, N.M.K.; Hossain, Z.; Islam, S.M.J. Schwannoma of the Base of the Tongue: A Case Report of a Rare Disease and Review of Literatures. *Case Rep. Surg.* **2020**, *2020*, 7942062. [CrossRef] [PubMed]
2. Damar, M.; Dinç, A.E.; Eliçora, S.; Bişkin, S.; Erten, G.; Biz, S. Facial Nerve Schwannoma of Parotid Gland: Difficulties in Diagnosis and Management. *Case Rep. Otolaryngol.* **2016**, *2016*, 3939685. [CrossRef] [PubMed]
3. Caughey, R.J.; May, M.; Schaitkin, B.M. Intraparotid Facial Nerve Schwannoma: Diagnosis and Management. *Otolaryngol. Neck Surg.* **2004**, *130*, 586–592. [CrossRef] [PubMed]
4. Pascual, P.M.; Maranillo, E.; Vázquez, T.; De Blas, C.S.; Lasso, J.M.; Sañudo, J.R. Extracranial Course of the Facial Nerve Revisited. *Anat. Rec.* **2019**, *302*, 599–608. [CrossRef]
5. Yang, H.-M.; Yoo, Y.-B. Anatomy of the Facial Nerve at the Condylar Area: Measurement Study and Clinical Implications. *Sci. World J.* **2014**, *2014*, 473568. [CrossRef] [PubMed]
6. Davis, R.A.; Anson, B.J.; Budinger, J.M.; Kurth, L.R. Surgical anatomy of the facial nerve and parotid gland based upon a study of 350 cervicofacial halves. *Surgery Gynecol. Obstet.* **1956**, *102*, 385–412.
7. Poutoglidis, A.; Paraskevas, G.K.; Lazaridis, N.; Georgalas, C.; Vlachtsis, K.; Markou, K.; Gougousis, S.; Fyrmpas, G.; Keramari, S.; Tsentemeidou, A.; et al. Extratemporal facial nerve branching patterns: Systematic review of 1497 cases. *J. Laryngol. Otol.* **2022**, *136*, 1170–1176. [CrossRef]
8. Martínez-Pascual, P.; Pérez-Lloret, P.; Alcaide, E.M.; Sanz-García, C.; de Blas, C.S.; Sanudo, J.; Konschake, M.; Porzionato, A.; De Caro, R.; Macchi, V. Connections between postparotid terminal branches of the facial nerve: An immunohistochemistry study. *Clin. Anat.* **2023**, *36*, 28–35. [CrossRef]
9. Jirawatnotai, S.; Kaewpichai, K.; Tirakotai, W.; Mothong, W.; Kaewsema, A.; Sriswadpong, P. Nerve to the zygomaticus major muscle for facial reanimation surgery: A cadaveric study for branching patterns and axonal count. *Asian J. Neurosurg.* **2020**, *15*, 516–520. [CrossRef] [PubMed]
10. Stankevicius, D.; Suchomlinov, A. Variations in Facial Nerve Branches and Anatomical Landmarks for Its Trunk Identification: A Pilot Cadaveric Study in the Lithuanian Population. *Cureus* **2019**, *11*, e6100. [CrossRef]
11. Piagkou, M.; Tzika, M.; Paraskevas, G.; Natsis, K. Anatomic variability in the relation between the retromandibular vein and the facial nerve: A case report, literature review and classification. *Folia Morphol.* **2013**, *72*, 371–375. [CrossRef] [PubMed]
12. Guinto, G.; Hernandez, E.; Gallardo-Ceja, D.; Gallegos-Hernandez, F.; Arechiga, N.; Guinto-Nishimura, G. Anatomical Basis of the Zygomatic-Transmandibular Approach: Operative Video. *J. Neurol. Surg. Part B Skull Base* **2021**, *83* (Suppl. 3), e646–e647. [CrossRef] [PubMed]
13. Liu, J.; Pinheiro-Neto, C.D.; Yang, D.; Wang, E.; Gardner, P.A.; Hirsch, B.E.; Snyderman, C.H.; Fernandez-Miranda, J.C. Comparison of Endoscopic Endonasal Approach and Lateral Microsurgical Infratemporal Fossa Approach to the Jugular Foramen: An Anatomical Study. *J. Neurol. Surg. Part B Skull Base* **2021**, *83* (Suppl. 2), e474–e483. [CrossRef]
14. Seo, B.F.; Choi, H.J.; Seo, K.J.; Jung, S.-N. Intraparotid facial nerve schwannomas. *Arch. Craniofacial Surg.* **2019**, *20*, 71–74. [CrossRef] [PubMed]
15. Gao, Y.; Shi, Z.; Wang, C.; Yu, Z. Facial nerve schwannoma mimicking chronic suppurative otitis media: A case report. *Medicine* **2019**, *98*, e16844. [CrossRef] [PubMed]
16. Bartindale, M.; Heiferman, J.; Joyce, C.; Balasubramanian, N.; Anderson, D.; Leonetti, J. The Natural History of Facial Schwannomas: A Meta-Analysis of Case Series. *J. Neurol. Surg. Part B Skull Base* **2019**, *80*, 458–468. [CrossRef]
17. Shimizu, K.; Iwai, H.; Ikeda, K.; Sakaida, N.; Sawada, S. Intraparotid Facial Nerve Schwannoma: A Report of Five Cases and an Analysis of MR Imaging Results. *AJNR Am. J. Neuroradiol.* **2005**, *26*, 1328–1330.
18. Jaiswal, A.; Mridha, A.R.; Nath, D.; Bhalla, A.S.; Thakkar, A. Intraparotid facial nerve schwannoma: A case report. *World J. Clin. Cases* **2015**, *3*, 322–326. [CrossRef]
19. Yamakami, I.; Ono, J.; Yamaura, A. Sigmoid Sinus Dural Arteriovenous Malformation Resulting from Jugular Foramen Schwannoma—Case Report. *Neurol. Med. Chir.* **1998**, *38*, 43–46. [CrossRef]
20. Kühn, J.P.; Wagner, M.; Bozzato, A.; Linxweiler, M. Multiple schwannomas of the facial nerve mimicking cervical lymphoma: A case report. *J. Med. Case Rep.* **2021**, *15*, 436. [CrossRef]
21. Simone, M.; Vesperini, E.; Viti, C.; Camaioni, A.; Lepanto, L.; Raso, F. Intraparotid facial nerve schwannoma: Two case reports and a review of the literature. *Acta Otorhinolaryngol. Ital.* **2018**, *38*, 73–77. [CrossRef] [PubMed]
22. Matsumine, H.; Sasaki, R.; Fujii, K.; Sakurai, H. Intramasseteric Schwannoma Derived from the Masseteric Nerve. *Plast. Reconstr. Surg. Glob. Open* **2019**, *7*, e2175. [CrossRef] [PubMed]
23. Chandra, S.R.; Karim, F.; Rawal, Y.B. Divergent Schwannoma-Like Phenotype in a Pleomorphic Adenoma. *Head Neck Pathol.* **2017**, *11*, 567–574. [CrossRef] [PubMed]

24. Bewley, A.F.; Azhdam, A.M.; Borrelli, M. Intraparotid Facial Nerve Schwannoma Mimicking Primary Parotid Neoplasm. *Ear, Nose Throat J.* **2021**, *100* (Suppl. 6), 881S–883S. [CrossRef] [PubMed]
25. Roth, S.H.; Faquin, W.C.; Gimenez, C.; Vadalia, B.; Frank, D.K.; Li, J.Y. Schwannoma-Like Pleomorphic Adenoma: Two Cases and a Review of the Literature. *Head Neck Pathol.* **2020**, *14*, 166–172. [CrossRef]
26. Osano, H.; Ioka, Y.; Okamoto, R.; Nakai, Y.; Hayashi, H.; Tsuchiya, Y.; Yamada, S. Angioleiomyoma of the cheek: A case report. *J. Oral Sci.* **2015**, *57*, 63–66. [CrossRef]
27. Bakar, B. The Jugular Foramen Schwannomas: Review of the Large Surgical Series. *J. Korean Neurosurg. Soc.* **2008**, *44*, 285–294. [CrossRef]
28. Shivhare, P.; Shankarnarayan, L.; Jambunath, U.; Basavaraju, S.M. Benign lymphoepithelial cysts of parotid and submandibular glands in a HIV-positive patient. *J. Oral Maxillofac. Pathol.* **2015**, *19*, 107. [CrossRef]
29. Galhotra, V.; Sheikh, S.; Jindal, S.; Singla, A. Segmental neurofibromatosis. *Indian J. Dent.* **2014**, *5*, 166–169. [CrossRef]
30. Kader, M.I.S.A.; Abdullah, A.; Yunus, M.R.M.; Jaafar, M.N.; Kew, T.Y. Preoperative Challenges in Managing Intraparotid Schwannoma. *Cureus* **2022**, *14*, e21392. [CrossRef]
31. Chowdhary, S.; Thangavel, S.; Ganesan, S.; Alexander, A. Extratemporal intraparotid facial nerve schwannoma. *BMJ Case Rep.* **2021**, *14*, e239407. [CrossRef] [PubMed]
32. Sim, L.; Yeoh, X.Y.; Tan, T.E.; Zakaria, Z.; Mohamad, I. Intracapsular Enucleation of Intraparotid Facial Nerve Schwannoma with Intratemporal Extension. *Medeni. Med. J.* **2022**, *37*, 113–118. [CrossRef] [PubMed]
33. Marchioni, D.; Ciufelli, M.A.; Presutti, L. Intraparotid facial nerve schwannoma: Literature review and classification proposal. *J. Laryngol. Otol.* **2007**, *121*, 707–712. [CrossRef] [PubMed]
34. Bagga, M.B.; Bhatnagar, D.; Katoch, S. Preauricular intraparotid schwannoma: A rare presentation with literature review. *Contemp. Clin. Dent.* **2021**, *12*, 191–194. [CrossRef]
35. Paolucci, T.; Cardarola, A.; Colonnelli, P.; Ferracuti, G.; Gonnella, R.; Murgia, M.; Santilli, V.; Paoloni, M.; Bernetti, A.; Agostini, F.; et al. Give me a kiss! An integrative rehabilitative training program with motor imagery and mirror therapy for recovery of facial palsy. *Eur. J. Phys. Rehabil. Med.* **2020**, *56*, 58–67. [CrossRef]
36. Sasaki, A.; Miyazaki, S.; Hori, T. Extracranial Facial Nerve Schwannoma Treated by Hypo-fractionated CyberKnife Radiosurgery. *Cureus* **2016**, *8*, e797. [CrossRef]
37. Cho, H.R.; Kwon, S.S.; Chung, S.; Choi, Y.J. Intraparotid Facial Nerve Schwannoma. *Arch. Craniofacial Surg.* **2014**, *15*, 28–31. [CrossRef]
38. Dumitru, M.; Berghi, O.N.; Taciuc, I.-A.; Vrinceanu, D.; Manole, F.; Costache, A. Could Artificial Intelligence Prevent Intraoperative Anaphylaxis? Reference Review and Proof of Concept. *Medicina* **2022**, *58*, 1530. [CrossRef]
39. Kang, G.C.; Soo, K.-C.; Lim, D.T. Extracranial Non-vestibular Head and Neck Schwannomas: A Ten-year Experience. *Ann. Acad. Med. Singap.* **2007**, *36*, 233–238. [CrossRef]
40. Rigante, M.; Petrelli, L.; de Corso, E.; Paludetti, G. Intracapsular microenucleation technique in a case of intraparotid facial nerve schwannoma. Technical notes for a conservative approach. *Acta Otorhinolaryngol. Ital.* **2015**, *35*, 49–52.

Disclaimer/Publisher's Note: The statements, opinions and data contained in all publications are solely those of the individual author(s) and contributor(s) and not of MDPI and/or the editor(s). MDPI and/or the editor(s) disclaim responsibility for any injury to people or property resulting from any ideas, methods, instructions or products referred to in the content.

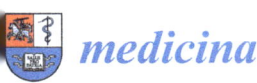

Case Report

Myoepithelial Carcinoma Arising in a Salivary Duct Cyst of the Parotid Gland: Case Presentation

Michał Gontarz [1,*], Jolanta Orłowska-Heitzman [2], Krzysztof Gąsiorowski [1], Jakub Bargiel [1], Tomasz Marecik [1], Paweł Szczurowski [1], Jan Zapała [1] and Grażyna Wyszyńska-Pawelec [1]

1. Department of Cranio-Maxillofacial Surgery, Jagiellonian University Medical College, 30-688 Cracow, Poland
2. Department of Pathomorphology, Jagiellonian University Medical College, University Hospital, 30-688 Cracow, Poland
* Correspondence: michal.gontarz@uj.edu.pl; Tel.: +48-12-4002800

Abstract: Cystic lesions observed in parotid glands are relatively rare and comprise 2–5% of all parotid primaries. A salivary duct cyst (SDC) is a true cyst representing 10% of all salivary gland cysts. The risk of malignant transformation of SDC's epithelium is extremely rare. In the literature, only three cases of carcinoma ex SDC of the parotid gland are described. This report presents the first in the literature case of myoepithelial carcinoma (MECA) arising from a parotid SDC. A 75-year-old male patient was referred to the Department of Cranio-Maxillofacial Surgery of the Jagiellonian University in Cracow, Poland due to a cystic tumor arising from the right parotid gland. Superficial parotidectomy with facial nerve preservation was performed. Histological examination confirmed a rare case of MECA emerging from the SDC. The immunohistochemical profile of MECA ex SDC was presented. During 6 months of the follow-up, local recurrence or distant metastasis was not observed.

Keywords: salivary duct cyst; parotid gland; myoepithelial carcinoma; parotid cyst; parotid cancer; malignant parotid cyst

1. Introduction

The World Health Organization (WHO) 2022 Classification of Head and Neck Tumours distinguishes tumors and tumor-like lesions, which include a variety of cysts [1]. Cystic lesions observed in parotid glands are relatively rare and comprise 2–5% of parotid primaries [2]. According to Takita et al., cystic lesions in the parotid gland can be all divided into non-neoplastic cysts, benign tumors with cystic formation (Warthin tumor, cystadenoma), and malignant tumors with macrocystic change (mucoepidermoid carcinoma, acinic cell carcinoma) [2]. Non-neoplastic cysts include salivary duct cysts (SDC), lymphoepithelial cysts, HIV-associated salivary gland disease, dermoid cysts, and lymphangioma [2]. SDC is a true cyst representing 10% of all salivary gland cysts [3]. SDCs develop from the cystic dilatation of the salivary gland duct and are observed in the superficial lobe of the parotid gland and minor salivary glands [4]. A SDC is an acquired cyst, which occurs following obstruction of the salivary duct. The main causes of salivary duct obstruction are sialoliths and mucous plaques, as well as postoperative, posttraumatic, or postinflammatory stenosis [5]. However, in most cases, the specific cause of the salivary duct obstruction is unknown. A SDC is lined with double- or multi-layered columnar and/or cuboid cells: sometimes squamous or oncocytic metaplasia might be observed [3,5]. The risk of malignant transformation of the SDC's epithelium is extremely rare. In the literature, only three cases of carcinoma ex SDC of the parotid gland are presented: undifferentiated carcinoma [6], adenocarcinoma [7], and mucoepidermoid carcinoma [8].

The current report describes the first in the literature case of myoepithelial carcinoma (MECA) arising from the parotid SDC.

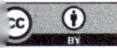

2. Case Report

In September 2021, a 75-year-old male patient was admitted to the Department of Cranio-Maxillofacial Surgery of the Jagiellonian University in Cracow, Poland, with a ten-year history of a slowly growing, painless cystic tumor of the left parotid gland. Progression in the last period was not observed. The patient suffered from arterial hypertension, and mitral and tricuspid valve regurgitation. In 2018, the patient had a stroke of the right hemisphere of the brain, with left-sided paresis and balance disorders. Physical examination revealed a soft, movable, and fluctuating cystic tumor of the parotid gland with unchanged skin above it. In fine needle aspiration cytology (FNAC), 15 mL of brown fluid content was obtained. Any signs of peripheral facial nerve paresis were not observed. Computed tomography (CT) showed a unilateral, solitary, well-defined, thin-walled, multilocular cystic lesion with dimensions of 49 mm (ax.) × 29 mm (cor.) × 37 mm (sag.) located in the superficial lobe of the parotid gland. In the distal part of the cystic lesion, a contrast-enhancing solid tumor 9 mm in diameter was revealed (Figure 1A). Imaging of the neck, chest, and abdomen excluded regional and distant metastases.

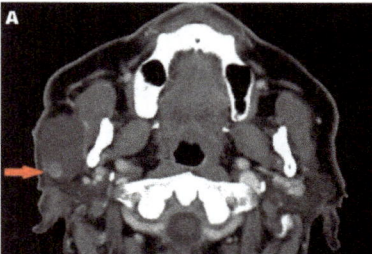
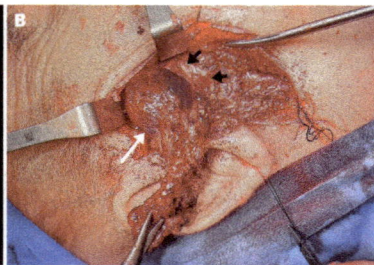
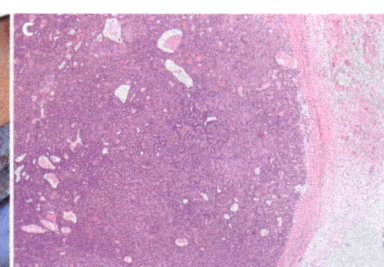

Figure 1. (**A**) Computed tomography (CT) scan at diagnosis showed a unilateral, solitary, well-defined, thin-walled, multilocular cystic lesion located in the superficial lobe of the right parotid gland. In the distal part of the cystic lesion, a contrast-enhancing solid tumor 9 mm in diameter was revealed (red arrow). (**B**) The thin-walled multilocular cyst (white arrow) with the superficial lobe of the parotid gland as a surgical specimen. The cyst was located directly on the lateral aspect of the temporal, zygomatic, and buccal branches of the facial nerve (black arrows). (**C**) The tumor was composed of mixed small cells, partially epithelioid, partially spindle without marked cytological atypia, with a tendency to form trabecular structures. HE, obj. magnification 200×.

2.1. Surgery

The patient was qualified for surgical treatment. A modified Blair incision was used to perform superficial parotidectomy with facial nerve preservation. During the surgery, intraoperative neuromonitoring was used to identify branches of the facial nerve (Inomed C2 Nerve Monitor). As an antibiotic prophylaxis, 1 g of Cefazolin was administrated. The superficial lobe of the parotid gland with the thin-walled cyst was excised. The tumor was located in the lumen of the cyst, which was situated in the superficial lobe, directly on the lateral aspect of the temporal, zygomatic, and buccal branches of the facial nerve (Figure 1B). The inferior pole of the parotid gland was intact. The great auricular nerve and parotid fascia were preserved. Active drainage was removed on the second day after surgery. Four days following surgery, the patient was discharged home. The healing process was uneventful with proper facial nerve function.

2.2. Pathology

The histopathological examination of the surgical specimen revealed a salivary gland with lobules separated by adipose tissue and preserved histological structure. Adjacent to the salivary gland a multilocular cyst with a diameter of 40 mm was found. The cyst was lined with mainly single-layered cuboid glandular cells, in some places with double-layered, and focal formation of small papillary outgrowths up to 0.1 mm in size.

One of the cyst's cavities included a tumor with an 8-mm diameter growing from the cyst's wall. The tumor was composed of mixed small cells, partially epithelioid, partially spindle without marked cytological atypia, with a tendency to form trabecular structures (Figure 1C). The tumor mass surrounded the glandular structures of the salivary gland with positive staining for cytokeratin 19 (CK19) (Figure 2A). The immunohistochemical profile of MECA ex SDC characterized positive staining for keratins AE1:AE3, S-100 protein, smooth muscle actin (SMA), p40, DOG1, and SOX10 (Figures 2B, 3 and 4A). Only limited staining for epithelial membrane antigen (EMA) was found. Immunoreactivity for chromogranin and thyroglobulin was negative (Figure 4B). The Ki-67 labeling index (LI) in the tumor was about 10% (Figure 4C).

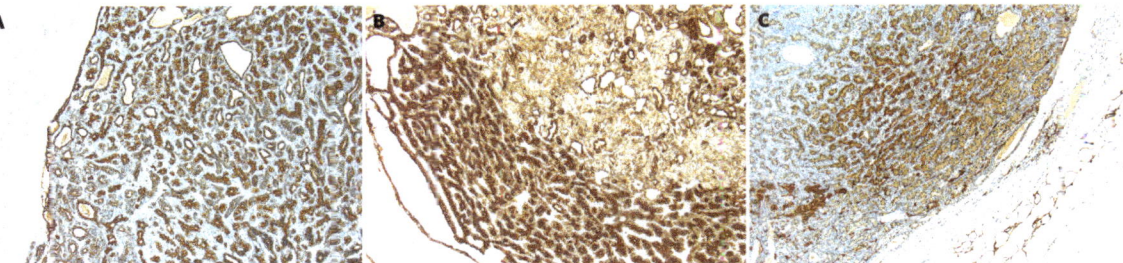

Figure 2. (**A**) The tumor mass surrounded the glandular structures of the salivary gland with positive staining for cytokeratin 19 (CK19). Obj. magnification 200× (**B**) The immunohistochemical profile of the tumor characterized positive staining for keratins AE1:AE3 and (**C**) S-100 protein Obj. magnification 200×.

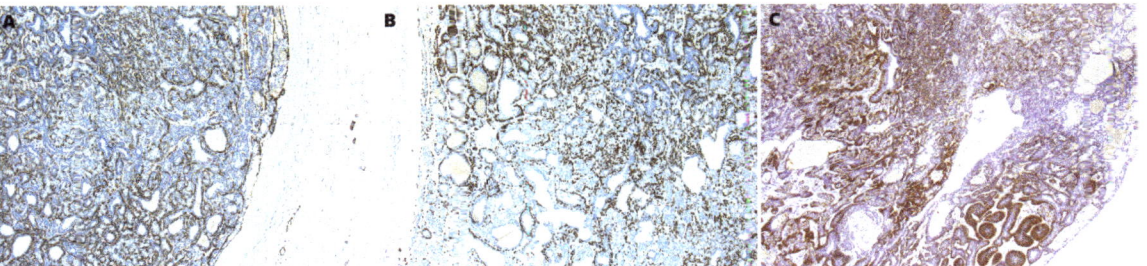

Figure 3. (**A**) Positive immunohistochemical staining for smooth muscle actin (SMA), (**B**) p40 and (**C**) DOG1. Obj. magnification 200×.

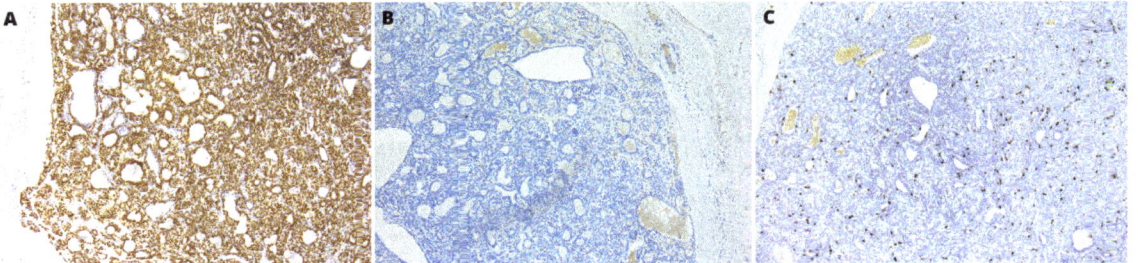

Figure 4. (**A**) Positive immunohistochemical staining for SOX10. (**B**) Negative immunoreactivity for chromogranin. (**C**) The Ki-67 labeling index (LI) in the tumor was about 10%. Obj. magnification 200×.

The entire histological picture supported the diagnosis of a low-grade myoepithelial carcinoma ex-salivary duct cyst. A cluster of cancer cells was found in the cyst wall except for the well-limited remains of the tumor tissue thrust into the lumen of the cyst. Minimally infiltrative growth through the cystic wall without surrounding tissue involvement was observed. Perineural and angiolymphatic invasion was not present. MECA ex SDC was resected with adequate surgical margins (>5 mm, R0 resection). Moreover, in the surgical specimen of the superficial lobe of the parotid gland, ten small lymph nodes with features of reactive changes without metastases were also found.

2.3. Follow Up

After tumor board consultation, due to the radical resection and early stage of low-grade cancer pT1N0, the patient was qualified for systematic oncological follow-up in accordance with the NCCN guidelines. A follow-up ultrasound examination 3 months after the procedure was performed without signs of locoregional recurrence. During 6 months of the follow-up, locoregional recurrence was not observed and the facial nerve function was preserved. Unfortunately, in February 2022, the patient died due to acute pancreatitis with peritonitis.

3. Discussion

Eighty percent of SDC occurs in the parotid gland and comprises about 1–2% of parotid lesions and 10% of all salivary gland cysts [2,3]. SDC is frequently observed in patients older than 30 years old without sex predilection [2,3]. Usually, SDC is a thin-walled, unilateral, solitary cyst situated in the superficial lobe of the parotid gland. Wall thickening might occur due to hemorrhage or infection as a result of FNAC. The differential diagnosis for SDC includes cystadenoma and low-grade mucoepidermoid carcinoma with cystic formation [4]. Surgical resection is the treatment of choice. However, after FNAC, the SDC can disappear completely and the surgery should be postponed until the recurrence of the cyst.

MECAs, also known as malignant myoepitheliomas, are rare entities and are composed of neoplastic myoepithelial cells with infiltrative growth. Myoepithelial cells are observed around the acinus and intercalated ducts of the saliva [9]. MECAs account for less than 2% of all salivary gland cancers and 0.1–0.45% of all salivary gland tumors [10–13]. The most common site of occurrence is the parotid gland (76.6%) followed by the submandibular gland [11]. This was also confirmed by our previous research, in which MECA was found in three cases localized in the parotid gland, which accounted for 1.3% of epithelial salivary gland cancers and 0.37% of all epithelial salivary gland tumors [14]. Etiological factors of MECAs origin are unknown and males and females are affected equally with an average age of around 60 years [13,15,16]. MECAs can either develop de novo or can arise in a pleomorphic adenoma and myoepithelioma [13,16]. Nevertheless, to the best of our knowledge, this case report describes the first case of MECA arising in the SDC of the parotid gland.

The pathological definition of myoepithelioma remains under discussion due to the morphological diversity of the neoplastic myoepithelial cells [16]. Differential diagnoses between benign and malignant myoepitheliomas can also be problematic. In some cases, MECA might be misclassified as a benign salivary gland tumor [10]. According to Nagao et al., MECAs are distinguished by >7 mitotic figures/10 high power fields (HPFs) or Ki-67 LI > 10%. According to Kane and Bagwan, MECAs of the parotid gland might have microscopically partial or complete encapsulation [17]. Histologically, MECAs are characterized by a wide range of morphologic tumor cell types: epithelioid, clear, hyaline, spindle, and mixed [15,17]. About 60% of MECAs are low-grade cancers with quite uniform small- to intermediate-size nuclei with gently distributed chromatin and inconspicuous nucleoli [15]. The immunohistochemical profile of MECA is characterized by the expression of Vimentin, S-100 protein, and the three antibodies against keratins (CAM5.2, AE1:AE3, and 34βE12) [15–19]. In addition, SMA and calponin are immunoreactive in 50% and 75% of tumors, respectively [15].

According to NCCN guidelines from 2022, surgery is the MECAs treatment of choice [20]. Low-grade MECAs with a clinically negative neck do not require elective neck dissection, unlike high-grade MECAs [20]. Xiao et al.'s study presented that occult metastases after elective neck dissection are observed in 15.2% of patients with cN0 neck. This study also confirmed that high-grade MECAs are independent, significant predictors of regional nodal disease in multivariate analysis (OR = 4.42) [21]. Clinically and/or in diagnostic imaging, enlarged lymph nodes should be treated with therapeutic neck dissection with primary MECA resection [20]. Postoperative radiotherapy or radiochemotherapy should be considered in cases of high-grade T3–4a MECAs with close or positive margins, perineural/angiolymphatic invasion, and lymph node metastases found in the surgical specimen [20].

Savera et al.'s study revealed that 29% of MECAs patients die from the disease after an average of 32 months. Only high-grade MECAs are strongly correlated with poor prognosis [15,21]. On the other hand, Luo in the cohort of 290 patients, reported 5-, 10-, and 15-year overall survival (OS) of 68.9%, 53%, and 38.1%, respectively. The independent prognostic factors influencing OS were TNM stage, grade, and postoperative radiotherapy [11]. The presented case of a low-grade MECA ex SDC consisted of mixed (epithelioid and spindle) tumor cell types. Radical resection of MECA ex SDC (R0 resection) and early stage of the disease indicated only observation without adjuvant treatment. Unfortunately, the follow-up period was only 6 months (with proper facial nerve function, without locoregional recurrence) due to the patient's death from another cause.

4. Conclusions

In conclusion, carcinoma ex SDC of the parotid gland is an extremely rare entity. To our knowledge, this is the first described case of the MECA arising from the parotid SDC. Surgery is the standard of care for both SDC and MECA. MECA emerging from SDC can be successfully treated with superficial parotidectomy with facial nerve preservation without recurrence. MECA, depending on the grade and stage, might require additional neck dissection as well as adjuvant treatment.

Author Contributions: Conceptualization, M.G., J.B, J.O.-H. and G.W.-P.; methodology, M.G., J.B., J.O.-H. and K.G.; software, M.G., T.M. and P.S.; validation, M.G., J.B. and K.G.; formal analysis, M.G., T.M., J.O.-H. and J.Z.; investigation, M.G., J.O.-H., J.B., K.G. and P.S.; resources, M.G., J.O.-H., J.Z. and G.W.-P.; data curation, M.G., T.M. and P.S.; writing—original draft preparation, M.G., T.M. J.O.-H. and G.W.-P.; writing—review and editing, M.G., J.O.-H. and G.W.-P.; visualization, M.G. and J.B.; supervision, J.Z. and G.W.-P.; project administration, M.G. and J.Z. All authors have read and agreed to the published version of the manuscript.

Funding: This research received no external funding

Institutional Review Board Statement: The study was conducted according to the guidelines of the Declaration of Helsinki and approved by the Institutional Review Board of Jagiellonian University (No: 122.6120.287.2016).

Informed Consent Statement: Patient consent was waived so long as all personal information remained confidential.

Data Availability Statement: Restrictions apply to the availability of these data. Data were obtained from patients treated at the Department of Cranio-Maxillofacial Surgery, Cracow, Poland, and cannot be shared, in accordance with the General Data Protection Regulation (EU) 2016/679.

Acknowledgments: We thank Krzysztof Śliwiński for technical assistance in clinical imaging.

Conflicts of Interest: The authors declare no conflict of interest.

References

1. WHO Classifcation of Tumours Editorial Board. Head and Neck Tumours. In *WHO Classifcation of Tumours Series*, 5th ed.; International Agency for Research on Cancer: Lyon, France, 2022; Volume 9. Available online: https://publications.iarc.fr/ (accessed on 5 December 2022).
2. Takita, H.; Takeshita, T.; Shimono, T.; Tanaka, H.; Iguchi, H.; Hashimoto, S.; Kuwae, Y.; Ohsawa, M.; Miki, Y. Cystic lesions of the parotid gland: Radiologic-pathologic correlation according to the latest World Health Organization 2017 Classification of Head and Neck Tumours. *Jpn. J. Radiol.* **2017**, *35*, 629–647. [CrossRef] [PubMed]
3. Kato, H.; Kawaguchi, M.; Ando, T.; Aoki, M.; Kuze, B.; Matsuo, M. CT and MR imaging findings of non-neoplastic cystic lesions of the parotid gland. *Jpn. J. Radiol.* **2019**, *37*, 627–635. [CrossRef] [PubMed]
4. Stojanov, I.J.; Malik, U.A.; Woo, S.B. Intraoral Salivary Duct Cyst: Clinical and Histopathologic Features of 177 Cases. *Head Neck Pathol.* **2017**, *11*, 469–476. [CrossRef] [PubMed]
5. Takeda, Y.; Yamamoto, H. Salivary duct cyst: Its frequency in a certain Japanese population group (Tohoku districts), with special reference to adenomatous proliferation of the epithelial lining. *J. Oral. Sci.* **2001**, *43*, 9–13. [CrossRef] [PubMed]
6. Minocha, V.R.; Verma, K.; Kapur, B.M. Malignant parotid cyst. *Aust. New Zealand J. Surg.* **1975**, *45*, 99–101. [CrossRef] [PubMed]
7. Schwetschke, O.; Zimmerer, A.; Bosch, F.X.; Maier, H. Salivary duct cyst of the parotid gland and adenocarcinoma. *HNO* **1994**, *42*, 441–445.
8. Seifert, G. Mucoepidermoid carcinoma in a salivary duct cyst of the parotid gland. Contribution to the development of tumours in salivary gland cysts. *Pathol. Res. Pract.* **1996**, *192*, 1211–1217. [CrossRef]
9. Myers, E.N.; Ferris, R.L. *Salivary Gland Disorders*; Springer: Berlin/Heidelberg, Germany, 2007.
10. Xu, B.; Mneimneh, W.; Torrence, D.E.; Higgins, K.; Klimstra, D.; Ghossein, R.; Katabi, N. Misinterpreted Myoepithelial Carcinoma of Salivary Gland: A Challenging and Potentially Significant Pitfall. *Am. J. Surg. Pathol.* **2019**, *43*, 601–609. [CrossRef] [PubMed]
11. Luo, Y. Myoepithelial carcinoma of major salivary glands: Analysis of population-based clinicopathologic and prognostic features *Transl. Oncol.* **2022**, *20*, 101410. [CrossRef]
12. Giridhar, P.; Gupta, P.; Mallick, S.; Upadhyay, A.D.; Rath, G.K. Impact of adjuvant therapy on survival in patients with myoepithelial carcinoma: A systematic review and individual patient data analysis of 691 patients. *Radiother. Oncol.* **2019**, *140*, 125–130. [CrossRef] [PubMed]
13. Cormier, C.; Agarwal, S. Myoepithelial Carcinoma Ex-Pleomorphic Adenoma: A Rare Pathology Misdiagnosed as Pleomorphic Adenoma; With a Novel TERT Promoter Mutation and High PD-L1 Expression. *Head Neck Pathol.* **2022**, *16*, 322–330. [CrossRef] [PubMed]
14. Gontarz, M.; Bargiel, J.; Gąsiorowski, K.; Marecik, T.; Szczurowski, P.; Zapała, J.; Wyszyńska-Pawelec, G. Epidemiology of Primary Epithelial Salivary Gland Tumors in Southern Poland-A 26-Year, Clinicopathologic, Retrospective Analysis. *J. Clin. Med.* **2021**, *10*, 1663. [CrossRef] [PubMed]
15. Savera, A.T.; Sloman, A.; Huvos, A.G.; Klimstra, D.S. Myoepithelial carcinoma of the salivary glands: A clinicopathologic study of 25 patients. *Am. J. Surg. Pathol.* **2000**, *24*, 761–774. [CrossRef] [PubMed]
16. Nagao, T.; Sugano, I.; Ishida, Y.; Tajima, Y.; Matsuzaki, O.; Konno, A.; Kondo, Y.; Nagao, K. Salivary gland malignant myoepithelioma: A clinicopathologic and immunohistochemical study of ten cases. *Cancer* **1998**, *83*, 1292–1299. [CrossRef]
17. Kane, S.V.; Bagwan, I.N. Myoepithelial carcinoma of the salivary glands: A clinicopathologic study of 51 cases in a tertiary cancer center. *Arch. Otolaryngol. Head Neck Surg.* **2010**, *136*, 702–712. [CrossRef] [PubMed]
18. Meyer, M.T.; Watermann, C.; Dreyer, T.; Ergün, S.; Karnati, S. 2021 Update on Diagnostic Markers and Translocation in Salivary Gland Tumors. *Int. J. Mol. Sci.* **2021**, *22*, 6771. [CrossRef] [PubMed]
19. Thompson, H.B.; Law, M.L.; Vasquez, R.V.; Fernandez, O.C. Parotid Myoepithelial Carcinoma in a Pediatric Patient with Multiple Recurrences: Case Report. *Case Rep. Oncol.* **2021**, *24*, 989–997. [CrossRef] [PubMed]
20. NCCN Guidelines. Available online: https://www.nccn.org/guidelines/guidelines-detail?category=1&id=1437 (accessed on 14 December 2022).
21. Xiao, C.C.; Baker, A.B.; White-Gilbertson, S.J.; Day, T.A. Prognostic Factors in Myoepithelial Carcinoma of the Major Salivary Glands. *Otolaryngol. Head Neck Surg.* **2016**, *154*, 1047–1053. [CrossRef] [PubMed]

Disclaimer/Publisher's Note: The statements, opinions and data contained in all publications are solely those of the individual author(s) and contributor(s) and not of MDPI and/or the editor(s). MDPI and/or the editor(s) disclaim responsibility for any injury to people or property resulting from any ideas, methods, instructions or products referred to in the content.

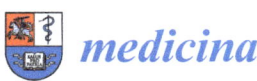

Case Report

Mixed Eccrine Cutaneous Tumor with Folliculo–Sebaceous Differentiation: Case Report and Literature Review

Dimitrinka Kisova [1,*], Tihomir Dikov [1], Vesela Ivanova [1], Hristo Stoyanov [2] and Greta Yordanova [3]

1 Department of General and Clinical Pathology, Faculty of Medicine, Medical University Sofia, 1431 Sofia, Bulgaria; tdikov@medfac.mu-sofia.bg (T.D.); vivanova@medfac.mu-sofia.bg (V.I.)
2 Department of Maxillofacial Surgery, Alexandrovska University Hospital, 1431 Sofia, Bulgaria; drhristostoyanov@gmail.com
3 Department of Orthodontics, Faculty of Dental Medicine, Medical University Sofia, 1431 Sofia, Bulgaria; g.yordanova@fdm.mu-sofia.bg
* Correspondence: d_kisova@medfac.mu-sofia.bg

Abstract: *Background/Introduction:* Cutaneous mixed tumor is a rare benign neoplasm that exhibits a wide range of metaplastic changes and differentiation in the epithelial, myoepithelial, and stromal components, which is often confused with various other skin lesions. *Case report:* We present an unusual case of a 58-year-old woman with a mixed tumor of the upper lip, previously misdiagnosed as adnexal carcinoma on a preoperative biopsy. The excision biopsy shows a well-circumscribed lesion composed of various cells and structures featuring folliculo–sebaceous differentiation embedded in a prominent chondromyxoid stroma. The immunohistochemical study proves the various lineages of differentiation and classifies the neoplasm as the less common eccrine subtype of cutaneous mixed tumor. *Discussion:* The common embryologic origin of the folliculo–sebaceous apocrine complex leads to a great histological variety of cellular components of mixed tumors and the formation of structures that resemble established types of adnexal neoplasms, which could be a diagnostic pitfall, especially on a small incision biopsy.

Keywords: skin; adnexal; tumors; eccrine mixed tumor; histopathology

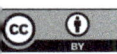

1. Background

Cutaneous mixed tumor, previously known as chondroid syringoma, is a rare benign adnexal/appendageal tumor considered to be the cutaneous analogue of pleomorphic adenoma. The most widely reported frequency is around 0.01% of all cutaneous neoplasms showing a preference for the head and neck region. Mixed tumors usually present as solitary well circumscribed lesions in middle-aged people with slight male predominance [1].

These tumors usually exhibit a wide range of metaplastic changes and differentiation in the epithelial, the myoepithelial, and the stromal components. Sometimes these changes are so prominent as to cause misdiagnosis with other adnexal or mesenchymal neoplasms [2].

Cutaneous mixed tumors are usually further subclassified into the more common apocrine type and the rare eccrine type. The apocrine cases are generally associated with folliculo–sebaceous differentiation, where the epithelial component is composed of branching tubular structures and cystic spaces embedded in a myxoid or chondromyxoid stroma. The tubules are composed of an outer myoepithelial cell layer and an inner epithelial cell layer, sometimes showing secretion by decapitation. Solid aggregates of epithelial cells, as well as isolated polygonal and plasmacytoid (hyaline) epithelial cells, may also be seen. The eccrine variety of mixed tumors by contrast shows an epithelial component represented by small tubules lined by a single layer of uniform cuboidal, oval, or round epithelial cells, having eosinophilic or hyalinized glassy cytoplasm and vesicular nuclei, without decapitation secretion. [3] These differences in the subtypes of mixed tumors are thought to be representative of the common embryologic origin of the folliculo–sebaceous apocrine complex, sometimes also referred as complex neoplasms of the primary epithelial germ, and the eccrine counterpart in contrast should be considered as a putative eccrine lesion [3–5].

2. Case Report

A 58-year-old woman presented with a several year history of a firm mass on the upper lip measuring 10/8/7 mm that had gradually become larger over time (Figure 1). Following a dermatologist consultation, a biopsy was performed with the diagnosis of a malignant trichoepithelioma.

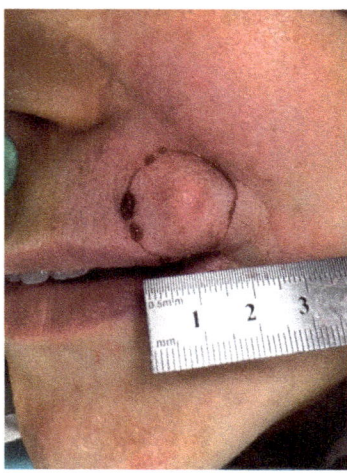

Figure 1. A firm nodule on the upper lip area.

Later, the histologic result was revised with the conclusive diagnosis of microcystic adnexal carcinoma, and the patient was referred for surgical excision. Based on the availability of the location and the well circumscribed properties of the neoplasm it was decided on a more cosmetic approach with a consecutive plastic reconstruction of the area (Figure 2). By the second postoperative week, a clean, neat, and thin scar was formed (Figure 3).

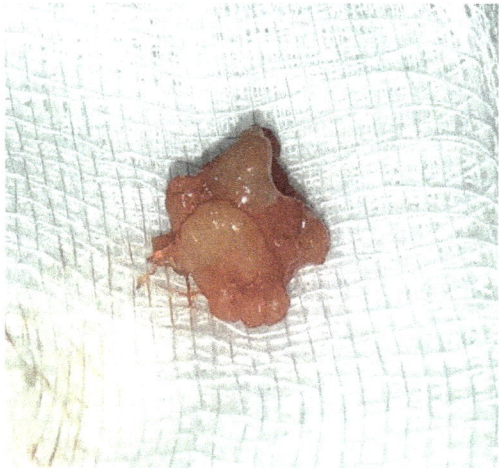

Figure 2. Well circumscribed subcutaneous tan lesion.

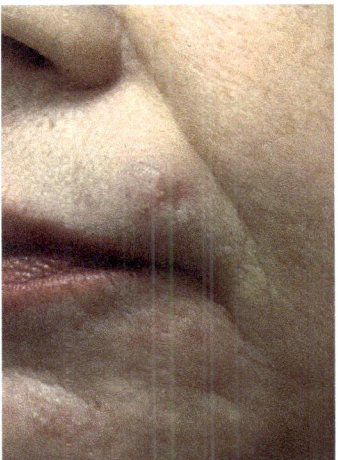

Figure 3 Two weeks after surgery.

3. Histopathologic Assessment

The histopathologic examination of the hematoxylin-and-eosin–stained slides revealed a well circumscribed unencapsulated lesion in the subcutis without clear connection to the epidermis or adnexal structures and scant inflammatory infiltrate. With respect to the epithelial component, the following patterns were observed: tubular structures lined by one or two layers of epithelial cells, strands/cords, single cell distribution, cribriform structures, syringomatoid tadpole-like structures, and small solid nests (Figure 4A,D). The epithelial component also showed variations in the cell appearance with the focal presence of plasmacytoid (hyaline) cells, shadow cells, physaliphorous-like cells, and intracellular vacuolization reminiscent of abortive luminal differentiation [1].

The follicular differentiation was determined by the presence of infundibular cysts (cystlike structures lined by a stratified squamous epithelium that contains a granular layer and corneocytes in lamellar pattern) (Figure 4B), basaloid metrical cells, trichchyalin granules, follicular germlike structures, and trichilemmal differentiation (palisaded pale or clear columnar cells often associated with a basal membrane, often with nuclei at the pole opposite to the basement membrane, indicating follicular differentiation toward the outer sheath at the bulb) (Figure 4C,E).

No other metaplastic or other cellular alterations involving the epithelial components were observed. The myoepithelial component consisted of strands/cords and small solid nests.

Sebaceous differentiation was determined by the presence of mature adipocytes with vacuolated cytoplasm and scalloped nuclei, some of which connected to trichilemmal cyst-like structures (Figure 5A).

No apocrine differentiation in the form of decapitation secretion was observed.

Apart from the typical myxohyaline and cartilaginous appearances of the stromal component, other variations were observed like lipomatous metaplasia consisting of small clusters of mature lipocytes, some of which contained intranuclear inclusions in the form of so-called Lochkern [1] (Figure 5).

Careful examination of the slides from the previous biopsy showed some of the same patterns: infundibular cysts, double-layered tubular structures, and trichilemmal and sebaceous elements, as well as some strands/cords of cells and clusters of mature adipocytes (Figure 6). The stromal component was mostly of the spindled cell variety, lacking the myxochondroid appearance of the excisional biopsy. These findings led us to deduct that this lesion was misdiagnosed as microcystic adnexal carcinoma for it in fact contains a lot of the hallmarks of cutaneous mixed tumor without the characteristic stomal appearance.

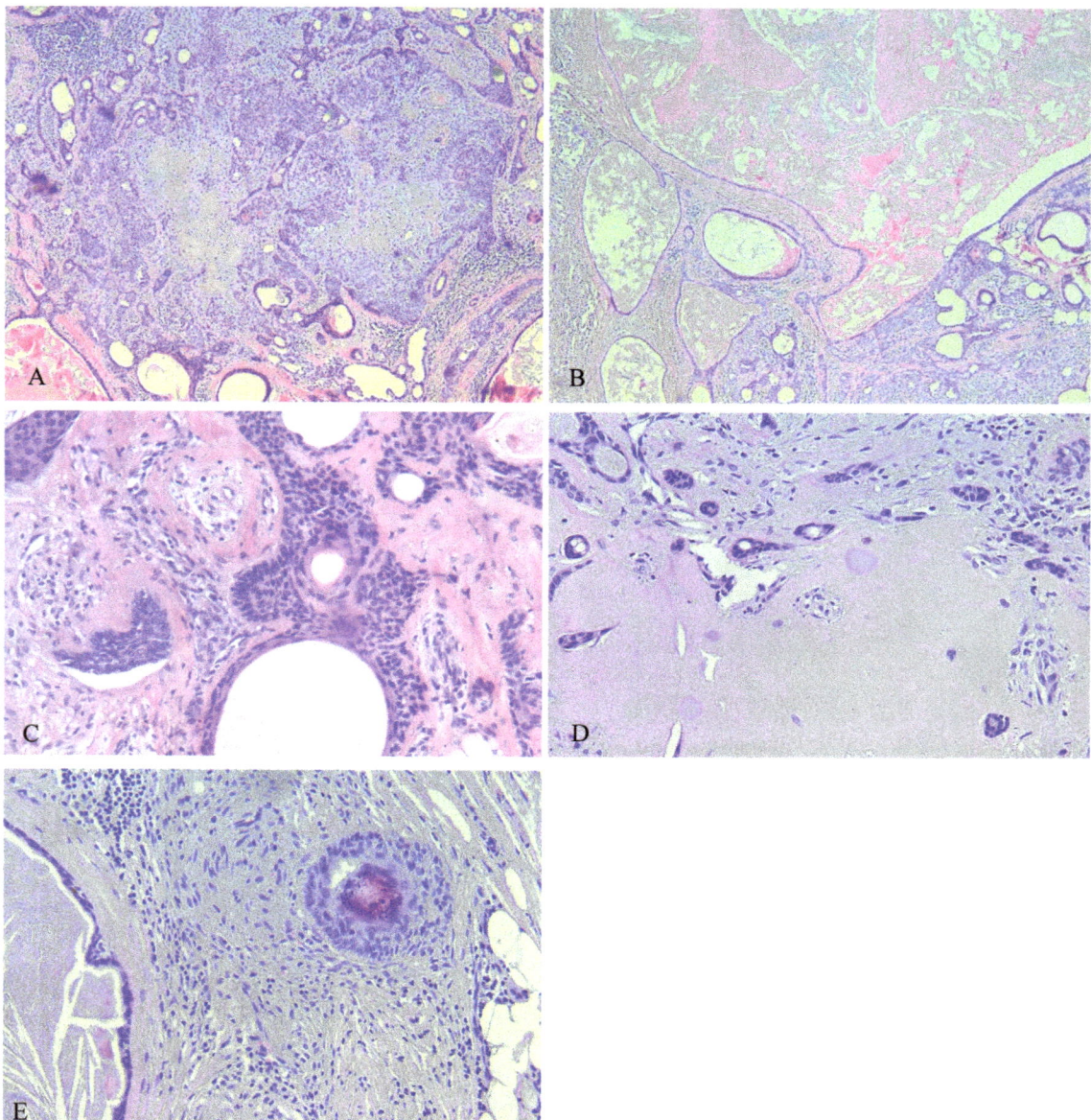

Figure 4. (**A**) Tubular structures and solid areas in a mixochondroid background. (**B**) Infundibular cysts in various sizes with corneocytes in lamellar pattern. (**C**) Follicular germlike structures, (small aggregations of germinative cells with peripheral palisading, with or without associated whorls of delicate collagen bundles and thin fibroblasts). (**D**) Comma/tadpole shaped ducts; syringoma like eccrine structures. (**E**) Cells resembling those of the internal epithelial sheath (trichohyalin granules).

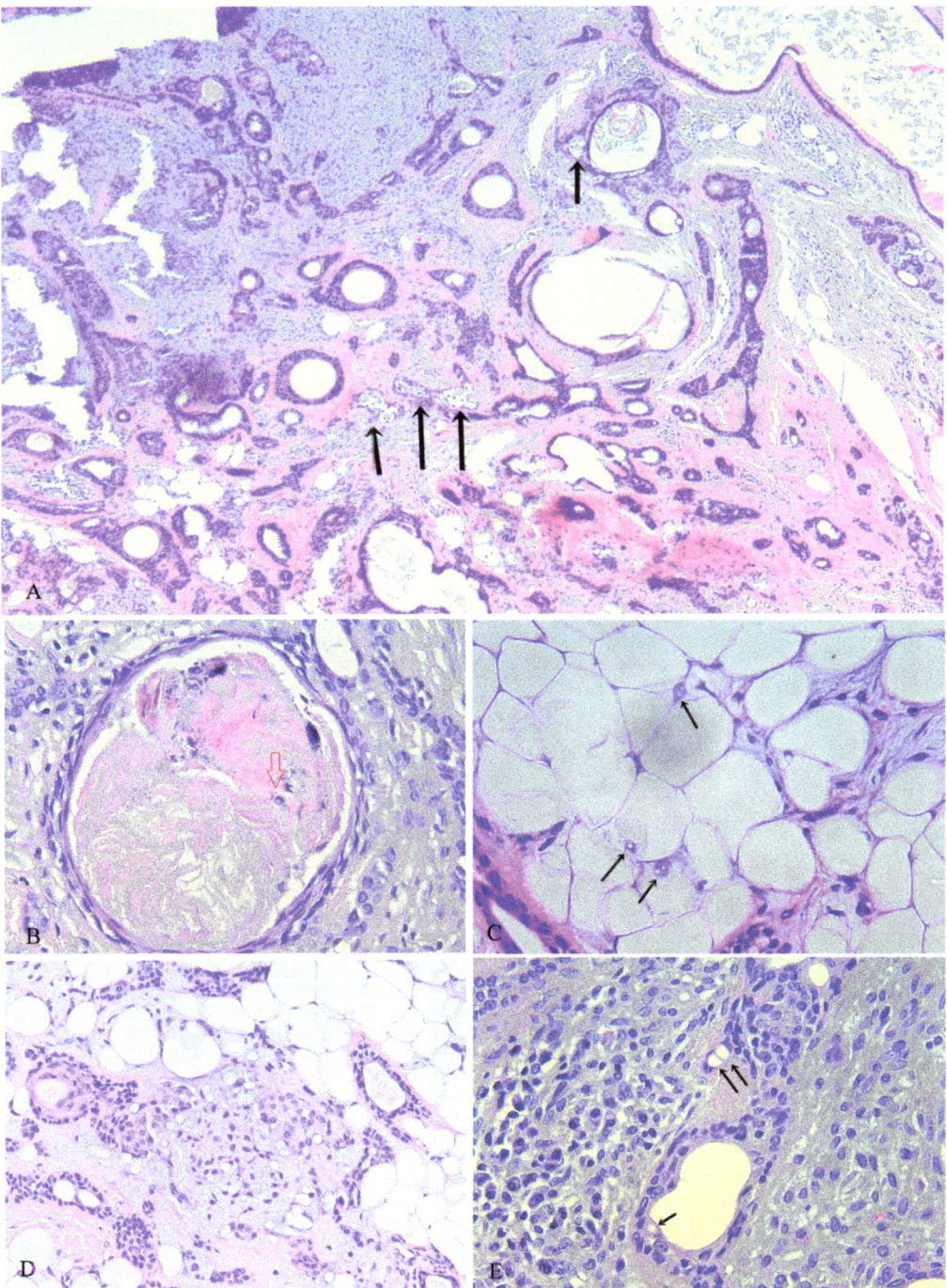

Figure 5. (**A**) Sebaceous gland elements (black arrows). (**B**) Shadow cells (red arrow). (**C**) Lipomatous metaplasia—mature adipocytes with intranuclear inclusions—Lochkern. (**D**) Physaliphorous-like cells. (**E**) Intracytoplasmic vacuoles.

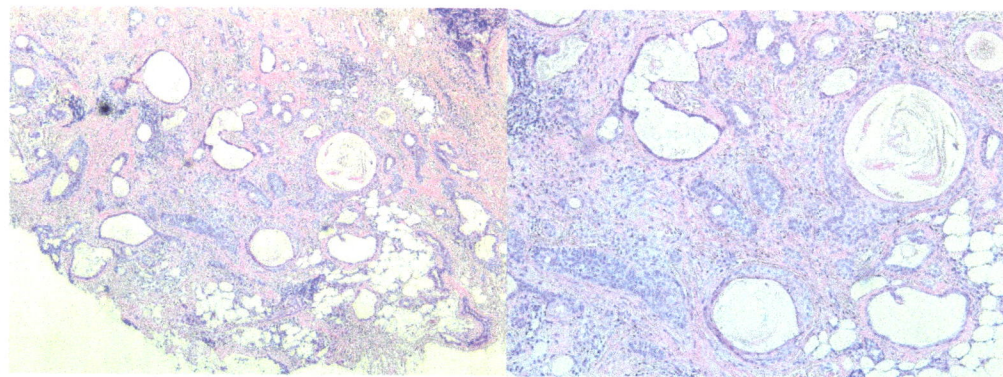

Figure 6. H&E stained slides from the first incisional biopsy of the patient.

4. Immunohistochemical Study

Immunohistochemical stains were performed on tissue sections from both the incisional and excisional biopsy. CEA and EMA were performed on the first specimen showing positive staining of the luminal cells of the neoplastic tubules, with occasional staining of the secretory material (Figure 7A,B). The epithelial cells were uniformly positive for CK14/5 confirming the eccrine nature of the mixed tumor, whereas GCDF15 was negative except for a single neoplastic tubular structure (Figure 7C,D). BerEP4 showed positive areas trichoblastic differentiation, and p63 was positive in the cells showing a myoepithelial morphologic phenotype (Figure 7E,F) [6].

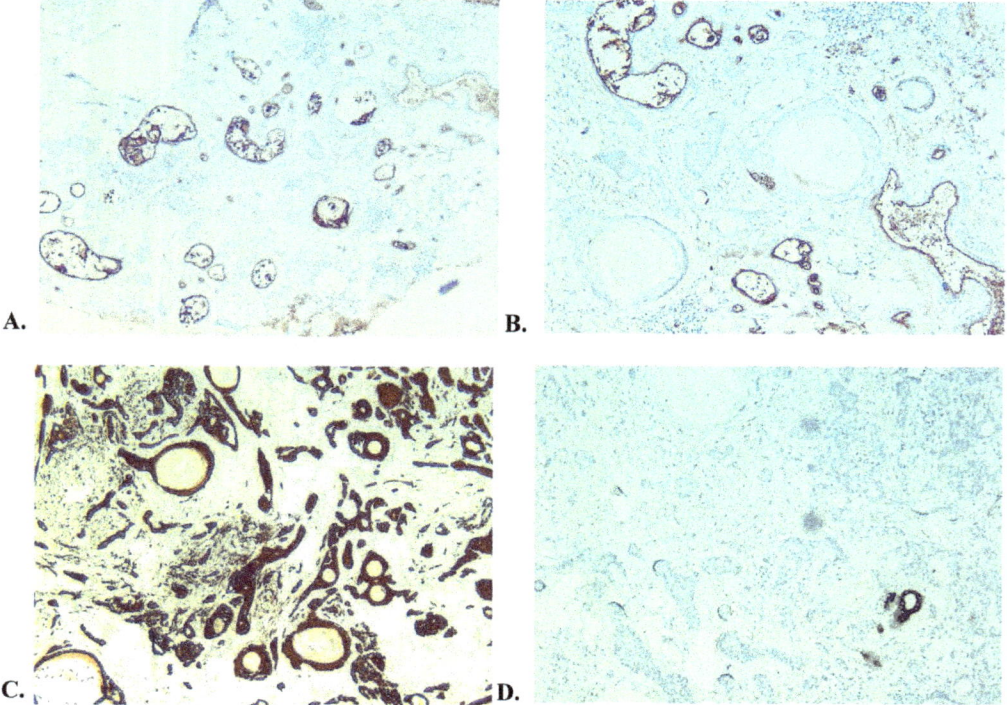

Figure 7. *Cont.*

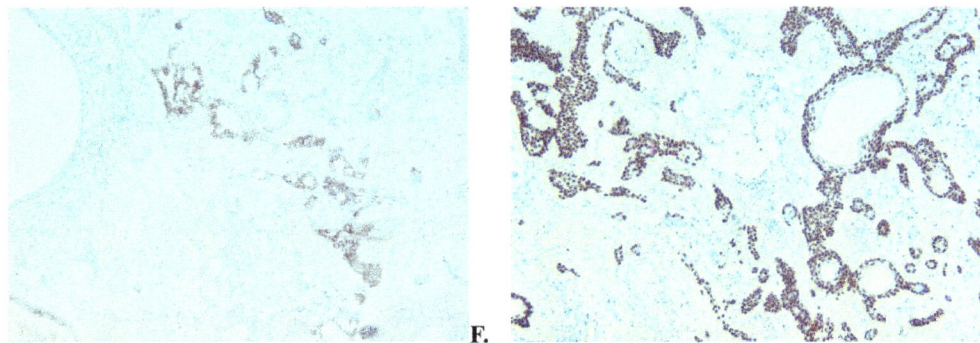

Figure 7. (**A**,**B**) CEA and EMA, respectively, showing positive staining in the luminal epithelial cells as well as in the secretory material but overall negativity in the neoplastic cells. (**C**) Positive expression of CK14/5 in the epithelial cells. (**D**) GCDFP15 positivity is a single neoplastic tubule. (**E**) BerEP4 positivity in a portion of the neoplastic tubules. (**F**) p63 positive staining is shown in the outer layer of the neoplastic tubules as part of the myoepithelial component.

5. Discussion

Mixed tumor of the skin, arguably referred to as chondroid syringoma, is a rare and mostly benign skin lesion, comprising epithelial, myoepithelial, and mesenchymal stromal-derived elements [7]. The most commonly reported location is in the head and neck region with a frequency of less than 0.1% [7,8]. Due to the wide variety of differentiation and metaplastic changes in these lesions, it may present a diagnostic pitfall as it could mimic various skin and adnexal neoplasms. Cutaneous mixed tumor may be a diagnosis more frequent than expected, as case studies show a high risk of misdiagnosis, especially on a preoperative biopsy material, most commonly confused with other benign lesions such as dermoid or sebaceous cysts, neurofibromas, dermatofibromas, histiocytomas, pilomatricomas, and seborrheic keratosis [8,9]. The epithelial component is comprised of neoplastic structures that resemble established types of adnexal neoplasms, some of which are recognized in syringoma and apocrine hidradenoma, as well as some malignant differential diagnoses: carcinomas with a mucinous stroma, carcinosarcoma, mucoepidermoid carcinoma, and not rarely basal cell carcinoma [10–12]. We as well are presenting a clinical case with the misdiagnosis of microcystic adenocarcinoma on the preoperative biopsy. In a limited biopsy, lesions of this nature could represent a diagnostic pitfall by potentially mimicking a metastatic carcinoma [3]. Another potential diagnostic pitfall is the presence of physaliphorous-like cells occasioning a resemblance to the cells of a chordoma [3]. Some authors have discussed the differential diagnosis of such tumors with some mesenchymal neoplasms, including osteoma cutis and cutaneous chondroma [11,13,14]. Mixed tumors may show a prominent myoepithelial component with changes such as collagenous spherulosis, a feature originally reported in the breast; this occurrence in the salivary glands has been reported in myoepitheliomas and pleomorphic adenomas [1].

Overall, most of the available cases report a definite association between the apocrine subtype of cutaneous mixed tumor and folliculo–sebaceous differentiation [15]. Our case represents an undeniable folliculo–sebaceous differentiation with immunohistochemically verified eccrine origin of the neoplastic tubular structures (CK14/5+), which broadcasts common histogenesis of the folliculo–sebaceous–apocrine complex and the eccrine glands. This proves further investigation is needed to determine the definite progenitor cell type of mixed tumor and the usefulness of ICH for determining the tumor subtype as either eccrine or apocrine.

The most effective method for definitive diagnosis of mixed tumor is total excision and histopathologic examination. Fine-needle aspiration cytology has also been described for the diagnosis of mixed tumor, but for such a small subcutaneous lesion, this remained ineffective [8].

Two distinct cytologic components are reported to be diagnostic by FNA: a mesenchymal element with a chondroid appearance and an epithelial component. Although FNA may be useful if it is necessary to determine the pathology prior to definitive excision, histologic examination of an excised specimen remains the definitive method of diagnosis [16,17].

Although this tumor may be treated with various methods, including electrodesiccation, dermabrasion, and vaporization with argon or CO_2 lasers, the treatment of choice is complete excision with a cuff of normal tissue in order to examine the histopathologic features [8,10]. As incidence of non-melanoma skin cancer is increasing, it is proving to be a public health problem, taking also into account the higher treatment costs, especially at the level of the face, as a more cosmetic approach is desired. Concluding the correct diagnosis is of utmost importance not only for patient prognosis, but it has also been observed that treatment costs differ according to the type of the neoplasm. [18]

The literature reviews suggest that recurrences were seen only when treatment consisted of electrodesiccation or incomplete excision. Lesions did not recur once they had been removed in toto [7]. Malignant transformation is exceptionally rare, with only a few cases reported where additionally a long term followup is recommended, as some authors even suggest adjuvant radiotherapy [19–21].

The heterogenicity of cutaneous mixed tumors highlights the importance of obtaining adequate tissue for histologic evaluation, as they can be confused with other skin neoplasms because of their clinically ambiguous presentations.

Author Contributions: All authors have contributed to the conceptualization of the manuscript. Methodology, V.I. and H.S.; resources, G.Y.; writing—original draft preparation, D.K. and T.D.; writing—review and editing, V.I. and G.Y. All authors have read and agreed to the published version of the manuscript.

Funding: This research received no external funding.

Institutional Review Board Statement: Ethical review and approval are not applicable as there were no experiments or tests run on human or animal subjects. The manuscript is a retrospective case report and is not a part of a study requiring ethical approval. Furthermore, no confidential patient information is disclosed.

Informed Consent Statement: The clinical procedures were carried out according to the guidelines of the World. Medical Association's Declaration of Helsinki and the Ministry of Health for Good Clinical Practice. Written informed consent has been obtained from the patient to publish this paper.

Data Availability Statement: The authors confirm that the data supporting the findings of this study are available within the article.

Conflicts of Interest: The authors declare no conflict of interest.

References

1. Wan, H.; Xu, M.; Xia, T. Clinical and pathological study on mixed tumors of the skin. *Medicine* **2018**, *97*, e12216. [CrossRef] [PubMed]
2. Kazakov, D.V.; Belousova, I.E.; Bisceglia, M.; Calonje, E.; Emberger, M.; Grayson, W.; Hantschke, M.; Kempf, W.; Kutzner, H.; Michal, M.; et al. Apocrine mixed tumor of the skin ("mixed tumor of the folliculosebaceous-apocrine complex"). Spectrum of differentiations and metaplastic changes in the epithelial, myoepithelial, and stromal components based on a histopathologic study of 244 cases. *J. Am. Acad. Dermatol.* **2007**, *57*, 467–483. [CrossRef] [PubMed]
3. Kazakov, D.V.; Kacerovska, D.; Hantschke, M.; Zelger, B.; Kutzner, H.; Requena, L.; Grayson, W.; Bisceglia, M.; Schaller, J.; Kempf, W.; et al. Cutaneous mixed tumor, eccrine variant: A clinicopathologic and immunohistochemical study of 50 cases, with emphasis on unusual histopathologic features. *Am. J. Dermatopathol.* **2011**, *33*, 557–568. [CrossRef]
4. Rodríguez-Díaz, E.; Armijo, M. Mixed tumors with follicular differentiation: Complex neoplasms of the primary epithelial germ. *Int. J. Dermatol.* **1995**, *34*, 782–785. [CrossRef]
5. Mills, S.E. Mixed tumor of the skin: A model of divergent differentiation. *J. Cutan. Pathol.* **1984**, *11*, 382–386. [CrossRef] [PubMed]

6. Ansai, S.; Takayama, R.; Kimura, T.; Kawana, S. Ber-EP4 is a useful marker for follicular germinative cell differentiation of cutaneous epithelial neoplasms. *J. Dermatol.* **2012**, *39*, 688–692. [CrossRef] [PubMed]
7. Hirsch, P.; Helwig, E.B. Chondroid Syringoma: Mixed Tumor of Skin, Salivary Gland Type. *Arch. Dermatol.* **1961**, *84*, 835–847. [CrossRef]
8. Yavuzer, R.; Başterzi, Y.; Sari, A.; Bir, F.; Sezer, C. Chondroid syringoma: A diagnosis more frequent than expected. *Dermatol. Surg.* **2003**, *29*, 179–181. [CrossRef]
9. Baran, J.L.; Hoang, M.P. Apocrine mixed tumor of the skin with a prominent pilomatricomal component. *J. Cutan. Pathol.* **2009**, *36*, 882–886. [CrossRef]
10. Chen, A.H.; Moreano, E.H.; Houston, B.; Funk, F.G. Chondroid syringoma of the head and neck: Clinical management and literature review. *Ear Nose Throat J.* **1996**, *75*, 104–108. [CrossRef]
11. Tirumalae, R.; Boer, A. Calcification and ossification in eccrine mixed tumors: Underrecognized feature and diagnostic pitfall. *Am. J. Dermatopathol.* **2009**, *31*, 772–777. [CrossRef] [PubMed]
12. Linares González, L.; Aguayo Carreras, P.; Rueda Villafranca, B.; Navarro-Triviño, F.J. Chondroid Syringoma Mimicking Basal Cell Carcinoma. *Actas Dermo-Sifiliográficas* **2020**, *111*, 341–343. [CrossRef]
13. Shimizu, S.; Han-Yaku, H.; Fukushima, S.; Shimizu, H. Immunohistochemical study of mixed tumor of the skin with marked ossification. *Dermatology* **1996**, *193*, 255–257. [CrossRef] [PubMed]
14. Thompson, J.; Squires, S.; Machan, M.; Fraga, G.R.; Aires, D. Cutaneous mixed tumor with extensive chondroid metaplasia: A potential mimic of cutaneous chondroma. *Dermatol. Online J.* **2012**, *18*, 9. [CrossRef] [PubMed]
15. Kazakov, D.V.; Bisceglia, M.; Spagnolo, D.V.; Kutzner, H.; Belousova, I.E.; Hes, O.; Sima, R.; Vanecek, T.; Yang, Y.; Michal, M. Apocrine mixed tumors of the skin with architectural and/or cytologic atypia: A retrospective clinicopathologic study of 18 cases. *Am. J. Surg. Pathol.* **2007**, *31*, 1094–1102. [CrossRef]
16. Gottschalk-Sabag, S.; Glick, T. Chondroid syringoma diagnosed by fine-needle aspiration: A case report. *Diagn. Cytopathol.* **1994**, *10*, 152–155. [CrossRef]
17. Srinivasan, R.; Rajwanshi, A.; Padmanabhan, Y.; Dey, P. Fine needle aspiration cytology of chondroid syringoma and syringocystadenoma papilliferum: A report of two cases. *Acta Cytol.* **1993**, *37*, 535–538.
18. Faur, C.I.; Moldovan, M.A.; Văleanu, M.; Rotar, H.; Filip, L.; Roman, R.C. The Prevalence and Treatment Costs of Non-Melanoma Skin Cancer in Cluj-Napoca Maxillofacial Center. *Medicina* **2023**, *59*, 220. [CrossRef]
19. Harrist, T.J.; Aretz, T.H.; Mihm, M.C., Jr.; Evans, G.W.; Rodriquez, F.L. Malignant chondroid syringoma. *Arch. Dermatol.* **1981**, *117*, 719–724. [CrossRef]
20. Lal, K.; Morrell, T.J.; Cunningham, M.; O'Donnell, P.; Levin, N.A.; Cornejo, K.M. A Case of a Malignant Cutaneous Mixed Tumor (Chondroid Syringoma) of the Scapula Treated With Staged Margin-Controlled Excision. *Am. J. Dermatopathol.* **2018**, *40*, 679–681. [CrossRef]
21. Lu, H.; Chen, L.F.; Chen, Q.; Shen, H.; Liu, Z. A rare large cutaneous chondroid syringoma involving a toe: A case report. *Medicine* **2018**, *97*, e9825. [CrossRef] [PubMed]

Disclaimer/Publisher's Note: The statements, opinions and data contained in all publications are solely those of the individual author(s) and contributor(s) and not of MDPI and/or the editor(s). MDPI and/or the editor(s) disclaim responsibility for any injury to people or property resulting from any ideas, methods, instructions or products referred to in the content.

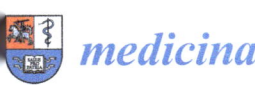

Article

The Prevalence and Treatment Costs of Non-Melanoma Skin Cancer in Cluj-Napoca Maxillofacial Center

Cosmin Ioan Faur [1], Mădălina Anca Moldovan [1,*], Mădălina Văleanu [2], Horațiu Rotar [1], Laura Filip [1] and Rareș Călin Roman [1]

[1] Department of Maxillofacial Surgery and Radiology, Oral and Cranio-Maxillofacial Surgery, "Iuliu Hațieganu" University of Medicine and Pharmacy, 33 Moților Street, 400001 Cluj-Napoca, Romania
[2] Department of Medical Informatics and Biostatistics, "Iuliu Hatieganu" University of Medicine and Pharmacy, 6 Pasteur Street, 400012 Cluj-Napoca, Romania
* Correspondence: madilazar@yahoo.com; Tel.: +40-742054108

Abstract: *Background and Objectives:* An increasing incidence of non-melanoma skin cancer (NMSC) is noted, as well as an increasing cost of the treatment, with NMSC becoming a public health problem. We aimed to investigate the prevalence and treatment costs of surgically treated NMSC from the Oral and Maxillofacial Surgery Department of Cluj-Napoca County Hospital. *Materials and Methods:* We retrospectively analyzed the clinical data and the charge data of hospitalization from the informatic system of Cluj-Napoca County Hospital. All patients benefited from standard surgical excision with the reconstruction of the post-excisional defect. A statistical analysis of the costs related to the patients' features, period and conditions of hospitalization, materials, medication, and paraclinical investigations was performed. *Results:* Between 2015 and 2019, 133 patients with NMSC were addressed to our department, with basal cell carcinoma (BCC) being four-fold higher than squamous cell carcinoma (SCC). Most NMSC cases were diagnosed in stage I or II, and they benefited from local reconstruction. The treatment costs progressively increased in the last five years, reaching a total cost of EUR ~13.000 in 2019. The treatment cost per episode was higher for SCC compared to BCC, while the total cost of treatment in 5 years was higher for BCC. Low income, immunosuppression, comorbidities, flap reconstruction option, long-lasting surgery, and prolonged hospitalization were associated with an increased cost of the treatment. *Conclusion:* The prevalence and treatment cost of surgically treated NMSC of the head and neck region increased in the last five years, with high-cost drivers being related to patients and treatment options.

Keywords: non-melanoma skin cancer; head and neck cancer; hospitalization costs

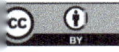

1. Introduction

Non-melanoma skin cancer (NMSC) is an important health problem due to increased incidence in the last years and the increased morbidity and costs of the treatment [1,2]. However, the real incidence of NMSC is unknown. The World Health Organization (WHO) estimates 2–3 million malignant skin tumors per year which are most likely under-reported, especially in light of a recent study that estimated 3.3 million people who suffered from 5.4 million NMSC cases, part of them presenting more than one skin tumor [3]. In addition, the GLOBOCAN project of the International Agency for Research on Cancer reported an incidence of 1,198,000 new cases of NMSC (excluding basal cell carcinoma) in all sites worldwide in 2020, which was four-fold higher than malignant melanoma (324.000 new cases) [1]. The incidence of NMSC in the European population varies depending on geographical area, histopathological type, and age [4]. The prevalence of head and neck NMSC reported in Northeastern Romania was 72.5% and in Poland was 90% [5,6].

Most histopathological variants of the NMSC are basal cell carcinoma (BCC) (75–80%) and squamous cell carcinoma (SCC) (20–25%), the remnant variants (1%) being Merkel cell carcinoma, sebaceous carcinoma, apocrine adenocarcinoma, and other rare tumors [7]. In Europe, BCC presents a high incidence in Western Europe, especially in the Netherlands (87.5/100,000 person-years), Switzerland, and Italy (70/100,000 person-years), and a low incidence in Central and Eastern Europe, with Croatia presenting the lowest incidence (33.6/100.000 person-years). In addition to BCC, SCC has a high incidence in Western Europe (Switzerland 28.9/100.000 person-years), followed by Northern Europe, and a low incidence in Central and Eastern Europe (Croatia 8.9/100,000 person-years) [1–4].

The risk factors for developing NMSC are fair skin, increased number of freckles, sunburns, sun exposure, radiation, and immunosuppression [4–8]. Owing to the UV-associated risk, Australia and New Zealand are the countries with the highest risk of developing NMSC [1]. In addition, aging is an independent risk factor for the occurrence of head and neck NMSC. The head and neck region is prone to developing NMSC, being a highly sun-exposed area [5,6].

BCC causes significant morbidity due to local destructive spread and high local recurrence risk but has low metastatic potential [9]. On the contrary, SCC has a high propensity for metastatic spread, and hence a poor prognosis. SCC mortality is usually associated with locoregional and distant metastases [10]. The 5-year survival rates of NMS depend on age, immunosuppression status, surgical margins, and tumor features being higher for BCC compared to SCC [11]. Overall, NMSC has a better prognostic than other skin cancers, such as malignant melanoma or Merkel carcinoma [12,13].

NMSC treatment can be conducted by standard surgical excision, Mohs micrographic surgery, or destructive methods, such as curettage, cautery, cryosurgery, photodynamic therapy, and the application of local drugs [14]. Surgical excision, which encompasses 85% of cases, reports a five-year cure rate of 99% for BCC and 97% for SCC [15]. The cost of cancer treatment is high, being an economic and clinical burden to the National Healthcare system, as well as an economic burden to individuals [13]. The NMSC diagnosis and treatment costs are more expensive than those of malignant melanoma, due to higher incidence, even though the cost of malignant melanoma is higher per person-year [16,17]. Moreover, the NMSC treatment costs increased in the last years more than other skin cancers, being four-fold more expensive than malignant melanoma treatment [15–18]. BCC has a higher total cost of treatment compared with SCC [19]. Generally, the costs of head and neck cancers are higher compared with other locations, and the patients tend to be poorer and to have accrued lower levels of education than patients with other cancers [13,15,20]. Moreover, head and neck NMSC treatment has a higher cost than other anatomical regions, with the highest cost in nose BCC and auricle SCC tumors [5,16,19]. The costs also vary in different geographical areas due to different incidence and treatment protocols [21].

NMSC is not usually reported to a cancer database, hence the incidence and cost of the treatment are difficult to assess. Moreover, there are a few studies that discuss the head and neck NMSC treatment costs, and from our knowledge, none are reported in Romania. We aim to evaluate the prevalence and the direct costs of surgical treatment of head and neck NMSC from the Maxillofacial Surgery Department of Cluj-Napoca County Hospital.

2. Materials and Methods

We conducted a retrospective study on patients who were addressed to the Oral and Maxillofacial Surgery Department of Cluj-Napoca County Hospital between the first of January 2015 to the 31st of December 2019. We enrolled the patients who were hospitalized for at least 24 h in our department and had a histopathological result of head and neck BCC or SCC and primary or recurrent tumors. All the patients were treated by surgical excision and reconstruction of the defect. We excluded the patients who had an inconclusive histopathologic result, melanoma, Merkel cell skin cancer, or other rare malignant skin tumors, as well as benign skin lesions and the patients that underwent oncological treatment. All the included patients were staged according to American Joint Committee on Cancer (eighth edition) [22,23]. The patients' comorbidities were classified based on the American Society of Anesthesiologists (ASA) risk stratification to have an objective assessment of the general health status [24]. Not all the patients responded to education formation and economical status at hospital admission. This study was approved by the Ethics Committee of "Iuliu Hatieganu" University of Medicine and Pharmacy (AVZ 20/03.02.2022), and it is in accordance with the updated Declaration of Helsinki.

2.1. Data Collection and Cost Analysis

We reviewed the clinical data and the charge data of hospitalization from the informatic system of Cluj-Napoca County Hospital. The data extracted from the electronic medical records included the following: patients' demographics and associated medical diagnoses; the results of histopathological examinations; tumor characteristics, such as site; clinical and pathologic stage; treatment modality; and the discharge bill. The histopathological subtypes were classified according to the major pattern present in the specimen, many of them (89%) having 2 or more histopathological variants in the same specimen. We categorized the treatment after standard surgical excision as per primam closure, skin graft, and local flap reconstruction.

We analyzed only the direct costs of care related to the hospitalization for NMSC surgical treatment (hospitalization accommodation costs, material costs, medication costs, and paraclinical examinations costs), without assessment of the direct costs of follow-up or the indirect (e.g., productivity costs) or intangible costs (e.g., monetary value of health loss and reduces the quality of life) [21,25]. The costs were presented as total treatment costs for NMSC, BCC, and SCC tumors and as individual mean costs of the tumors' treatment related to the number of patients or episodes of cancer. A patient is defined as a person that suffered from at least one malignant skin tumor in the time interval. An episode (of cancer) is defined as a malignant skin tumor of a patient treated in one setting appointment (hospitalization). Hence, the means of cost per episode and per patient were constructed.

The costs are reported in Euros, with an exchange medium rate calculated after the Romanian National Bank rank (e.g., 5-year medium exchange rate Euro-RON). In addition, the costs are adjusted to the inflation rate up to 2022, according to the Romanian National Bank.

2.2. Statistical Analysis

The SPSS 25.0 software (SPSS Inc, Chicago, IL, USA) was used for statistical analysis and data description. The level of statistical significance was set at $\alpha = 0.05$. Mean $\pm$ standard deviation was used to describe normally distributed continuous quantitative data and absolute and relative frequencies (%) were used for qualitative data.

The comparison of the means was performed by the Student t-test for normally distributed data of two independent groups. The non-parametric Mann–Whitney and Kruskal–Wallis tests were used to compare the means of two independent groups with non-normal distribution. The Kruskal–Wallis test was also used for the comparison between more than two groups with non-normal distribution, and then the Tukey HSD test was used for post hoc analysis. Chi-Square or Fisher Exact tests were used to compare qualitative variables. Univariate regression analysis was used to estimate costs.

3. Results

3.1. Demographical and Epidemiological Consideration of the Population

From a total of 195 patients who were addressed for skin tumors to our service between 2015 and 2019, 144 patients presented malignant tumors, including 133 (92%) BCC and SCC patients (Figure 1). This study enrolled 102 (76%) BCC patients, 27 (20%) SCC patients, and 4 (4%) patients with both skin cancers, which presented 152 episodes of cancer. Most of the BCC tumors were nodular (66 tumors), infiltrative (33 tumors), or basosquamous (13 tumors) differentiated, the rest (8 tumors) being less frequent histopathological BCC variants. SCC grading revealed 11 well-differentiated, 18 intermediate-differentiated, and 3 poorly differentiated tumors, with only 5 of the SCC tumors (15%) being non-keratinizing lesions. Sixteen patients had two NMSCs with different localizations, excised during the 5-year period (eleven BCC patients, one SCC, and four patients had one BCC and one SCC).

One 74-year-old female patient presented four hospitalizations between 2018 and 2019 for BCC tumors located in different head and neck regions.

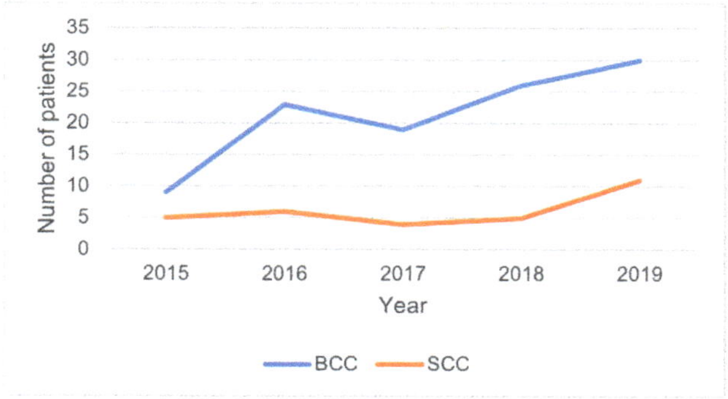

Figure 1. Year distribution of the skin cancer patients.

The mean ± standard deviation age of the NMSC patients was 67 ± 13 years, being slightly increased for SCC subpopulations (69 ± 15 years) compared to SCC ones (67 ± 13 years). The maximum prevalence of NMSC episodes was in the seventh decade of life, as can be seen in Table 1. The male-to-female ratio was 1.3:1 and most of the patients (60.53%) had an urban place of residence. In addition, most of the patients (61 subjects) that responded to the admission questionnaire did have any education following high school, and only 32 patients had university studies. In addition, many of these patients had low-income economic status.

Table 1. Non-melanoma skin cancer epidemiology and treatment costs.

		Malignant Skin Cancer Episodes				NMSC Treatment Cost Per Episode	
	NMSC n = episodes (n%)	BCC n = episodes (n%)	SCC n = episodes (n%)	p value (BCC vs. SCC among subsets) *		Mean ± standard deviation (Euro) **	p Value (costs comparison among subsets) ***
			Age decade distribution				
20–30	2 (1.31%)	1 (0.83%)	1 (3.13%)			110 ± 9	
30–40	5 (3.27%)	4 (3.33%)	1 (3.13%)			177 ± 67	
40–50	18 (11.76%)	15 (12.5%)	3 (9.38%)			205 ± 90	
50–60	5 (3.27%)	4 (3.33%)	1 (3.13%)	0.31		226 ± 42	0.04
60–70	37 (24.18%)	33 (27.5%)	4 (12.5%)			248 ± 150	
70–80	54 (35.29%)	41 (34.17%)	13 (40.63%)			281 ± 224	
80–90	30 (19.61%)	22 (18.33%)	8 (25%)			352 ± 210	
90–100	1 (0.65%)	-	1 (3.13%)			-	
			Sex				
Female	64 (42.1%)	49 (40.83%)	15 (46.85%)	0.53		323 ± 271	0.17
Male	88 (57.9%)	71 (59.17%)	17 (53.13%)			271 ± 245	
			Place of living				
Rural	60 (39.47%)	45 (37.5%)	15 (46.88%)	0.33		331 ± 327	0.44
Urban	92 (60.53%)	75 (62.5%)	17 (53.13%)			266 ± 190	
			Educational formation				
Elementary school	5 (3.76%)	2 (1.87%)	3 (9.68%)			331 ± 329	
Medium school	24 (18.05%)	21 (19.63%)	3 (9.68%)			242 ± 159	
Technical school	9 (6.77%)	8 (7.48%)	1 (3.23%)	0.13		523 ± 622	0.16
High School	19 (14.29%)	16 (14.95%)	3 (9.68%)			258 ± 293	
College	15 (11.28%)	11 (10.28%)	4 (12.9%)			214 ± 163	

Table 1. *Cont.*

	Malignant Skin Cancer Episodes				NMSC Treatment Cost Per Episode	
	NMSC n = episodes (n%)	BCC n = episodes (n%)	SCC n = episodes (n%)	p value (BCC vs. SCC among subsets) *	Mean ± standard deviation (Euro) **	p Value (costs comparison among subsets) ***
Economic status						
Low income	42 (27.45%)	23 (19.17%)	10 (31.25%)	0.66	300 ± 331	<0.01
Medium income	26 (16.99%)	47 (39.16%)	3 (9.38%)		283 ± 282	
Upper income	4 (2.61%)	3 (2.5%)	1 (3.13%)		103 ± 4	
Immunosuppression						
Yes	6 (3.95%)	3 (2.5%)	3 (9.38%)	0.07	419 ± 212	0.04
No	146 (96.05%)	117 (97.5%)	29 (90.63%)		277 ± 213	
ASA risk classification						
I	50 (32.89%)	40 (33.33%)	10 (31.25%)	0.91	242 ± 219	0.03
II	54 (35.53%)	42 (35%)	12 (37.5%)		333 ± 106	
III	48 (31.58%)	38 (31.67%)	10 (31.25%)		339 ± 142	
Tumor's location (head and neck regions)						
Auricular	11 (7.24%)	5 (5%)	5 (15.63%)	0.14	214 ± 113	0.14
Cervical	2 (1.32%)	1 (0.83%)	1 (3.13%)		215 ± 49	
Frontal	17 (11.18%)	11 (9.17%)	6 (18.75%)		332 ± 303	
Cheek	29 (19.08%)	24 (20%)	5 (15.63%)		329 ± 225	
Infraorbital	7 (4.61%)	5 (5%)	1 (3.13%)		203 ± 61	
Labial	5 (3.29%)	4 (3.33%)	1 (3.13%)		376 ± 225	
Mental	3 (1.97%)	3 (2.5%)	-		143 ± 33	
Orbital	14 (9.21%)	13 (10.83%)	1 (3.13%)		421 ± 340	
Nasal	46 (30.26%)	40 (33.33%)	6 (18.75%)		256 ± 154	
Temporal	18 (11.84%)	12 (10%)	6 (18.75%)		301 ± 456	
Stage of the disease						
I	97 (63.82%)	83 (69.17%)	14 (43.75%)	0.002	253 ± 151	0.65
II	31 (20.39%)	25 (20.83%)	6 (18.75%)		307 ± 184	
III	21 (13.82%)	11 (9.17%)	10 (31.25%)		371 ± 446	
IV	3 (1.97%)	1 (0.83%)	2 (6.25%)		974 ± 715	
Type of reconstruction						
Primary closure	50 (32.68%)	37 (30.83%)	13 (40.63%)	0.52	198 ± 116	<0.01
Skin graft	8 (5.23%)	5 (5%)	2 (6.25%)		220 ± 134	
Local flap	94 (61.44%)	77 (64.17%)	17 (53.13%)		352 ± 315	
Time needed for surgical procedure						
<1 h	66 (43.42%)	53 (44.16%)	13 (40.62%)	-	257 ± 177	<0.01
1–2 h	66 (43.42%)	52 (43.33%)	14 (43.75%)		340 ± 155	
>2 h	20 (13.16%)	15 (12.5%)	5 (15.62%)		647 ± 581	
Days of hospitalization						
1	69 (45.39%)	56 (46.66%)	13 (40.62%)	0.53	139 ± 31	<0.01
2	36 (23.68%)	31 (25.83%)	5 (15.62%)		281 ± 190	
3	18 (11.84%)	13 (10.83)	5 (15.62%)		357 ± 46	
4	14 (9.21%)	9 (7.5%)	5 (15.62%)		475 ± 58	
5	4 (2.63%)	3 (2.5%)	1 (3.12%)		596 ± 29	
6	5 (3.28%)	4 (3.33%)	1 (3.12%)		627 ± 70	
7>	6 (3.94%)	4 (3.33%)	2 (6.25%)		1177 ± 526	

* Statistical analysis of episode comparison between BCC and SCC subsets; ** average treatment costs of NMSC related to the cancer episodes; *** statistical analysis of NMSC cost between different subsets.

We found 148 primary tumor excisions of NMSC (117 BCC and 31 SCC) and 4 recurrence tumor excisions (3 BCC and 1 SCC). The tumor distribution in the head and neck regions is seen in Table 1. The nasal and cheek regions were highly involved by NMSC tumors. The skin malignant tumors were diagnosed frequently in stage I (97 tumors) or II (31 tumors) and were frequently managed by radical excision (146 tumors) with flap reconstruction (84 cases) or primary closure (50 cases) (Table 1). The surgical defects located in nasal, cheek, and orbital regions often required flap reconstructions, and the ones located in frontal and temporal areas had more primary closures than flap reconstructions ($p < 0.05$) (Figure 2).

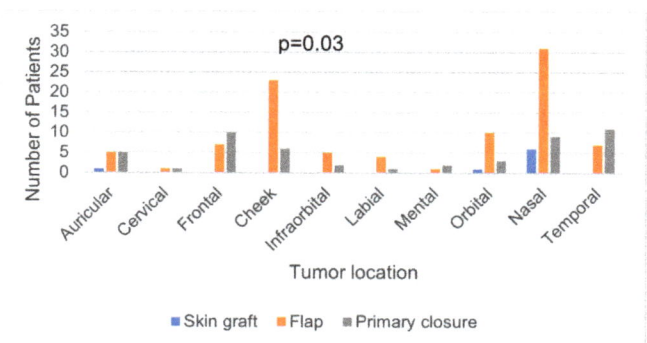

Figure 2. Correlation between tumor location and type of reconstruction used to repair the surgical defect.

The surgical excisions and reconstructions last less than 1 h or between 1 and 2 h for most of the tumors (Table 1). The patients were hospitalized between 1 (61 patients) and 10 days (1 stage IV patient), with a median (Q1, Q3) of 2 (1;3) days of hospital staying. A total of 342 days (264 BCC and 78 SCC) were needed for the head and neck skin cancer treatment in the 5 years.

Even if the first stage of NMSC cases were frequently surgically treated in less than one hour, there was no statistical significance regarding the correlation between the tumor stage and the time required by surgery to be performed (Figure 3). However, there was a statistically significant correlation between the tumor stage and the hospitalization days. Stages I and II were mostly treated within one to three days of hospitalization (Figure 4). In addition, the days of hospitalization were statistically correlated with the type of reconstruction, with primary closure and skin grafts requiring fewer hospitalization days than local flap reconstruction (Figure 5). On the contrary, the hospitalization days were not statistically correlated with ASA risk, even though most ASA risk I patients required one to three days of hospitalization (Figure 6).

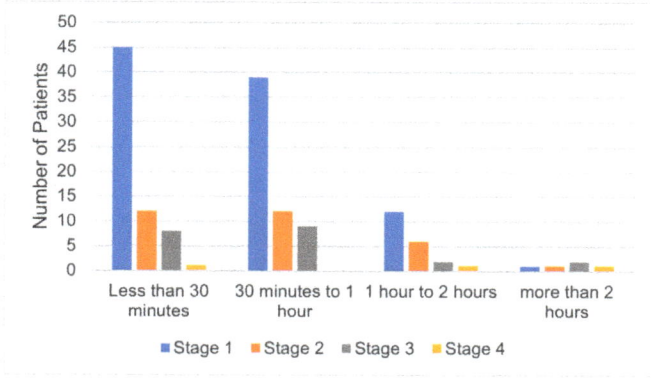

Figure 3. Correlation between tumor stage and time required to perform surgery.

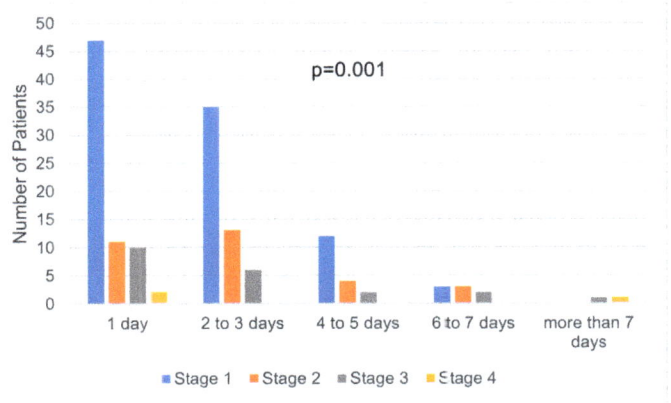

Figure 4. Correlation between tumor stage and days of hospitalization.

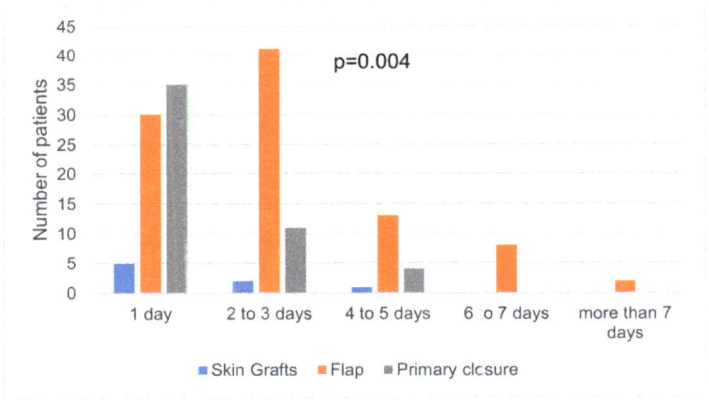

Figure 5. Correlation between days of hospitalization and type of reconstruction.

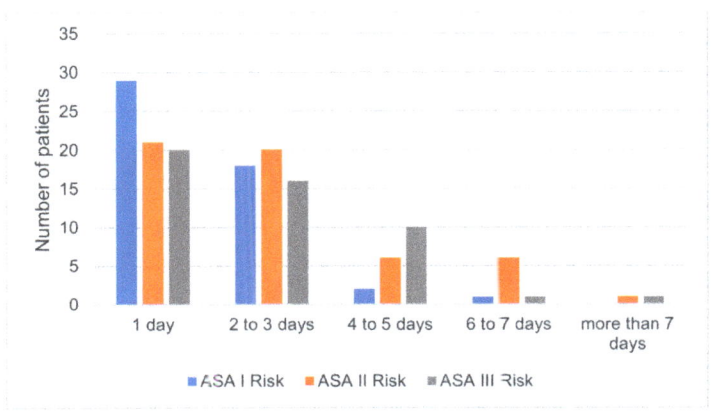

Figure 6. Correlation between days of hospitalization and ASA risk.

3.2. The Cost of NMSC Treatment

The direct costs of NMSC in 5 years of treatment were approximately EUR 45.000, with an average cost/patient and cost/episode of EUR 336 and EUR 294, respectively. The costs of treatment/episode had a statistically significant increase ($p = 0.03$) from EUR 228 in 2015 to EUR 352 in 2019, with a mean increase of approximately 28 EUR/year (Figure 7). The total treatment cost/5 years was more expensive (approximately EUR 34.000) for BCC than SCC (approximately EUR 11.300). However, the average treatment cost/patient was higher for SCC (EUR 352) than for BCC (EUR 316). The most expensive treatment (EUR 2064) was applied to a temporal BCC patient that was hospitalized for 10 days in 2017.

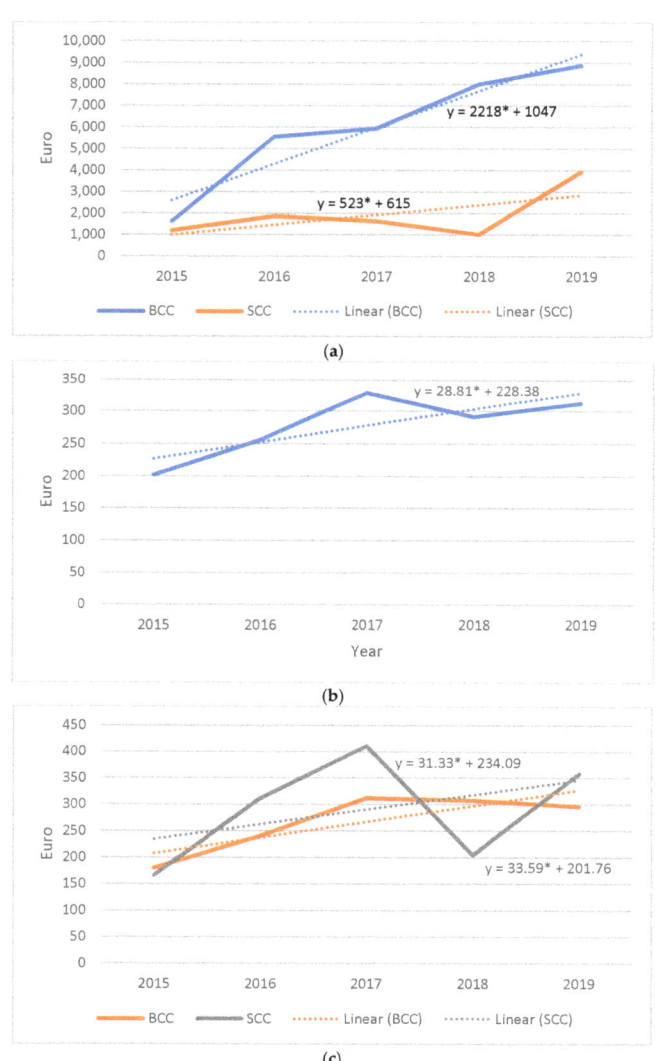

Figure 7. Direct treatment costs of NMSC: (**a**) total costs/5 years for SCC and BCC; (**b**) the increasing NMSC treatment costs/episode during 5 years of analysis; (**c**) the increasing BCC and SCC treatment costs/episode during 5 years of analysis.

Additional to the costs of the surgery and the accommodation, the total direct costs of treatment included EUR 2774 for the drugs administrated during the hospitalization, EUR 2384 for the supplies, and EUR 5670 for the paraclinical examinations for the 5 years of analysis. However, the costs of the surgery and the accommodation cannot be differentiated and individually assessed due to the lack of data illustrated in the informatic system of the hospital. The details of the treatment costs are seen in Table 2. Except for the medication, the medium cost of the supplies and paraclinical examination was higher for SCC in comparison with BCC.

Table 2. Averages of direct cost details of head and neck skin cancers for five years of treatment related to patient and episode of cancer.

Costs (EUR)	NMSC	BCC	SCC
Total direct costs			
Average cost per patient	336	317	252
Average cost per episode	294	282	341
Drug costs			
Average cost per patient	20	22	13
Average cost per episode	18	19	12
Paraclinical examination costs			
Average cost per patient	42	38	49
Average cost per episode	37	33	48
Supply costs			
Average cost per patient	18	17	17
Average cost per episode	15	15	17

The average cost per day of treatment for NMSC was EUR 131, with SCC being more expensive to treat (EUR 138) in comparison with BCC (EUR 127). However, the cost increased with the days of hospitalization, being 9-fold higher for more than 7 days of hospital staying than for 1 day of hospitalization.

3.3. Cost of NMSC Treatment Related to the Demographical and Clinical Features

Starting from the third decade of life, the treatment cost of NMSC statistically significantly increased ($t = 0.04$) by approximately 10% to 25% per decade (Table 1). The male patients and the subjects that had a rural place of living presented higher costs of treatment, however, without any statistical significance. Moreover, the patients that underwent technical schools and subjects with lower income presented higher costs of treatment, with the economic status classification being the only statistically significant result ($p = 0.004$).

Immunosuppression was a general status-related factor that influenced the treatment costs, with immunosuppressed patients presenting a statistically significant higher cost of treatment compared with the non-immunosuppressed subjects (Table 1). ASA risk classification also statistically increased the cost of NMSC, with the third class presenting a 39% higher cost compared to the first class.

The orbital region presented the highest cost of NMSC treatment. In addition to tumor location, the tumor stage did not present statistical significance, even if stage IV had approximately 4-fold increased treatment costs compared to stage I.

Re-excision costs were 1.57-fold higher than radical treatment of a primary tumor, without any statistical significance. In addition, standard excision surgery associated with flap reconstruction or surgery that lasts more than two hours presented the highest treatment cost ($p < 0.001$).

4. Discussion

The prevalence of NMSC tumors of the head and neck region in our study (approximately 90% of the malignant skin tumors) was higher than that reported in northeastern

Romania, however, the BCC to SCC ratio (4:1) was in accordance with the literature [1,5,6]. In addition, we had similar results regarding the age-related risk for NMSC development, with approximately 80% of the episodes of cancer in our research occurring in subjects older than 60 years, with a slightly increased age of SCC subjects [21,26]. We found that the nose was the most frequent tumor site for NMSC lesion development.

We identified increasing costs of NMSC treatment per year in the last 5 years, which could be attributed to the increasing number of patients and to the treatment costs of cancer episodes, expected to be much higher in the next years as the costs were constantly raising by 28 EUR/year. The increasing costs of the treatment rely on the new technologies and better quality of life offered by the new therapies [27]. However, our findings underestimate the real total costs of NMSC treatment, which has a complex calculation [20,26]. The direct cost of treatment represents approximately 72% of the total cost related to NMSC treatment, without including the oncological treatment, follow-up, patients' loss of income, quality-of-life changes, and economic reintegration [21,25]

We included only patients that were addressed to a Maxillofacial hospital, without subjects that were treated by other specialists, such as Plastic Surgery or Dermatology physicians, where the treatment options and the associated costs may be different from our standard surgical excision [15,21,26]. In addition, this research was limited to the hospitalized patients and charge data, aiming to identify the economic burden of the healthcare system and to observe the cost distribution patterns and high-cost drivers. However, the costs of hospitalized patients are higher than ambulatory-treated patients [15]. Still, the cost of NMSC treatment in Romania is cheaper than in other countries, such as Australia or other Northern or Western European countries [21,26].

Different from other studies, we could not find an association between the place of living or sex and NMSC increased cost. In the research of Tran et al. and Doran et al., urban place of residence or female patients presented higher costs of NMSC treatment compared with rural place of living and male patients [19,21]. Elderly patients presented a higher cost of treatment compared to young adults due to various arguments. Firstly, the prevalence of NMSC in senior people is higher compared to young adults [21,26]. Secondly, elderly people require special medical attention due to the increased prevalence of comorbidities, quantified in our study by the ASA risk. The patients classified as high ASA risk had a significantly higher cost compared to the low-risk subjects [20]. However, our results did not indicate a statistical correlation between the increased number of hospitalization and advanced ASA risk. In addition, immunosuppressed patients had a higher cost of treatment compared with non-immunosuppressed ones, with five out of the six immunosuppressed patients included in this study being aged more than 60 years old.

The increased costs of NMSC treatment for technical school and low-income patients were consistent with other research. The subjects that are exposed more to professional emissions and have low income are prone to developing NMSC cancers, and the treatment costs are higher compared with patients of other education and economic status [6,20]. However, we found a statistical significance of increasing costs related only to educational formation.

The head and neck NMSC treatment is more expensive than other anatomical regions, such as the thorax and limbs, but it is lower compared with head and neck mucosal malignancies (e.g., SCC of oral cavity or oropharynx) [19,20]. However, 19% of head and neck cancers are located on the skin [25]. Particularly, the orbital region had the highest cost of treatment per episode, which may be due to the difficulty of local reconstruction of this anatomical area [28,29]. These results are different from other research, where nasal and auricle NMSC had the highest treatment costs [5,16,19]. In our research, the nasal region presented an average cost of treatment per episode lower than the orbital region, but the total cost of treatment was the highest compared with other anatomical regions, due to the highest number of NMSC episodes.

Although the treatment cost of BCC per 5 years was higher compared to SCC, the BCC treatment cost per episode was cheaper than SCC, similar to other research [19,26]. These findings may be explained by the increased rates of BCC tumors and the more radical treatment required by SCC tumors, as well as the more paraclinical examinations needed perioperatively by SCC tumors to evaluate the locoregional or distant metastasis [17,20,31].

Different from the study by Chen et al. that observed a significant increase in treatment costs in the advanced stages of the disease, we observed an approximately 4-fold increase in the treatment costs of stage IV compared with stage I, but our results had no statistical significance [15]. However, the costs may be related to the more complex surgical procedure and to the more careful postoperative medical attention in advanced stages compared to early stages [32].

The local flap was approximately 60% more expensive than the skin graft. The result of this type of reconstruction is more aesthetic compared to the skin graft due to its similar color and texture to the adjacent facial tissues [33]. Both variants of reconstruction are used for tumors of increased dimensions, where the primary closure is not possible. However, the local flaps require an increased procedure time compared to other types of reconstruction, with the time needed to perform the surgery also being a factor that increased the costs [25]. A procedure that lasts longer than 2 h has more than double the costs compared with surgeries that can be performed faster (1 h). In addition, the local flap required more days of hospitalization than the primary closure or skin graft.

In our study, the high length of hospitalization was associated with higher costs of treatment. This finding may rely on the general health status of the patient or on the complex surgical procedure that requires many days of medical attention [31]. However, we found a statistical correlation between the hospital stay and the reconstruction type and tumor stage, without ASA risk. The median length the hospitalization for NMSC patients was 2 days, indicating that the surgical treatment of NMSC can be performed as a fast-track surgery, especially for patients with low ASA risk and early stages of cancer.

We enrolled a limited number of patients, which may influence the statistical analysis. Due to COVID-19 lockdowns, the number of patients that were addressed to Oral and Maxillofacial Surgery for head and neck skin tumors was reduced, hence, we limited the inclusion criteria to the 31st of December 2019 [34]. However, the majority of included patients were clustered in stage I or II, similar to other research [35].

Another limitation of our study was the lack of capacity to particularly assess the cost of the surgical procedure due to the lack of specific data in our hospital's informatic system.

5. Conclusions

Non-melanoma skin cancers are an important health problem due to increasing prevalence and treatment costs in the last years. The factors that can increase the costs of the treatment are related to the patient, such as age, low income, immunosuppression, and comorbidities, and to the procedure, such as flap reconstruction option, long-lasting surgery, and prolonged hospitalization.

Author Contributions: C.I.F., M.A.M., H.R., L.F. and R.C.R. conceptualized the study design and wrote part of the manuscript; C.I.F., M.A.M. and R.C.R. collected the patients' medical history from the informatic system; M.V. performed the data analysis. All authors have read and agreed to the published version of the manuscript.

Funding: This research received no external funding.

Institutional Review Board Statement: This study was approved by the Ethics Committee of "Iuliu Hatieganu" University of Medicine and Pharmacy (AVZ 20/03.02.2022), and it is in accordance with the updated Declaration of Helsinki.

Informed Consent Statement: Not applicable.

Data Availability Statement: Not applicable.

Acknowledgments: All authors read and agreed on the submission form of the manuscript.

Conflicts of Interest: The authors declare no conflict of interest.

References

1. Sung, H.; Ferlay, J.; Siegel, R.L.; Laversanne, M.; Soerjomataram, I.; Jemal, A.; Bray, F. Global Cancer Statistics 2020: GLOBOCAN Estimates of Incidence and Mortality Worldwide for 36 Cancers in 185 Countries. *CA Cancer J. Clin.* **2021**, *71*, 209–249. [CrossRef]
2. Eisemann, N.; Waldmann, A.; Geller, A.C.; Weinstock, M.A.; Volkmer, B.; Greinert, R.; Breitbart, E.W.; Katalinic, A. Non-Melanoma Skin Cancer Incidence and Impact of Skin Cancer Screening on Incidence. *J. Investig. Dermatol.* **2014**, *134*, 43–50. [CrossRef]
3. Cancer.Net Editorial Board. Skin Cancer (Non-Melanoma): Statistics. Available online: https://www.cancer.net/cancer-types/skin-cancer-non-melanoma/statistics (accessed on 1 October 2022).
4. Lomas, A.; Leonardi-Bee, J.; Bath-Hextall, F. A systematic review of worldwide incidence of nonmelanoma skin cancer. *Br. J. Dermatol.* **2012**, *166*, 1069–1080. [CrossRef] [PubMed]
5. Fijałkowska, M.; Koziej, M.; Antoszewski, B. Detailed Head Localization and Incidence of Skin Cancers. *Sci. Rep.* **2021**, *11*, 12391. [CrossRef]
6. Andrese, E.; Solovăstru, L.G.; Taranu, T.; Iancu, T.S. Epidemiological and pathological aspects of skin cancer in North East of Romania. *Rev. Med. Chir. Soc. Med. Nat.* **2014**, *118*, 457–462.
7. Ciążyńska, M.; Kamińska-Winciorek, G.; Lange, D.; Lewandowski, B.; Reich, A.; Sławińska, M.; Pabianek, M.; Szczepaniak, K.; Hankiewicz, A.; Ułańska, M.; et al. The Incidence and Clinical Analysis of Non-Melanoma Skin Cancer. *Sci. Rep.* **2021**, *11*, 4337. [CrossRef]
8. Kasumagic-Halilovic, E.; Hasic, M.; Ovcina-Kurtovic, N. A Clinical Study of Basal Cell Carcinoma 394 A Clinical Study of Basal Cell Carcinoma. *Med Arch.* **2019**, *73*, 394–398. [CrossRef] [PubMed]
9. Marzuka, S.B. Basal cell carcinoma: Pathogenesis, epidemiology, clinical features, diagnosis, histopathology, and management. *Yale J. Biol. Med.* **2015**, *88*, 167–179.
10. Riihilä, P.; Nissinen, L.; Knuutila, J.; Nezhad, P.R.; Viiklepp, K.; Kähäri, V.M. Complement System in Cutaneous Squamous Cell Carcinoma. *Int. J. Mol. Sci.* **2019**, *20*, 3550. [CrossRef] [PubMed]
11. Lubov, J.; Labbé, M.; Sioufi, K.; Morand, G.B.; Hier, M.P.; Khanna, M.; Sultanem, K.; Mlynarek, A.M. Prognostic Factors of Head and Neck Cutaneous Squamous Cell Carcinoma: A Systematic Review. *J. Otolaryngol.—Head Neck Surg.* **2021**, *50*, 54. [CrossRef]
12. Steding-Jessen, M.; Birch-Johansen, F.; Jensen, A.; Schüz, J.; Kjær, S.K.; Dalton, S.O. Socioeconomic Status and Non-Melanoma Skin Cancer: A Nationwide Cohort Study of Incidence and Survival in Denmark. *Cancer Epidemiol.* **2010**, *34*, 689–695. [CrossRef] [PubMed]
13. Mariotto, A.B.; Robin Yabroff, K.; Shao, Y.; Feuer, E.J.; Brown, M.L. Projections of the Cost of Cancer Care in the United States: 2010–2020. *JNCI J. Natl. Cancer Inst.* **2011**, *103*, 117. [CrossRef] [PubMed]
14. Newlands, C.; Currie, R.; Memon, A.; Whitaker, S.; Woolford, T. Non-Melanoma Skin Cancer: United Kingdom National Multidisciplinary Guidelines. *J. Laryngol. Otol.* **2016**, *130*, S125. [CrossRef] [PubMed]
15. Chen, J.T.; Kempton, S.J.; Rao, V.K. The Economics of Skin Cancer: An Analysis of Medicare Payment Data. *Plast. Reconstr. Surg.–Glob. Open* **2016**, *4*, 9. [CrossRef]
16. Duarte, A.F.; Sousa-Pinto, B.; Freitas, A.; Delgado, L.; Costa-Pereira, A.; Correia, O. Skin Cancer Healthcare Impact: A Nation-Wide Assessment of an Administrative Database. *Cancer Epidemiol.* **2018**, *56*, 154–160. [CrossRef]
17. Ruiz, E.S.; Morgan, F.C.; Zigler, C.M.; Besaw, R.J.; Schmults, C.D. Analysis of National Skin Cancer Expenditures in the United States Medicare Population, 2013. *J. Am. Acad. Dermatol.* **2019**, *80*, 275–278. [CrossRef]
18. Guy, G.P.; Machlin, S.R.; Ekwueme, D.U.; Yabroff, K.R. Prevalence and Costs of Skin Cancer Treatment in the U.S., 2002−2006 and 2007−2011. *Am. J. Prev. Med.* **2015**, *48*, 183–187. [CrossRef]
19. Tran, D.A.; Coronado, A.C.; Sarker, S.; Alvi, R. Estimating the Health Care Costs of Non-Melanoma Skin Cancer in Saskatchewan Using Physician Billing Data. *Curr. Oncol.* **2019**, *26*, 114. [CrossRef]
20. Massa, S.T.; Osazuwa-Peters, N.; Adjei Boakye, E.; Walker, R.J.; Ward, G.M. Comparison of the Financial Burden of Survivors of Head and Neck Cancer with Other Cancer Survivors. *JAMA Otolaryngol. Head Neck Surg.* **2019**, *145*, 239–249. [CrossRef]
21. Doran, C.M.; Ling, R.; Byrnes, J.; Crane, M.; Searles, A.; Perez, D.; Shakeshaft, A. Estimating the Economic Costs of Skin Cancer in New South Wales, Australia. *BMC Public Health* **2015**, *15*, 952. [CrossRef]
22. Zanoni, D.K.; Patel, S.G.; Shah, J.P. Changes in the 8th Edition of the American Joint Committee on Cancer (AJCC) Staging of Head and Neck Cancer: Rationale and Implications. *Curr. Oncol. Rep.* **2019**, *21*, 52. [CrossRef]
23. Amin, M.B.; Edge, S.B.; Greene, F.L.; Schilsky, R.L.; Brookland, R.K.; Washington, M.K.; Gershenwald, J.E.; Compton, C.C.; Hess, K.R.; Sullivan, D.C.; et al. *AJCC Cancer Staging Manual*; American Joint Committee on Cancer (AJCC): Chicago, IL, USA, 2017; ISBN 9783319406176.
24. Mayhew, D.; Mendonca, V.; Murthy, B.V.S. A Review of ASA Physical Status—Historical Perspectives and Modern Developments. *Anaesthesia* **2019**, *74*, 373–379. [CrossRef] [PubMed]
25. Pang, J.; Crawford, K.; Faraji, F.; Ramsey, C.; Kemp, A.; Califano, J.A. An Analysis of 1-Year Charges for Head and Neck Cancer: Targets for Value-Based Interventions. *Otolaryng.—Head Neck Surg.* **2020**, *163*, 546–553. [CrossRef] [PubMed]
26. Mofidi, A.; Tompa, E.; Spencer, J.; Kalcevich, C.; Peters, C.E.; Kim, J.; Song, C.; Mortazavi, S.B.; Demers, P.A. The Economic Burden of Occupational Non-Melanoma Skin Cancer Due to Solar Radiation. *J. Occup. Environ. Hyg.* **2018**, *15*, 481–491. [CrossRef] [PubMed]
27. Tangka, F.K.; Trogdon, J.G.; Richardson, L.C.; Howard, D.; Sabatino, S.A.; Finkelstein, E.A. Cancer Treatment Cost in the United States. *Cancer* **2010**, *116*, 3477–3484. [CrossRef] [PubMed]

8. Iglesias, M.E.; Santesteban, R.; Larumbe, A. Oncologic Surgery of the Eyelid and Orbital Region. *Actas Dermo-Sifiliogr. (Engl. Ed.)* **2015**, *106*, 365–375. [CrossRef]
9. Yüce, S.; Demir, Z.; Selçuk, C.T.; Çelebioğlu, S. Reconstruction of Periorbital Region Defects: A Retrospective Study. *Ann. Maxillofac. Surg.* **2014**, *4*, 45. [CrossRef]
10. Dacosta Byfield, S.; Chen, D.; Yim, Y.M.; Reyes, C. Age Distribution of Patients with Advanced Non-Melanoma Skin Cancer in the United States. *Arch. Dermatol. Res.* **2013**, *305*, 845–850. [CrossRef]
11. Whitney, R.L.; Bell, J.F.; Tancredi, D.J.; Romano, P.S.; Bold, R.J.; Joseph, J.G. Hospitalization Rates and Predictors of Rehospitalization among Individuals with Advanced Cancer in the Year After Diagnosis. *J. Clin. Oncol.* **2017**, *35*, 3610. [CrossRef]
12. Brambullo, T.; Azzena, G.P.; Toninello, P.; Masciopinto, G.; De Lazzari, A.; Biffoli, B.; Vindigni, V.; Bassetto, F. Current Surgical Therapy of Locally Advanced CSCC: From Patient Selection to Microsurgical Tissue Transplant. Review. *Front. Oncol.* **2021**, *11*, 5185. [CrossRef]
13. Egeler, S.A.; Huang, A.; Johnson, A.R.; Ibrahim, A.; Bucknor, A.; Peymani, A.; Mureau, M.A.M.; Lin, S.J. Regional Incidence of and Reconstructive Management Patterns in Melanoma and Nonmelanoma Skin Cancer of the Head and Neck: A 3-Year Analysis in the Inpatient Setting. *J. Plast. Reconstr. Aesthetic Surg.* **2020**, *73*, 507–515. [CrossRef] [PubMed]
14. Asai, Y.; Nguyen, P.; Hanna, T.P. Impact of the COVID-19 Pandemic on Skin Cancer Diagnosis: A Population-Based Study. *PLoS ONE* **2021**, *16*, e0248492. [CrossRef] [PubMed]
15. Jambusaria-Pahlajani, A.; Kanetsky, P.A.; Karia, P.S.; Hwang, W.T.; Gelfand, J.M.; Whalen, F.M.; Elenitsas, R.; Xu, X.; Schmults, C.D. Evaluation of AJCC Tumor Staging for Cutaneous Squamous Cell Carcinoma and a Proposed Alternative Tumor Staging System. *JAMA Dermatol.* **2013**, *149*, 402–410. [CrossRef] [PubMed]

Disclaimer/Publisher's Note: The statements, opinions and data contained in all publications are solely those of the individual author(s) and contributor(s) and not of MDPI and/or the editor(s). MDPI and/or the editor(s) disclaim responsibility for any injury to people or property resulting from any ideas, methods, instructions or products referred to in the content.

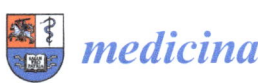

Case Report

Tongue Base Ectopic Thyroid Tissue—Is It a Rare Encounter?

Balica Nicolae Constantin [1,2], Trandafir Cornelia Marina [1,2,*], Stefanescu Horatiu Eugen [1,2], Enatescu Ileana [3] and Gluhovschi Adrian [4]

1. ENT Department, Victor Babeş University of Medicine and Pharmacy, Bd. Revolutiei No. 6, 300054 Timisoara, Romania
2. Victor Babes University of Medicine and Pharmacy Timisoara, Piața Eftimie Murgu Nr. 2, 300041 Timisoara, Romania
3. NeoNatology Department, University of Medicine and Pharmacy Timisoara, 300041 Timisoara, Romania
4. Gynecology Department, University of Medicine and Pharmacy Timisoara, 300041 Timisoara, Romania
* Correspondence: trandafir.cornelia@gmail.com

Abstract: Failure in the embryological development of the thyroid in adults is rarely seen. We present the case of a 79-year-old female patient who complained of dysphagia and progressive upper respiratory obstruction, which started 12 months prior to her admission. An ENT clinical exam revealed a tongue base, spherical, well-defined tumour covered by normal mucosa. Further assessments established the diagnosis of the tongue base ectopic thyroid tissue. Due to the patient's symptoms, a transhyoid tongue base tumour removal was performed. The selected patient gave consent for participation and inclusion in this paper, in compliance with the 1964 Helsinki declaration.

Keywords: tongue base; ectopic thyroid tissue; dysphagia; upper airway obstruction

1. Introduction

Ectopic thyroid tissue is an embryologic defect. The disease involves the aberrant development of the thyroid gland from the foramen caecum to its inferior cervical position [1,2]. The causes and exact mechanism of this aberrant defect have not been clearly elucidated, even though some transcription factors seem to playa role in the migration of the thyroid [3]. Its prevalence is about 1 per 100,000–300,000 people, increasing to 1 per 4000–8000 in patients with thyroid disease [1,2]. It is mostly diagnosed in childhood, adolescence, and around menopause, with a slight prevalence in females [4].

Ectopic thyroid tissue can be found anywhere along the course of the thyroglossal duct [5]. The base of the tongue represents the most frequent location [6]. Other sites involved are the anterior tongue, the submandibular or sublingual region, the larynx, the trachea, the mediastinum, and the heart [7,8]. The differential diagnosis of ectopic thyroid tissue must include metastatic thyroid carcinoma [9].

Most ectopic thyroids are asymptomatic. The symptoms are related to the sites of the ectopic tissue and can cause dysphagia, dysphonia, bleeding, or even upper respiratory obstruction, and, therefore, patients are referred to an ENT specialist for their diagnosis and treatment.

The combination of diagnostic imaging techniques and hormonal biological examinations correlating with the clinical ENT examination plays a fundamental role in the diagnosis of an ectopic thyroid tissue.

There is no consensus for the optimal treatment of ectopic thyroid tissue due its rarity. Some authors recommend a "wait-and-see" policy to ascertain whether the patient is in a euthyroid status or if the asymptomatic ectopic tumour is small. If the tumour continues to enlarge, leading to the compression of surrounding structures with consecutive occurrences of algia, dysphagia, dysphonia, or upper respiratory obstruction, surgical treatment can be proposed. Conventionally, various external approaches have been described in the literature; recently, transoral surgery has gained increasing popularity as an alternative

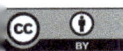

to external surgical treatment. Suppressive hormone therapy and ablative radioiodine therapy are described as alternative treatments for patients with lingual thyroid by some authors [3,4,10].

It is important to establish the periodic follow-up of patients with an endocrinologist specialist due to the post-operative hypothyroidism risk.

2. Case Report

A 79-year-old female patient with dysphagia and respiratory insufficiency was admitted to the ENT department. The symptomatology started twelve months prior to her admission to the hospital. She had no history of smoking and no alcohol intake. She was under medical treatment for hypercholesterolemia and high blood pressure.

The clinical ENT examination revealed no cervical adenopathy. The endoscopic examination (with a 70 degree rigid hypopharyngoscope) revealed a tongue base, spherical, solid, well-defined tumour covered by normal mucosa and obstructing the visualisation of the larynx (Figure 1).

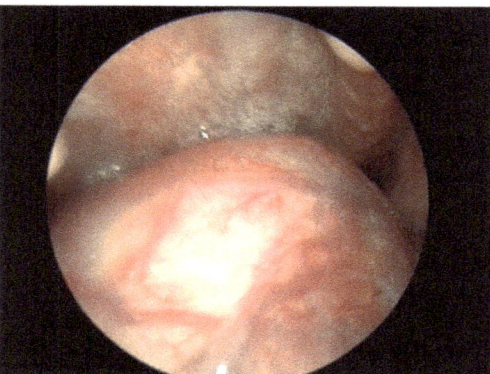

Figure 1. 70 degrees rigid hypopharyngoscope shows the mass in the sublingual region.

By comparing the further assessments (neck ultrasonography, thyroid scintigraphy, and cervical region Magnetic Resonance Imaging MRI (Figure 2)), the diagnosis of a tongue base ectopic thyroid tissue was established.

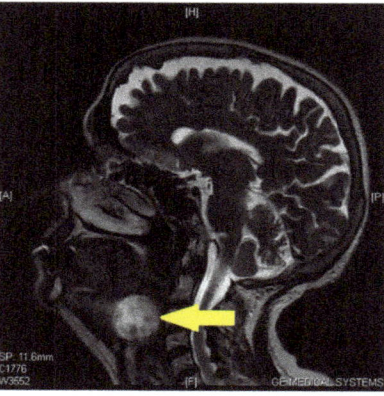

Figure 2. Magnetic Resonance Imaging (MRI) imaging shows a mass in the sublingual region (arrow).

Due to the patient's symptomatology, the decision was made to perform surgical treatment with an external approach. Under general anaesthesia, we performed a tracheotomy and a transversal superior incision at the level of the hyoid bone, externally excising the tongue base tumour (Figure 3).

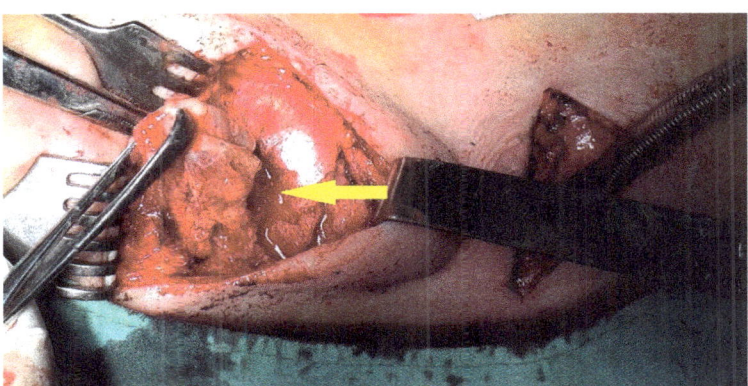

Figure 3. Intraoperatory imaging (Arrow—Tumor).

The tracheotomy was performed for airway control following surgery. Nutrition was delivered via a naso-gastric feeding tube. The post-operative treatment included a large spectrum of antibiotics for prophylaxis, anti-reflux medical treatment, and non-opioid analgesics. The post-operative evolution was unremarkable. The tracheotomy cannula and the feeding tube were both maintained for seven days, and deglutition was normal after the removal of the feeding tube. The patient was free of symptoms two weeks after the surgical procedure. The patient was referred to an endocrinologist before and after the surgery for hormonal substitutive treatment. Circulating levels of thyroid hormones at baseline were thyroid stimulating hormone TSH 12.8 µU/mL, FT3 1.9 pg/mL, and FT4 8.9 pg/mL.

The patient started L-T4 replacement therapy 5–7 days after the surgery. The value of L-T4 was 100 µg per day. After two month under L-T4 replacement therapy, the TSH was 3.0 µU/mL; FT 3 was 4.1 pg/mL; and FT4 was 11.5 pg/mL.

The anatomo-pathological exam revealed the ectopic thyroid tissue.

Six years after the surgery, there was no evidence of recurrence and no symptomatology.

3. Discussion

The first endocrine gland that occurs during foetal development is the thyroid gland [11].

The embryologic development implies an endodermal diverticulum (third or fourth week of gestation), which descends from the foramen caecum to the thyroid gland's final location (24th day) through the thyroglossal duct. The latter undergoes atrophy prior to the definitive formation of the thyroid [1,12,13]. Failure in thyroid migration along the path from the original region of the thyroid to its final cervical location causes ectopic thyroid tissue, which can be commonly found at any location from the tongue base to the mediastinum [14,15].

Many causes have been linked to the failure of thyroid migration, as well as to atypical morphological aspects of the thyroid, notably molecular, genetic, or epigenetic disorders [16,17].

In 70–90% of cases of ectopic foci of thyroid tissue, the ectopic tissue is the only thyroid tissue present, and the thyroid gland is absent [3,6,18]. It may occur at any age, from 5 months to 40 years, being more common at younger ages, with a high prevalence in females [1,2,19,20]. In the literature, only a few cases of a dual ectopic thyroid gland along with a cervical thyroid gland have been described [21]. In the literature, half of patients are euthyroid, and the rest are hypothyroid [3,6]. In our case the patient was referred to an endocrinologist for the supplementation hormonal treatment and follow-up.

The presence of an ectopic thyroid tissue can be asymptomatic, can cause local symptoms such as dysphagia, and can be the leading cause of death as described by Dr Hickman in a case report of a new-born with a lingual thyroid who died from severe respiratory distress [7]. All diseases that can affect a normal thyroid can affect the ectopic thyroid tissue (adenoma, hyperplasia, inflammation, and rarely malignancy) [6,22]. The incidence of malignancy is estimated at 1% [19,23,24].

Massine et al. described a case of a 57-year-old patient with the diagnosis of a papillary carcinoma arising from a lingual thyroid and an invasive keratinising poorly differentiated squamous cell carcinoma from adjacent structures. The patient was treated by a total glossectomy, with a left elective neck dissection, supraglottic laryngectomy, and midline mandibulotomy with a rectus free flap [24].

The presence of an ectopic thyroid tissue is less frequently encountered in other anatomical spaces: the pancreas [25], porta hepatis [26], submucosa of the duodenum [27], and the iris [28]. In these cases, it is important for the clinician to rule out metastases from a thyroid carcinoma [29].

Sometimes the thyroid malignancy is excluded, but the ectopic tissue is confirmed at a distance from its normal path of embryological development. In those cases, the congenital defect is difficult to explain. Many theories are present in the literature. For example, the common origin of the intra-abdominal organs and the thyroid are from the endodermal germ layer. The presence of an ectopic thyroid tissue was found by Aiwen Ma et al. below the diaphragm, in a retroperitoneal mass between the superior border of the kidney, having a close interaction with the pancreatic hook [23,30].

However, the theory described previously does not explain the presence of the ectopic tissue in the adrenal gland because the adrenal cortex originates from the mesodermal layer while the medulla originates from the ectodermal layer. Many other explanations can be found in the literature: teratoma, metaplasia, and choristoma [23,31].

When a basilingual mass is found, a complete Ear, nose and throat examination (ENT) exam should be performed, and uncommon diseases should be kept in mind when examining any patient [32]. A cervical ultrasound is a valuable tool for identifying an ectopic thyroid tissue. Computed Tomography (CT) scans and MRI imaging are widely used to assess the exact location and extension of ectopic thyroid foci. Scintigraphy is highly sensitive in detecting thyroid tissue, which is used for the differentiation of the thyroid from other differential diagnoses. As has been previously described in the literature, a biochemical thyroid profile may be necessary in adult patients and in new-borns, as some studies suggest that hypothyroidism can be diagnosed in patients with ectopic thyroid tissue due to the absence of a functioning thyroid gland [11].

Differential diagnoses should include thyroglossal duct cysts without thyroid tissue, midline branchial cysts, lymphangioma, haemangioma, and minor salivary gland tumours [2,33].

If the diagnosis of an ectopic lingual thyroid is established and the patient presents obstructive symptomatology or a malignant disease is suspected, surgical treatment must be performed after a multidisciplinary examination of the patient.

The patients with an airway obstruction may include a tracheostomy as an emergency procedure or for airway control following surgery, as described in our report (severe postoperative oedema is frequent). Even though a tracheostomy is considered a routine surgical procedure, there area number of potential vessels that can be accidentally injured during the procedure. Injuries of the thyroidea-ima were described in some cases of percutaneous tracheostomy [34,35].A study by Laphatrada Yurasakpong et al. revealed the presence of the thyroidea-ima in approximately 3.8% population, with a decline in the prevalence of the thyroidea-ima over the generations. Awareness of this normal variant of neck anatomy is important when performing a tracheostomy [36]. In our report, this variant was not present.

The treatment of an ectopic lingual thyroid depends on several factors. In cases with no clinical symptoms, a substitutive therapy with thyroid hormones can be proposed. Ablative radioiodine therapy is reserved for cases when surgical therapy is contraindicated, and it is not usually used for young patients [13,24]. However, in our report, the size of the lesion, the presence of local symptoms, and the presence of complications made us perform the surgical therapy.

The excision of a lingual ectopic thyroid tissue may be performed with a variety of approaches from intensive surgical procedures (Sistrunk technique, lateral pharyngotomy, and trahnsyoid incision) to simpler and more cost-effective procedures [24,37]. Extensive surgeries offer good results, but complications such as fistula formation, infection, and the presence of a cervical/facial scar may be unsatisfactory for patients with higher cosmetic requirements.

The intraoperatory risk of bleeding during a tongue base surgery is high. However, external surgeries offer better visualisation, especially for large masses, and the bleedings are easy to control during an open surgery. Some authors use midline mandibulotomy and tongue splitting techniques to achieve a good exposure and minimise the risk of injuries [38,39].

Initially used to excise all thyroglossal tract tissue involved in thyroglossal cyst, the Sistrunk technique can be used for the management of an ectopic lingual tissue. It can offer a satisfactory removal, and the majority of the post-operative course is surgically uneventful [40,41].

In our days there has been a progressive trend to approach thyroid ectopic tissue using transoral surgery/laser methods. A Korean team demonstrated the feasibility of a Sistrunk procedure by robot-assisted surgery via a retroarticular incision for a thyroglossal cyst [42].

Trans-oral robotic surgery (TORS) is known as a minimally invasive surgical technique, approved in 2009 by the Food and Drug Administration (FDA) for head and neck surgery [43]. It improves access and visualisation, avoiding the classical invasive open techniques (midline labiotomy, tongue splitting, and mandibulotomy) [44–46]. Compared to traditional surgeries techniques, it has a different anatomic perspective. It understands the muscular landmarks and vascular anatomy and it is important for minimising the surgical risks, notably the bleeding one. The development of TORS allows for less morbidity and offers better cosmesis post-operatively [47].

In order to avoid substitutive lifelong hormone therapy, in the literature a transplantation of the lingual thyroid tissue in the muscles of the neck has been described [48].

Clearly, there remain certain situations in which minimally invasive methods are not possible. Patient factors and the availability of surgical skills and technologies should be taken into account when managing a patient with a thyroid ectopic tissue.

In our ENT department, there are more than 2500 patients admitted annually. The incidence of an ectopic thyroid among the admitted patients is roughly one case every five years.

As with many previous case reports, we acknowledge that the present article has some limitations. The rarity of this entity in our centre is likely subject to variations in clinical practice outcomes, linked to the hospital turnover of patients and the resources available.

4. Conclusions

Ectopic thyroid tissue is a rare developmental anomaly. An accurate ENT evaluation and differential diagnoses should increase the suspicion of an ectopic thyroid tissue. In cases with mild symptoms, substitutive hormone treatment might be implied, while in cases with deglutition or respiratory impairment, surgical treatment seems to be the best option.

Author Contributions Conceptualisation and methodology, B.N.C.; software, T.C.M.; validation, B.N.C. and S.H.E.; formal analysis, E.I.; investigation, T.C.M.; writing—original draft, B.N.C.; draft preparation, T.C.M.; writing—review and editing, G.A.; visualisation, S.H.E. All authors have read and agreed to the published version of the manuscript.

Funding: This research received no external funding.

Institutional Review Board Statement: The study was conducted in accordance with the Declaration of Helsinki and was approved by the ethical committee of the institution, CECS 55/25.11.2022 (2014 rev), and received Institutional SCMUT Approval: E-6701/24.11.2022.

Informed Consent Statement: Written informed consent was obtained from the patient to publish this paper.

Conflicts of Interest: The authors declare no conflict of interest.

References

1. Babazade, F.; Mortazavi, H.; Jalalian, H.; Shahvali, E. Thyroid tissue as a submandibular mass: A case report. *J. Oral Sci.* **2009**, *51*, 655–657. [CrossRef] [PubMed]
2. Di Benedetto, V. Ectopic thyroid gland in the submandibular region simulating a thyroglossal duct cyst: A case report. *J. Pediatr. Surg.* **1997**, *32*, 1745–1746. [CrossRef] [PubMed]
3. Noussios, G.; Anagnostis, P.; Goulis, D.G.; Lappas, D.; Natsis, K. Ectopic thyroid tissue: Anatomical, clinical, and surgical implications of a rare entity. *Eur. J. Endocrinol.* **2011**, *165*, 375–382. [CrossRef] [PubMed]
4. Toso, A.; Colombani, F.; Averono, G.; Aluffi, P.; Pia, F. Lingual thyroid causing dysphagia and dyspnoea. Case reports and review of the literature. *ACTA Otorhinolaryngol.* **2009**, *29*, 213–217.
5. Adelchi, C.; Mara, P.; Melissa, L.; De Stefano, A.; Cesare, M. Ectopic thyroid tissue in the head and neck: A case series. *BMC Res. Notes* **2014**, *7*, 790. [CrossRef]
6. Saito, M.; Banno, H.; Ito, Y.; Ido, M.; Goto, M.; Ando, T.; Kousaka, J.; Mouri, Y.; Fujii, K.; Imai, T.; et al. Case report: Surgical management of symptomatic pretracheal thyroid gland in a patient with dual ectopic thyroid. *Thyroid. Res.* **2022**, *15*, 23. [CrossRef]
7. Choudhury, B.K.; Saikia, U.K.; Sarma, D.; Saikia, M.; Choudhury, S.D.; Barua, S.; Dewri, S. Dual ectopic thyroid with normally located thyroid: A case report. *J. Thyroid. Res.* **2011**, *2011*, 159703. [CrossRef]
8. Eli, S.U.; Marnane, C.; Peter, R.; Winter, S. Ectopic, submandibular thyroid causing hyperthyroidism. *J. Laryngol. Otol.* **2011**, *125*, 1091–1093. [CrossRef]
9. Mace, A.T.M.; Mclaughlin, I.; Gibson, I.W.; Clark, L.J. Benign ectopic submandibular thyroid with a normotopic multinodular goitre. *J. Laryngol. Otol.* **2003**, *117*, 739–740. [CrossRef]
10. Alderson, D.J.; Lannigan, F.J. Lingual thyroid presenting after previous thyroglossal cyst excision. *J. Laryngol. Otol.* **1994**, *108*, 341–343. [CrossRef]
11. Alanazi, S.M.; Limaiem, F. Ectopic Thyroid. In *StatPearls*; StatPearls Publishing: Treasure Island, FL, USA, 2022. [PubMed]
12. DeFelice, M.; Lauro, R. Thyroid development and its disorders: Genetics and molecular mechanisms. *Endocr. Rev.* **2004**, *25*, 722–746. [CrossRef]
13. Gallo, A.; Leonetti, F.; Torri, E.; Manciocco, V.; Simonelli, M.; De Vincentiis, M. Ectopic lingual thyroid as unusual cause of severe dysphagia. *Dysphagia* **2001**, *16*, 220–223. [CrossRef]
14. Cassol, C.A.; Noria, D.; Asa, S. Ectopic thyroid tissue within the gall bladder: Case report and brief review of the literature. *Endocr. Pathol.* **2010**, *21*, 263–265. [CrossRef]
15. Shuno, Y.; Kobayashi, T.; Morita, K.; Shimizu, S.; Nishio, Y.; Ito, A.; Kobayashi, K.; Kawahara, M.; Teruya, M. Ectopic thyroid in the adrenal gland presenting as cystic lesion. *Surgery* **2006**, *139*, 580–582. [CrossRef]
16. Nettore, I.C.; Cacace, V.; De Fusco, C.; Colao, A.; Macchia, P.E. The molecular causes of thyroid dysgenesis: A systematic review. *J. Endocrinol. Investig.* **2013**, *36*, 654–664.
17. Abu-Khudir, R.; Paquette, J.; Lefort, A.; Libert, F.; Chanoine, J.P.; Vassart, G.; Deladoëy, J. Transcriptome, methylome and genomic variations analysis of ectopic thyroid glands. *PLoS ONE* **2010**, *5*, e13420. [CrossRef]
18. Kumar, R.; Sharma, S.; Marwah, A.; Moorthy, D.; Dhanwal, D.; Malhotra, A. Ectopic goiter masquerading as submandibular gland swelling: A case report and review of the literature. *Clin. Nucl. Med.* **2001**, *26*, 306–309. [CrossRef]
19. Kousta, E.; Konstantinidis, K.; Michalakis, C.; Vorias, M.; Sambalis, G.; Georgiou, M.; Theodoropoulos, G.E. Ectopic thyroid tissue in the lower neck with a coexisting normally located multinodular goiter and brief literature review. *Hormones* **2005**, *4*, 231–234. [CrossRef]
20. Bersaneti, J.A.; Silva, R.; Ramos, P.; Matsushita, M.; Souto, L. Ectopic thyroid presenting as a submandibular mass. *Head Neck Pathol.* **2011**, *5*, 63–66. [CrossRef]
21. Sood, A.; Sood, V.; Sharma, D.R.; Seam, R.K.; Kumar, R. Thyroid scintigraphy in detecting dual ectopic thyroid: A review. *Eur. J. Nucl. Med.* **2008**, *35*, 843–846. [CrossRef]
22. Jha, P.S.; Rote-Kaginalkar, V.; Titare, P.; Jadhav, M.B. Hemiagenesisofthyroidwithdualthyroidectopia:Ararecasereport. *Indian J. Radiol. Imaging* **2018**, *28*, 4–17.
23. Ma, A.; Liu, H. Ectopicthyroidofthepancreas:Acasereportandliteraturereview. *Medicine* **2017**, *96*, e8707. [CrossRef] [PubMed]
24. Massine, R.E.; Durning, S.J.; Koroscil, T.M. Lingual thyroid carcinoma: A case report and review of the literature. *Thyroid* **2001**, *11*, 1191–1196. [CrossRef] [PubMed]
25. Eyüboğlu, E.; Kapan, M.; Ipek, T.; Ersan, Y.; Oz, F. Ectopic thyroid in the abdomen: Report of a case. *Surg. Today* **1999**, *29*, 472–474. [CrossRef] [PubMed]
26. Ghanem, N.; Bley, T.; Altehoefer, C.; Högerle, S.; Langer, M. Ectopic thyroid gland in the porta hepatis and lingua. *Thyroid* **2003**, *13*, 503–507. [CrossRef]
27. Takahashi, T.; Ishikura, H.; Kato, H.; Tanabe, T.; Yoshiki, T. Ectopic thyroid follicles in the submucosa of the duodenum. *Virchows Arch. A Pathol. Anat. Histopathol.* **1991**, *418*, 547–550. [CrossRef]

8. Wagner, H.; Auw-Hädrich, C.; Werner, M.; Reinhard, T. Ectopic thyroid tissue in the iris: A case report. *BMC Ophthalmol.* **2021**, *21*, 314. [CrossRef]
9. Kondo, T.; Katoh, R.; Omata, K.; Oyama, T.; Yagawa, A.; Kawaoi, A. Incidentally detected liver metastasis of well-differentiated follicular carcinoma of the thyroid, mimicking ectopic thyroid. *Pathol. Int.* **2000**, *50*, 509–513. [CrossRef]
10. Campora, M.; Antonelli, C.T.; Mastracci, L.; Pigozzi, S.; Grillo, F. A Never Ending Journey: Ectopic Thyroid. *Int. J. Surg. Pathol.* **2017**, *25*, 241–242. [CrossRef]
11. Romero-Rojas, A.; Bella-Cueto, M.R.; Meza-Cabrera, I.A.; Cabezuelo-Hernández, A.; García-Rojo, D.; Vargas-Uricoechea, H.; Cameselle-Teijeiro, J. Ectopic thyroid tissue in the adrenal gland: A report of two cases with pathogenetic implications. *Thyroid* **2013**, *23*, 1644–1650. [CrossRef]
12. Sarău, C.A.; Poenaru, M.; Balica, N.C.; Baderca, F. Rare sinonasal lesions. *Rom. J. Morphol. Embryol.* **2017**, *58*, 1541–1547.
13. Hazarika, P.; Siddiqui, S.A.; Pujary, K.; Shah, P.; Nayak, D.R.; Balakrishnan, R. Dual ectopic thyroid: A report of two cases. *J. Laryngol. Otol.* **1998**, *112*, 393–395. [CrossRef]
14. Kamparoudi, P.; Paliouras, D.; Gogakos, A.S.; Rallis, T.; Schizas, N.C.; Lazopoulos, A.; Chatzinikolaou, F.; Sarafis, P.; Serchan, P.; Katsikogiannis, N.; et al. Percutaneous tracheostomy—Beware of the thyroidea-ima artery. *Ann. Transl. Med.* **2016**, *4*, 449. [CrossRef]
15. Gwilym, S.; Cooney, A. Acute fatal haemorrhage during percutaneous dilatational tracheostomy. *BJA Br. J. Anaesth.* **2004**, *92*, 298. [CrossRef]
16. Yurasakpong, L.; Nantasenamat, C.; Janta, S.; Eiamratchanee, P.; Coey, J.; Chaiyamoon, A.; Kruepunga, N.; Senarai, T.; Langer, M.F.; Meemon, K.; et al. The decreasing prevalence of the thyroid ima artery: A systematic review and machine learning assisted meta-analysis. *Ann. Anat.* **2022**, *239*, 151803. [CrossRef]
17. Prasad, K.C.; Bhat, V. Surgical management of lingual thyroid: A report of four cases. *J. Oral Maxillofac. Surg.* **2000**, *58*, 223–227. [CrossRef]
18. Wu, Z.X.; Zheng, L.W.; Dong, Y.J.; Li, Z.B.; Zhang, W.F.; Zhao, Y.F. Modified approach for lingual thyroid transposition: Report of two cases. *Thyroid* **2008**, *18*, 465–468. [CrossRef]
19. Guerra, G.; Cinelli, M.; Mesolella, M.; Tafuri, D.; Rocca, A.; Amato, B.; Rengo, S.; Testa, D. Morphological, diagnostic and surgical features of ectopic thyroid gland: A review of literature. *Int. J. Surg.* **2014**, *12*, S3–S11. [CrossRef]
20. Elechi, H.A. Hypothyroidism following sistrunk procedure: Thyroglossal duct cyst or ectopic thyroid? *Afr. J. Paediatr. Surg.* **2021**, *18*, 231–234. [CrossRef]
21. Lim, L.X.; Kwok, G.T.; Wong, E.; Morgan, G.J. Dual thyroid ectopia with submental thyroid excision using Sistrunk procedure: A case report. *Int. J. Surg. Case Rep.* **2021**, *82*, 105909. [CrossRef]
22. Kim, C.H.; Byeon, H.K.; Shin, Y.S.; Koh, Y.W.; Choi, E.C. Robot-assisted Sistrunk operation via a retroauricular approach for thyroglossal duct cyst. *Head Neck* **2014**, *36*, 456–458. [CrossRef] [PubMed]
23. Poon, H.; Li, C.; Gao, W.; Ren, H.; Lim, C.M. Evolution of robotic systems for transoral head and neck surgery. *Oral Oncol.* **2018**, *87*, 82–88. [CrossRef] [PubMed]
24. Atiyeh, B.S.; Abdelnour, A.; Haddad, F.F.; Ahmad, H. Lingual thyroid: Tongue-splitting incision for transoral excision. *J. Laryngol. Otol.* **1995**, *109*, 520–524. [CrossRef] [PubMed]
25. Vairaktaris, E.; Semergidis, T.; Christopoulou, P.; Papadogeorgakis, N.; Martis, C. Lingual thyroid: A new surgical approach—A case report. *J. Craniomaxillofac. Surg.* **1994**, *22*, 307–310. [CrossRef] [PubMed]
26. Prisman, E.; Patsias, A.; Genden, E.M. Transoral robotic excision of ectopic lingual thyroid: Case series and literature review. *Head Neck* **2015**, *37*, E88–E91. [CrossRef]
27. Vincent, A.; Jategaonkar, A.; Kadakia, S.; Ducic, Y. TORS excision of lingual thyroid carcinoma: Technique and systematic review. *Am. J. Otolaryngol.* **2019**, *40*, 435–439. [CrossRef]
28. Huang, H.; Lin, Y.H. Lingual thyroid with severe hypothyroidism: A case report. *Medicine* **2021**, *100*, e27612. [CrossRef]

Disclaimer/Publisher's Note: The statements, opinions and data contained in all publications are solely those of the individual author(s) and contributor(s) and not of MDPI and/or the editor(s). MDPI and/or the editor(s) disclaim responsibility for any injury to people or property resulting from any ideas, methods, instructions or products referred to in the content.

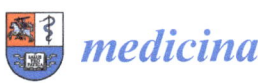 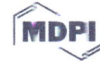

Article

Sheep's Head as an Anatomic Model for Basic Training in Endoscopic Sinus Surgery

Constantin Stan [1,2], Laszlo Peter Ujvary [1,*], Cristina Maria Blebea [1], Doinița Vesa [2,*], Mihai Ionuț Tănase [1], Mara Tănase [1], Septimiu Sever Pop [1], Doinel Gheorghe Rădeanu [1], Alma Aurelia Maniu [1] and Marcel Cosgarea [1]

[1] Department of ENT, "Iuliu Hațieganu" University of Medicine and Pharmacy, 400012 Cluj-Napoca, Romania; const.stan@ugal.ro (C.S.); cristina_blebea@yahoo.com (C.M.B.); dr.mihaitanase@gmail.com (M.I.T.); maratulmaci@yahoo.com (M.T.); severpop@me.com (S.S.P.); dr.radeanu@gmail.com (D.G.R.); almaciro@yahoo.com (A.A.M.); rcosgarea@yahoo.com (M.C.)

[2] Department of Surgical Clinic, Faculty of Medicine and Pharmacy, "Dunărea de Jos" University, 800008 Galați, Romania

* Correspondence: ujvarypeter@outlook.com (L.P.U.); vesa_doina@yahoo.com (D.V.); Tel.: +40-746-403-264 (L.P.U.); +40-723-350-166 (D.V.)

Abstract: *Background and Objectives*: This study aims to establish the sheep head as a viable anatomical model for training in functional endoscopic sinus surgery through comprehensive anatomical examination and training-based assessment of participants' satisfaction. *Materials and Methods*: Participants were divided into three groups according to their prior experience in endoscopic sinus surgery; in total, 24 participants were included. Each participant in the study was assigned to perform the designated procedures on a single sheep's head. Following the completion of the procedures, each participant was provided with a 14-item comprehensive satisfaction questionnaire with a scale attributed from 1 to 5. The normality of distribution was checked by applying the Shapiro–Wilk Test. The Kruskal–Wallis test was applied to compare study group sentiment of agreement towards individual procedures. *Results*: No significant differences were noted between the answers of the different groups. For the resident group, the average satisfaction score was 4.09 ± 0.54; junior specialist group 4.00 ± 0.55; for the senior specialist group overall satisfaction average score was 4.2 ± 0.77. *Conclusions*: The sheep's head can be successfully used for learning and practicing manual skills and the use of instruments specific to functional endoscopic sinus surgery. Moreover, the sheep head model can be used for training in other diagnostic or surgical procedures in the field of otorhinolaryngology, such as endoscopy of the salivary glands, open laryngotracheal surgery, or in otologic surgery, but also in other different surgical fields such as neurosurgery, ophthalmology or plastic surgery. Despite the differences between the ovine model and human anatomy, it provides a resourceful and cost-effective model for beginners in endoscopic nasal surgery.

Keywords: surgical training; simulation; sinus surgery; animal model; FESS

1. Introduction

The process of surgical training in Functional Endoscopic Sinus Surgery (FESS) heavily relies on the availability and accessibility of well-equipped laboratories that facilitate endoscopic dissection on cadaveric heads. However, the limited availability of cadavers due to medical, ethical, and moral considerations has led to the exploration of alternative methods, specifically the utilization of anatomical models that closely resemble the human head [1]. In order to achieve this objective, efforts have been made to develop techniques that can ease the learning process. One proposed approach involves using sheep heads as anatomical ex vivo models, although the literature on this subject is currently scarce and lacks comprehensive studies [2].

For endoscopic sinus surgery training, both the in-vivo ovine model and cadaveric simulations offer high handling fidelity. In certain countries, in-vivo animal simulation is prohibited, making animal cadaveric simulation a more accessible substitute [3,4]. The ovine sinus model allows the acquisition of endoscopic surgical skills using video endoscopic techniques. It is cost-effective, portable, and adaptable for use in various settings [5]. Moreover, the ex-vivo ovine model for training does not require institutional review committee approval and raises fewer ethical concerns compared to live animal models [5,6].

This study aims to establish the sheep head as a viable anatomical model for training in functional endoscopic sinus surgery through comprehensive anatomical examination and training-based assessment of participants' satisfaction.

2. Materials and Methods

2.1. Image Acquisition for Anatomical Description and Anatomical Sectioning

After ethical approval was granted (AV258/28.02.2022), an anatomical feasibility study was undertaken regarding the sheep head as an alternative for FESS training. For the anatomical study, 26 fresh-frozen adult sheep heads (Native Romanian Turcana sheep) were procured from the local slaughterhouse (veterinary clearance was obtained), at a price of 10 Romanian lei (RON) a piece, roughly the equivalent of two euros a piece. One head was defrosted and used as a sample for imaging acquisition and endoscopy and the other head was used to provide sectional anatomical details. The second head (frozen at $-20\ °C$) was serially sectioned in sagittal and transverse planes. The sagittal plane was paramedian to the septum, dividing the skull into two equal parts. The transverse sections were 2.5 cm in thickness. Sectional photographs were taken, and important anatomical elements were digitally labeled. The obtained information was presented to the participants through oral presentations and written handouts.

2.2. Model Preparation for Surgery and Instrumentation

Prior to the initiation of the maneuvers, a preparatory phase was undertaken, during which the fresh frozen sheep heads were allowed to undergo a gradual thawing process at room temperature for a duration of approximately 14 h. As a subsequent step in the preparatory process, the nasal cavities of the sheep heads were irrigated with a saline solution. Ultimately, before beginning the evaluation process, the tip of the nose was sectioned to facilitate endoscopic maneuvering, a useful aspect also presented by other authors [7]. Table 1 lists the equipment and instruments used for training.

Table 1. Equipment and instruments used for endoscopic maneuvers.

Nr	Equipment (Germany—KARL STORZ SE & Co. KG, Tuttlingen)
1.	Karl Storz TelePack X
2.	Karl Storz rigid Hopkins telescopes 0° and 30°
3.	Mladina head holder (Karl Storz®)
4.	Blakesley nasal forceps (Karl Storz®)
5.	Backbiter antrum punch (Karl Storz®)
6.	Cottle dorsal scissors (Karl Storz®)
7.	Freer elevator (Karl Storz®)
8.	Sickle knife (Karl Storz®)
9.	Straight and curved curette (Karl Storz®)
10.	Frazier suction tube (Karl Storz®)
11.	Scalpel handle with no. 11 blade (Karl Storz®)

The support was innovated by Mladina and Karl Storz Gmbh to fix in position and secure the lamb's head (Figure 1) [7,8]. In our study, we used it for the sheep's head, which, although it is more voluminous, could be fixed without problems.

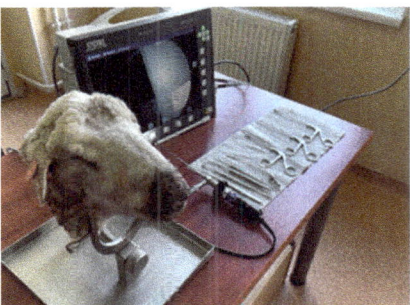

Figure 1. View of the sheep's head secured in the Karl Storz® special head holder.

A series of basic endoscopic maneuvers using the sheep's head as a model was performed by 24 participants. Each participant was allocated one sheep head (Table 2).

Table 2. Surgical steps undertaken by participants.

Nr	Surgical Step
1.	Foreign body removal (round plastic, popcorn)
2.	Endoscopic septal resection
3.	Endoscopic turbinoplasty
4.	Maxillary anthrostomy
5.	Ethmoidectomy

2.3. Participant Selection

Participants were divided into three groups according to their prior experience in endoscopic sinus surgery. The first group was formed by 10 first-year otolaryngology resident doctors with minimal or no experience in endoscopic sinus surgery. The second group consisted of 10 junior otolaryngology specialists with 3–5 years of exposure to rhinology procedures. The third group was formed by four senior otolaryngologists with over 20 years of experience.

2.4. Participant Assessment—Satisfaction Questionnaire

Each participant in the study was assigned to perform the designated procedures on a single sheep's head, targeting both nasal fossae. Following the completion of the procedures, each participant was provided with a 14-item comprehensive satisfaction questionnaire (File S1). For each answer, a scale from 1–5 was attributed, 1 denoting "totally disagree", and 5 signifying "completely agree". This allowed participants to provide nuanced feedback, enabling a comprehensive assessment of their overall satisfaction and perception of the performed procedures.

2.5. Statistical Analysis

For statistical analysis, Statistical Package for the Social Sciences (SPSS) 26.0 (Armonk, NY, USA: IBM Corp) was used. Data from the questionnaire was collected as numerical variables (1–5). For each group, mean and standard deviation were calculated for an individual answer within the questionnaire. The normality of distribution was checked by applying the Shapiro–Wilk Test. The Kruskal–Wallis test was applied to compare study group sentiment of agreement towards individual procedures.

3. Results

3.1. Basic Endoscopic Anatomy

Relevant anatomical structures regarding the endoscopic dissection can be seen in Figures 2–4. Opposed to humans, the inferior turbinate is comprised of two parts.

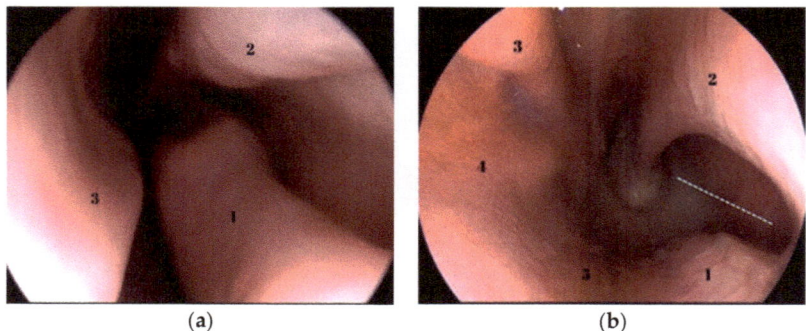

Figure 2. (**a**) Endoscopic view of the sheep's left nasal fossa. 1—inferior part of inferior turbinate; 2—superior part of inferior turbinate; 3—nasal septum; (**b**) endoscopic view of the posterior septal defect specific to the ovine model described by Mladina [7]—dotted white line. Right nasal fossa, 1—the lower limit of the septal defect; 2—the superior limit of the septal defect; 3—inferior turbinate; 4—lateral nasal wall; 5—nasal floor.

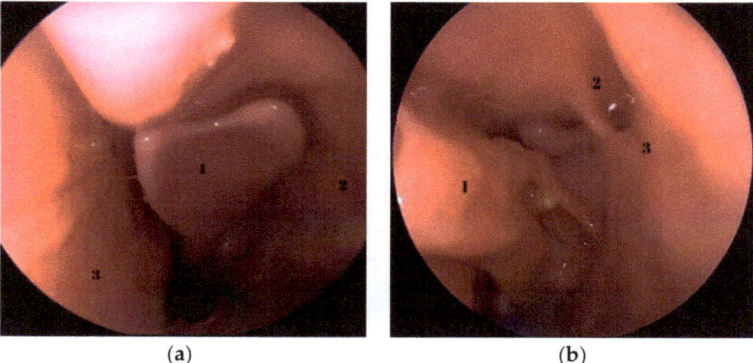

Figure 3. (**a**) Endoscopic view—left nasal fossa—1—middle turbinate; 2—lateral nasal wall; 3—septum. (**b**) Endoscopic view—left nasal fossa; 1—medialized middle turbinate; 2—natural ostium of the maxillary sinus; 3—uncinate process.

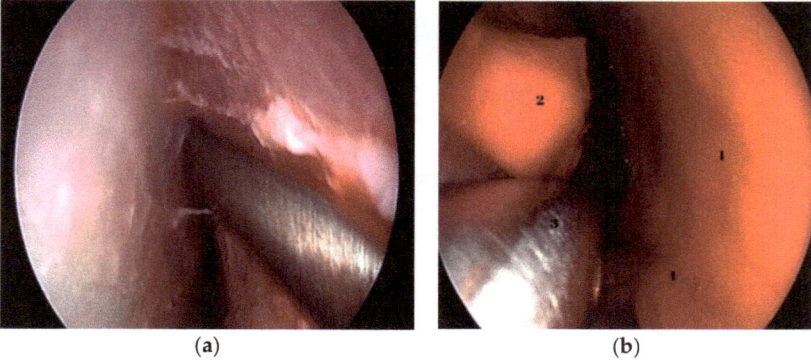

Figure 4. Endoscopic images of sub-perichondral dissection of the septum and turbinate fracture. (**a**) Sub-perichondral dissection of the septum, (**b**) Instrumental lateral fracture of the inferior turbinate. 1—lateral nasal wall; 2—inferior turbinate; 3—Cottle dorsal scissors; 4—insertion of the inferior turbinate to the lateral nasal wall.

The excision of the inferior turbinate permits the visualization of the middle turbinate. By gently and medially displacing it using an elevator, the natural ostium of the maxillary sinus becomes visible. To further enhance access and facilitate surgical intervention, the backbiter antrum punch can be employed to enlarge the natural ostium, resulting in the creation of a broad middle antrostomy.

3.2. Procedures and Evaluation

Following the extraction of a foreign body, attention was directed to raising the mucosal flap, bone resection and repositioning of the mucosal flap to mimic the maneuver performed during an actual turbinoplasty. Endoscopic septoplasty was undertaken as shown in Figure 4a. Following the initial procedures, the inferior turbinate was resected as a whole to facilitate the visualization of the middle turbinate—Figure 4b.

By medializing the middle turbinate, the natural ostium of the maxillary sinus is also pointed out, which was widened with the help of the backbiter antrum punch to create an anthrostomy. The last procedure undertaken was the ethmoidectomy—Figure 5a,b

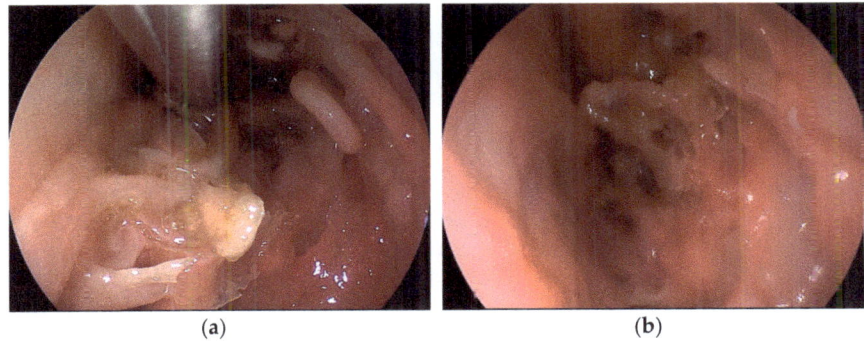

(a) (b)

Figure 5. (a,b) Endoscopic images of instrumental removal of ethmoidal cells.

The assessment of the overall satisfaction and perception of the performed procedures was as follows in Table 3.

Table 3. Satisfaction questionnaire assessment.

Questions	ENT Resident Mean (SD)	ENT Junior Mean (SD)	ENT Senior Mean (SD)	p Value [1]
The similarity of anatomical structures to humans	3.1 (0.7)	3.2 (0.6)	3.0 (0)	0.943
Realistic perception of the mucosa	4.7 (0.45)	4.4 (0.8)	4.33 (0.47)	0.386
Realistic perception of bone tissue	4.4 (0.66)	4.1 (0.83)	4 (0)	0.486
Good depth perception	4.2 (0.74)	4.4 (0.48)	5 (0)	0.391
Good applicability of the basic FESS instruments	4.1 (0.94)	4.4 (0.66)	4 (0)	0.475
Useful to improve hand-eye coordination	4.2 (0.6)	4.4 (0.48)	5 (0)	0.660
Useful to improve surgical technique	4.1 (0.83)	3.6 (0.66)	4.33 (0.47)	0.317
Generally useful for basic endoscopic sinus surgery training	4.1 (0.53)	3.8 (0.6)	4.33 (0.47)	0.130
Useful for endoscopic examination of the nasal cavities	4.4 (0.48)	4.5 (0.5)	5 (0)	0.340
Useful for extraction of a foreign body	4.8 (0.4)	4.5 (0.5)	4.66 (0.47)	0.511
Useful for the maxillary antrostomy	3.6 (0.8)	3.6 (0.48)	3.66 (0.47)	0.342
Useful for the ethmoidectomy	3 (0.73)	2.6 (0.66)	2.2 (0.4)	0.191
Useful for the septoplasty	4.8 (0.4)	4.2 (0.4)	4.66 (0.47)	0.582
Useful for the lower turbinoplasty	3.8 (0.4)	4.4 (0.48)	4.66 (0.47)	0.083

[1] = Kruskal–Wallis test; ENT = otolaryngology; SD = standard deviation; Values for each question and for each group are presented as mean and standard deviation. For most of the answers, no significant difference were noted between the answers of the different groups.

For the resident group, the average satisfaction score was 4.09 ± 0.54; junior specialist group 4.00 ± 0.55; for the senior specialist group overall satisfaction average score was 4.2 ± 0.77 (Figure 6). Considering the average score for all responses noted for each individual group, no statistical differences can be noted, with a *p*-value of 0.598.

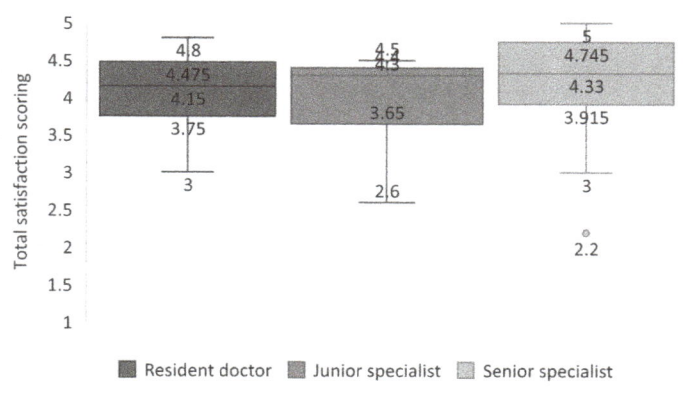

Figure 6. Total satisfaction scoring regarding participant groups.

4. Discussion

Overall satisfaction in all groups was equal to or above 4 out of 5, meaning that a strong agreement has been reached in all groups, regardless of previous experience, in favor of considering the sheep's head as a useful model for endoscopic endonasal surgical training.

The extraction of a foreign body from the nasal fossae necessitates hand–eye coordination, particularly due to the utilization of a 2D endoscopy image, which requires accurate depth perception and spatial orientation. Participants in all groups agreed that simulating foreign body extraction is a good procedure to learn utilizing this model.

Although other authors [7,8] recommend the complete removal of the anterior septal portion for better endoscopic visualization, we chose to keep a part of the anterior septum, considering the advantage it offers us for practicing septoplasty. Even so, this specific modification was advantageous in facilitating the accessibility and maneuverability required during endoscopic procedures. All study group participants were in strong agreement with the benefits offered by the sheep model in endoscopic septal resection training, with no statistical differences noted between groups.

The training scenario simulating a turbinoplasty provided a learning experience to enhance participants' endonasal tissue handling skills. This exercise proved to be particularly advantageous for beginners, as it offered a controlled environment in which to refine their skills.

The deliberate and controlled execution of partial resection and mucosal flap manipulation within the nasal cavity proved to be an invaluable training tool. By carefully excising a segment of the inferior turbinate, it becomes possible to accentuate the prominence of the middle turbinate, which serves to identify the natural ostium of the maxillary sinus.

Although the overall satisfaction was high in all groups there are a few drawbacks when considering the anatomical similarities. Similarity of anatomical landmarks compared to humans received an average score of 3.1. Also, procedures like ethmoidectomy and maxillary anthrostomy did not receive an overall high satisfaction score, averaging 2.6 for ethmoidectomy and 3.6 for anthrostomy.

There are few studies that have highlighted the utility of the ovine model as a viable substitute for surgical training in the field of functional endoscopic sinus surgery.

Gardiner [9] was the first author to propose the sheep's head for training in endoscopic sinus surgery, proposing both simple and more complex maneuvers. Awad et al. [5,6]

also proposed the sheep's head for surgical training in endoscopic rhino-sinusal surgery, showing clear advantages of its use, demonstrating the face, content and construct validation of this anatomic model. Mladina et al. [7,8,10] in their studies chose the lamb's head, due to its smaller size, which allows the use of standard endoscopic rhino-sinusal surgery instruments. He implemented a training program in endoscopic rhino-sinusal surgery using the lamb's head, which proved to be useful for the trainees and allowed the transition to the next level in endoscopic sinus surgery training, i.e., human cadaver training.

Although 3D printing technology has been frequently used for preoperative assessment in endoscopic sinus surgery [11], it is also used to create anatomical models for surgical training in FESS, with the possibility of creating high-fidelity models, being able to simulate certain sinus pathologies, benefiting from validation in this sense, but without benefiting from the real feeling of the tissues, an important disadvantage compared to the sheep's head training.

Even with the mentioned drawbacks, we consider that the ovine FESS model can be an integrative part of surgical training alongside artificial models. Combining the precise anatomy of the artificial models with the feel and overall experience of the ovine model, a more complex teaching experience could be achieved, considering the importance of functional endoscopic sinus surgery [12].

Otologic surgery is another field where the ovine model has been successfully implemented in the training and preparation of young doctors. Anschuetz et al. [13] carried out a study that developed and validated the ovine model for surgical training in endoscopic ear surgery. The anatomy of the sheep's ear was compared with that of humans and was used to perform a series of otological surgical procedures such as canaloplasty, myringoplasty, and ossiculoplasty. Procedures were subjectively evaluated using a postoperative questionnaire, using a scale from 1 to 10. Mean procedure times were as follows: canaloplasty (29.7 ± 13.2 min), middle ear dissection (7.7 ± 2.6 min), myringoplasty (7.7 ± 4.3 min), and ossiculoplasty (10.4 ± 2.7 min). Canaloplasty and flap elevation time decreased from 46.4 to 16.2 min over the study (absolute difference: 30.2 min, 95% CI 22.28–38.12). Subjective ratings were high: tissue quality (8.9/10), overall satisfaction (8.3), and learning experience (8.8). Beckmann et al. [14] carried out a study in which, using the ovine model, they evaluated the learning curve of laser stapedotomy for trainees, with considerable improvement of operative times once the maneuver is repeated. The experienced surgeon maintained a steady average time of 15:01 min throughout the training without any intraoperative issues. The fellow reduced surgical time gradually from 27:21 (first five cases) to 24:10 min (last five cases), and the resident also reduced this time from 42:38 to 21:08 min. Training methods in otosclerosis surgery are very limited, which is why the ovine model proved to be more than useful for this purpose.

Fernandez et al. [15] using eight lamb heads simulated rare situations that may occur intraoperatively in stapes surgery. Thus, floating footplate, footplate fracture, luxation of the incus or necrosis of the long process, overhanging facial nerve, and obliterative otosclerosis could be simulated. A subjective questionnaire with a scale from 1 to 10 was used to determine the satisfaction of the study participants. Taking into account that the options for surgical training in stapes surgery are very limited, the ovine model used in this regard proved to be an excellent learning method for young otologists.

The sheep model was also used for the training of plastic surgery fellows. Isaacson et al. [16] evaluated the possibility of surgical training using the sheep's head for a series of plastic surgery techniques performed for pathologies of the eyelids and the orbit. They harvested 10 sheep heads after the completion of an in vivo study. They evaluated a series of procedures such as upper eyelid blepharoplasty, ptosis repair, upper eyelid repair procedure in facial paralysis, lateral canthotomy, lower acantholysis, narrowing of the lower eyelid, and transconjunctival approach to the floor of the orbit. The overall utility was excellent but remarks were made for limitations due to anatomical variations, one of which is the anatomy of the lacrimal system.

In the field of laryngology the ovine model was used for training in open laryngotracheal surgery. The head and neck were used to simulate a series of surgical procedures, such as tracheotomy, laryngoplasty, tracheal resection with tracheal sutures, and laryngectomy with pharyngeal sutures. This time, the ovine model could be successfully implemented for the training of open surgical techniques, having the advantage of the learning of surgical skills and tissue handling on a model close to humans [17].

The ovine model was also described in the field of dentistry to aid in the learning curve of sinus augmentation. Valboneti et al. analyzed the sheep and human maxillary sinuses anatomy using cone beam computed tomography and histology. Obvious maxillary sinus differences were identified between the human head and ovine model, which were taken into account in order to carry out the experimental procedures [18].

The ovine model was also successfully used for training in sialendoscopy, Borner et al. [19] implemented such a training program in salivary gland endoscopy using the sheep's head, a novelty in the field considering that, for training in these procedures, pig's head was used for several years. The Stenson and Wharton ducts could be successfully visualized endoscopically and therapeutic maneuvers were also simulated by removing a stone from the Stenson duct.

The ovine head was also frequently used for training in different neurosurgical procedures. Kamp et al. [20] simulated a brain tumor model using agar-agar solution injected into fresh sheep brains. The tumor model would vary depending on the concentration of the injected solution, so a high concentration could cause the appearance of well-defined tissue masses, simulating possible brain metastases, while a solution with a lower concentration could cause the appearance of a diffuse infiltrative tissue, thus simulating a primary tumor formation at the level of the brain tissue. This model made it possible to simulate different intraoperative scenarios for young neurosurgeons, with the advantage of learning manual skills and obtaining a haptic sense, in a much more relaxed environment and without the pressure of real intraoperative scenarios.

Korotkov et al. [21] looked for an accessible anatomical model for the training of anterior clinoidectomy, the procedure performed in the case of vascular and tumoral conditions located at the frontotemporal level, which requires a high level of surgical training. Five formalized sheep heads were evaluated, at the level of which, through silicone injection, the presence of dural and extradural lesions was simulated. All the procedures were carried out successfully, thus demonstrating the fact that the sheep head model can be a good alternative to the human cadaver.

Another use of the sheep head model belongs to Altunrende et al. [22], who used the sheep skull for the training of neurosurgeons and ophthalmology residents in performing orbitotomy and frontal craniotomy using dissection under the microscope with good results and with satisfaction in the training of microsurgical techniques for the approach of the optic nerve and optic canal.

Limitations of this study include a small number of participants who belonged to a single training institution. Moreover, our study did not evaluate the transfer of skills acquired using this anatomical model in real endoscopic sinus surgery. Although effective in preparation, the ovine model has a major disadvantage compared to medical practice due to the lack of vascularization and the lack of inflammatory reaction of the rhino-sinusal mucosa often encountered in surgical practice.

In this sense, to extend our research and to eliminate this limitation, in vivo training sessions for endoscopic sinus surgery could be performed using sheep under general anesthesia with orotracheal intubation. In this way, participants can also face intraoperative bleeding, an essential aspect of the surgical training of young doctors. After performing the surgical procedures, in order to avoid their possible suffering, the sheep would be euthanized in accordance with ethical aspects.

At the moment, the training of young doctors in endoscopic sinus surgery is done through the residency program, which involves practicing directly on the live patient, in the operating room under the direct supervision of an experienced guiding surgeon.

However, this determines the limitation of the surgical gestures that can be performed by the young doctor, to avoid possible intra- and post-operative complications. Regarding surgical training in FESS using alternative anatomical models, there is still no organized framework in many countries, leaving room to extend the solutions to this particular ovine model too. To the best of our knowledge, there are various courses organized in university centers in our country, on synthetic anatomical models or even on the ovine model, as is otherwise organized in our center. In this sense, we want to improve the simulation conditions by using in the future the in vivo ovine model, which comes with a series of clear advantages.

5. Conclusions

The sheep's head can be successfully used for learning and practicing manual skills in the use of instruments specific to functional endoscopic sinus surgery, but also for learning some basic endoscopic sinus procedures. Moreover, the sheep head model can be used for training in other diagnostic or surgical procedures in the field of otorhinolaryngology, such as endoscopy of the salivary glands, open laryngotracheal surgery, or in otologic surgery, but also in other different surgical fields, such as neurosurgery, ophthalmology or plastic surgery. Despite the differences between the ovine model and human rhino-sinusal anatomy, it provides resources and minimal cost for beginners who want to develop skills applicable to their practice accuracy.

Similar data from the literature are quite limited, which is why this study should have an important role in the implementation of an anatomical model of a sheep's head for the training in functional endoscopic sinus surgery in our training center and others, considering the accessibility, reliability, and viability of the sheep's head and very good results obtained from its use.

Supplementary Materials: The following supporting information can be downloaded at: https://www.mdpi.com/article/10.3390/medicina59101792/s1, File S1. Satisfaction Questionnaire.

Author Contributions: Conceptualization, C.S., A.A.M. and M.C.; methodology, C.S. and M.C.; software, C.S., L.P.U and C.M.B.; validation, M.C., A.A.M. and C.S.; formal analysis, C.S.. S S.P., D.G.R. and D.V.; investigation, C.S., M.T., M.I.T. and D.V.; resources, C.S., D.G.R. and L.P.U.; data curation, L.P.U. and C.M.B.; writing—original draft preparation, C.S., M.I.T. and M.T.; writing—review and editing, C.S., S.S.P. and L.P.U.; visualization, M.T., D.V. and C.M.B.; supervision, M.C. All authors have read and agreed to the published version of the manuscript.

Funding: This research received no external funding.

Institutional Review Board Statement: The study was conducted in accordance with the Declaration of Helsinki, and approved by the Institutional Review Board of the "Iuliu Hatieganu" University of Medicine and Pharmacy. Registration number AV258/28.02.2022.

Informed Consent Statement: Informed consent was obtained from all subjects involved in the study.

Data Availability Statement: The data presented in this study are available on request from the corresponding author. The data are not publicly available due to privacy and ethical reasons.

Conflicts of Interest: The authors declare no conflict of interest.

References

1. Mallmann, L.B.; Piltcher, O.B.; Isolan, G.R. The Lamb's Head as a Model for Surgical Skills Development in Endonasal Surgery. *J. Neurol. Surg. B Skull Base* **2016**, *77*, 466–472. [CrossRef] [PubMed]
2. Stan, C.; Vesa, D.; Tănase, M.I.; Bulmaci, M.; Pop, S.; Rădeanu, D.G.; Cosgarea, M.; Maniu, A. Can Non-Virtual Reality Simulation Improve Surgical Training in Endoscopic Sinus Surgery? A Literature Review. *Adv. Med. Educ. Pract.* **2023**, *14*, 637–646. [CrossRef] [PubMed]
3. Stew, B.; Ooi, E. The role of simulation in endoscopic sinus surgery training. In *Paranasal Sinuses*; IntechOpen: London, UK, 2017 [CrossRef]
4. Mills, R.; Lee, P. Surgical skills training in middle-ear surgery. *J. Laryngol. Otol.* **2003**, *117*, 159–163. [CrossRef] [PubMed]

5. Awad, Z.; Touska, P.; Arora, A.; Ziprin, P.; Darzi, A.; Tolley, N.S. Face and content validity of sheep heads in endoscopic rhinology training. *Int. Forum. Allergy Rhinol.* **2014**, *4*, 851–858. [CrossRef] [PubMed]
6. Awad, Z.; Taghi, A.; Sethukumar, P.; Tolley, N.S. Construct validity of the ovine model in endoscopic sinus surgery training. *Laryngoscope* **2015**, *125*, 539–543. [CrossRef] [PubMed]
7. Mladina, R. *Endoscopic Surgical Anatomy of the Lamb's Head*; Storz Endo PressTM: Tuttlingen, Germany, 2011.
8. Skitarelić, N.; Mladina, R. Lamb's head: The model for novice education in endoscopic sinus surgery. *World J. Methodol.* **2015**, *5*, 144–148. [CrossRef] [PubMed]
9. Gardiner, Q.; Oluwole, M.; Tan, L.; White, P.S. An animal model for training in endoscopic nasal and sinus surgery. *J. Laryngol. Otol.* **1996**, *110*, 425–428. [CrossRef]
10. Mladina, R.; Vuković, K.; Štern Padovan, R.; Skitarelić, N. An animal model for endoscopic endonasal surgery and dacryocystorhinostomy training: Uses and limitations of the lamb's head. *J. Laryngol. Otol.* **2011**, *125*, 696–700. [CrossRef] [PubMed]
11. Radeanu, D.; Stan, C.; Maniu, A.A. Utility of 3D Reconstructions for Preoperative Planning in Functional Endoscopic Sinus Surgery (FESS). In Proceedings of the 6th International Conference on Advancements of Medicine And Health Care through Technology, Meditech 2018, Cluj Napoca, Romania, 17–20 October 2018.
12. Radeanu, D.; Marin, A.; Stan, C.; Maniu, A. FESS Role in Oral Surgery Rehabilitation. In Proceedings of the National Ent, Head and Neck Surgery Conference, Sibiu, Romania, 17–20 May 2017.
13. Anschuetz, L.; Bonali, M.; Ghirelli, M.; Mattioli, F.; Villari, D.; Caversaccio, M.; Presutti, L. An Ovine Model for Exclusive Endoscopic Ear Surgery. *JAMA Otolaryngol. Head Neck Surg.* **2017**, *143*, 247–252. [CrossRef] [PubMed]
14. Beckmann, S.; Yacoub, A.; Fernandez, I.J.; Niederhauser, L.; Fermi, M.; Caversaccio, M.; Marco, B.; Anschuetz, L. Exclusive Endoscopic Laser-Stapedotomy: Feasibility of an Ovine Training Model. *Otol. Neurotol.* **2021**, *42*, 994–1000. [CrossRef]
15. Fernandez, I.J.; Bonali, M.; Yacoub, A.; Ghirelli, M.; Fermi, M.; Presutti, L.; Caversaccio, M.; Anschuetz, L. Training model for salvage procedures in endoscopic stapes surgery. *Eur. Arch. Otorhinolaryngol.* **2021**, *278*, 987–995. [CrossRef] [PubMed]
16. Isaacson, G.; Wulc, A.E. Applicability of a sheep model for training in plastic surgery of eyelids and orbit. *Ear Nose Throat J.* **2022**, *101* (Suppl. S2), 43S–49S. [CrossRef] [PubMed]
17. Soliman, A.M.S.; Ianacone, D.C.; Isaacson, G.C. Ex vivo ovine model for teaching open laryngotracheal surgery. *World J. Otorhinolaryngol. Head Neck Surg.* **2018**, *4*, 140–144. [CrossRef]
18. Valbonetti, L.; Berardinelli, P.; Scarano, A.; Piattelli, A.; Mattioli, M.; Barboni, B.; Vulpiani, M.P.; Muttini, A. Translational Value of Sheep as Animal Model to Study Sinus Augmentation. *J. Craniofacial Surg.* **2015**, *26*, 737–740. [CrossRef] [PubMed]
19. Borner, U.; Caversaccio, M.; Wagner, F.; Marchal, F.; Anschuetz, L. First evaluation of an ovine training model for sialendoscopy. *Laryngoscope Investig. Otolaryngol.* **2023**, *8*, 903–911. [CrossRef] [PubMed]
20. Kamp, M.A.; Knipps, J.; Steiger, H.J.; Rapp, M.; Cornelius, J.F.; Folke-Sabel, S.; Sabel, M. Training for brain tumour resection: A realistic model with easy accessibility. *Acta Neurochir.* **2015**, *157*, 1975–1981. [CrossRef] [PubMed]
21. Korotkov, D.; Abramyan, A.; Wuo-Silva, R.; Chaddad-Neto, F. Cadaveric Sheep Head Model for Anterior Clinoidectomy in Neurosurgical Training. *World Neurosurg.* **2023**, *175*, e481–e491. [CrossRef] [PubMed]
22. Altunrende, M.E.; Hamamcioglu, M.K.; Hıcdonmez, T.; Akcakaya, M.O.; Bırgılı, B.; Cobanoglu, S. Microsurgical training model for residents to approach to the orbit and the optic nerve in fresh cadaveric sheep cranium. *J. Neurosci. Rural. Pract.* **2014**, *5*, 151–154. [CrossRef] [PubMed]

Disclaimer/Publisher's Note: The statements, opinions and data contained in all publications are solely those of the individual author(s) and contributor(s) and not of MDPI and/or the editor(s). MDPI and/or the editor(s) disclaim responsibility for any injury to people or property resulting from any ideas, methods, instructions or products referred to in the content.

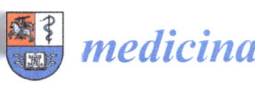

Article

Management of Capillary Hemangioma of the Sphenoid Sinus

Irina-Gabriela Ionita [1,2], Viorel Zainea [1,2], Catalina Voiosu [1,2], Cristian Dragos Stefanescu [1,2,*], Cristina Aura Panea [1,3], Adrian Vasile Dumitru [1,4], Ruxandra Oana Alius [2] and Razvan Hainarosie [1,2]

1. ENT Department, Faculty of Medicine, "Carol Davila" University of Medicine and Pharmacy, 8th Eroii Sanitari Boulevard, 050474 Bucharest, Romania
2. "Prof. Dr. D. Hociota" Institute of Phonoaudiology and Functional ENT Surgery, 21st Mihail Cioranu Street, 061344 Bucharest, Romania
3. Neurology Department, Elias Emergency University Hospital, 17th Marasti Boulevard, 011461 Bucharest, Romania
4. Pathology Department, Emergency University Hospital, 169th Independence Street, 050098 Bucharest, Romania
* Correspondence: dragos.stefanescu@umfcd.ro; Tel.: +40-730-047-455

Abstract: *Background and objectives:* Capillary hemangiomas are rare, benign vascular tumors that mainly affect the skin and soft tissue, with scarce appearance within the nasal cavities and paranasal sinuses. *Materials and methods:* We present a case report of capillary hemangioma of the sphenoid sinus and a review of the literature in the last ten years. *Results:* Clinical and endoscopic examination of the nose, radiologic assessment and particular histologic features contribute to the correct diagnosis of capillary hemangioma of the nose and paranasal sinuses. *Conclusions:* Transnasal endoscopic resection of capillary hemangioma located in the nose and paranasal sinuses is a valuable treatment method with good outcomes.

Keywords: capillary hemangioma sinus; endoscopic surgery; sphenoid tumor

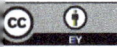

1. Introduction

Capillary hemangiomas are rare, benign vascular tumors that mainly affect the skin and soft tissue. These tumors are frequently encountered in infants and children, more common in the female population, and are rarely diagnosed in adults [1].

Hemangiomas are vascular tumors that appear due to endothelial cell growth. Proliferation of regular (with normal architecture) endothelial cells is characteristic for hemangiomas. They should not be mistaken for vascular malformation, which occurs due to defects of vascular morphogenesis [2]. Vascular malformations are lesion defined by vascular anomalies determined by the alteration of embryogenesis and vasculogenesis [2].

Most hemangiomas appear on the skin in the head and neck region, but only 12% occur in the nose and paranasal sinuses with a predominance of the nasal cavity location [3,4]. Hemangiomas in the paranasal sinuses are rare findings, and most cases are reported in the maxillary sinus. Kim S.J. and Kwon S.H. reported maxillary sinus involvement in only 8% of hemangiomas affecting the sinonasal epithelium; no sphenoid sinus involvement was described in this study [4]. The same authors state that the nasal septum and inferior turbinate were the most common sites affected by hemangiomas with 40.5% and 29.7% of all cases, respectively [4,5], but other sites such as the nasal vestibule, middle turbinate and uncinate process have been reported [6]. The presence of a capillary hemangioma within the sphenoid sinus is rare, and there are limited scientific papers regarding this specific site of appearance [1].

Intracranial hemangiomas are also rare cases, with a female predilection in adult patients, but with a possible rapid evolution, especially in pregnant women or women in the peripartum period [1,7,8]. Some authors state that pregnancy (due to all its hormonal changes) triggers the tumor's progression and can cause recurrence of the hemangioma [8].

The location and size of the tumor will determine the clinical manifestation, but headache and visual impairment are the most frequent symptoms.

2. Materials and Methods

The aim of this manuscript is to present a case report of capillary hemangiomas of the left sphenoid sinus and a review of the literature in the last ten years.

We reviewed English articles published in 2013–2023 on PubMed and the Wiley Online Library. An interrogation was made on specific terms "capillary hemangioma sinus", "capillary hemangioma nose", and "capillary hemangioma sphenoid". On PubMed, the search using the specific terms mentioned above revealed 35 articles, but only 14 were related to the nose and paranasal sinuses. In the Wiley Online Library, the investigation revealed 23 manuscripts with capillary hemangioma, but only 6 articles referred to the nose and paranasal sinuses. During the interrogation, we found no series of sphenoid sinus capillary hemangiomas. The articles presenting this specific localization were case reports. The included case series regarding capillary hemangioma consisted of a limited number of patients and were usually retrospective studies.

The aim of this paper is to present the case of a 31-year-old female patient referred to our clinic by a regional ENT specialist for an excruciating headache (eight out of ten on the Numeric Pain Rating Scale) experienced during a flight, which partially resolved after oral analgesic intake. She was first treated by her otolaryngologist with oral antibiotics, oral steroids, and nasal drops with improvement of the severe headache, but a computed tomography of the paranasal sinuses was recommended. There is no personal history of allergies or other medical associated conditions, no ENT- specific symptoms such as nose bleeding or rhinorrhea, and no neurologic or ophthalmologic manifestations. The patient also denied any history of head trauma or previous nasal and sinus surgery or pregnancy.

Complete physical examination and flexible optic examination of the nasal cavities, pharynx, and larynx (with white light and narrow-band imaging) revealed a nasal septum deviated to the left side, inferior turbinate hypertrophy grade III, and a pulsatile area at the level of the left sphenoethmoidal recess with an atypical vascular pattern on narrow-band imaging examination, without abnormal nasal or sinus discharge. The nasopharynx was mass-free, without signs of inflammation or secretions. On flexible endoscopy, no mass was visible within the nasal cavity or the left sphenoethmoidal recess. The rest of the specific ENT examination was normal.

The computed tomographic (CT) examination described a 32 × 28 mm pseudo-cystic lesion in the left sphenoid sinus that occupied approximately 80% of the sinus cavity, in close relation with its posterior wall. The lesion was located within the sinus cavity without extension into the sphenoethmoidal recess or the nasopharynx. No bone erosions were visible on the imaging. All other paranasal sinuses appeared well aerated and tumor-free (Figure 1a–c). The CT assessment also highlighted the nasal obstruction with left posterior nasal septum deviation that determines blockage of the left sphenoethmoidal recess and bilateral inferior turbinate hypertrophy.

Upon admission to the hospital, the standard blood tests were carried out in order to establish any systemic impairment caused by the intrasinusal lesion. All blood work came back negative for any signs of inflammation or infection. Internal medicine assessment was also performed as part of the preoperative anesthesiology protocol. Written informed consent was obtained. During preoperative discussions, the goals of the surgery and the potential risks and complications, both intraoperative and postoperative, were explained to the patient. After preanesthetic assessments were checked, the patient underwent endoscopic sinus surgery to address the left sphenoid sinus under general anesthesia with orotracheal intubation. Septoplasty and inferior turbinate resection were performed to allow adequate access to the left sphenoethmoidal recess. The left sphenoid sinus was opened under endoscopic control with a zero-degree endoscope, and a reddish mass occupying approximately one-third of the sinus was identified. To adequately approach the lesion, a large opening of the sphenoid sinus was performed, and the mass was carefully detached from the posterior wall of the sphenoid sinus, ablated (Figure 2), and sent for histopathology examination. The dissection of the lesion from the wall of the left sphenoid sinus was carried out cautiously in order to avoid iatrogenic incidents. In the course of the dissection, the bleeding was limited. After removal of the tumor, the posterior wall of the left sphenoid sinus was assessed, and no bone discontinuities were observed. During surgery, we were able to appreciate the size of the intra-sphenoidal lesion as being smaller than the size measured on the computed tomography assessment. At the end of surgery, bilateral nasal packing with Merocell No. 8 was performed. The nasal packing was maintained for 48 h. Then, the nasal packing was removed with no bleeding, and nasal saline instillation was recommended at discharge. The patient did not suffer any intraoperative and postoperative complications, and the recovery was uneventful. After the surgery, all symptoms subsided, and the patient was discharged with no complaints and scheduled for follow up in one week.

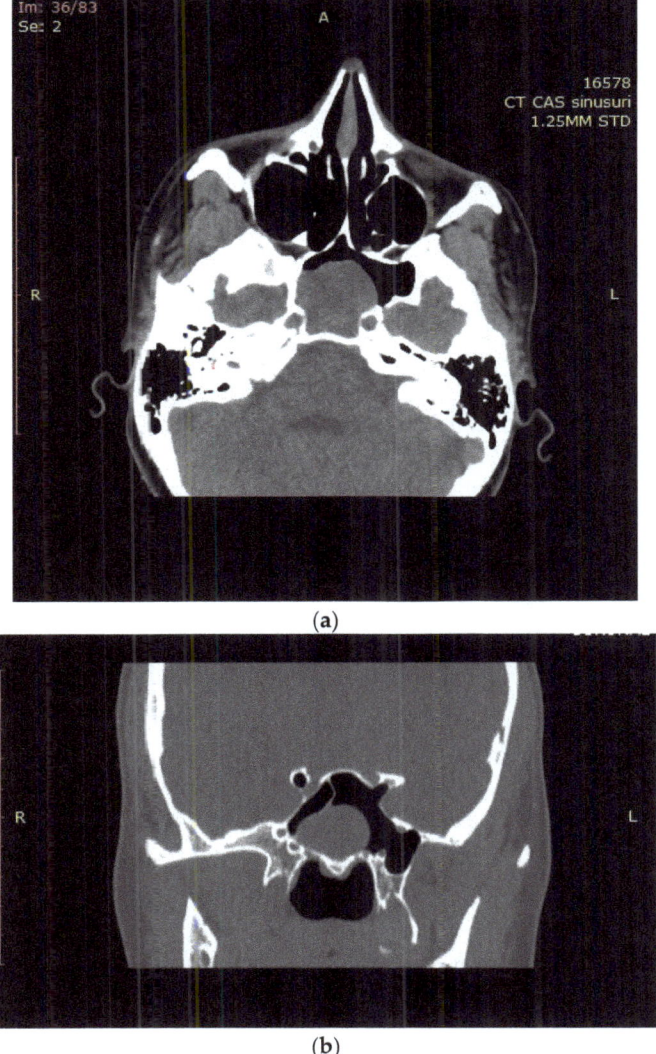

Figure 1. Cont.

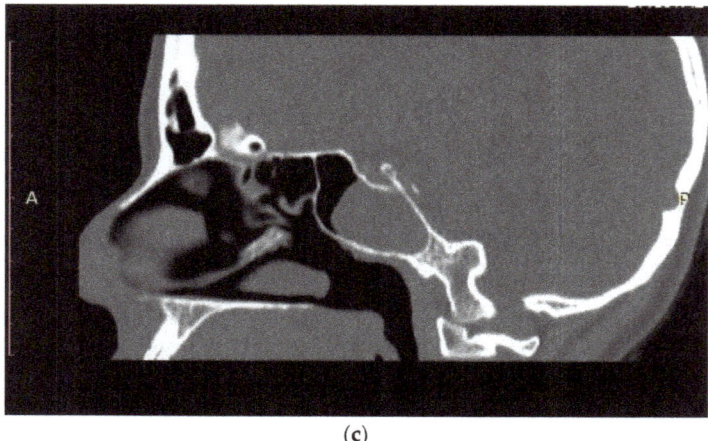

(c)

Figure 1. CT of the paranasal sinuses - (**a**) axial, (**b**) coronal, and (**c**) sagittal planes—lesion in the left sphenoid sinus.

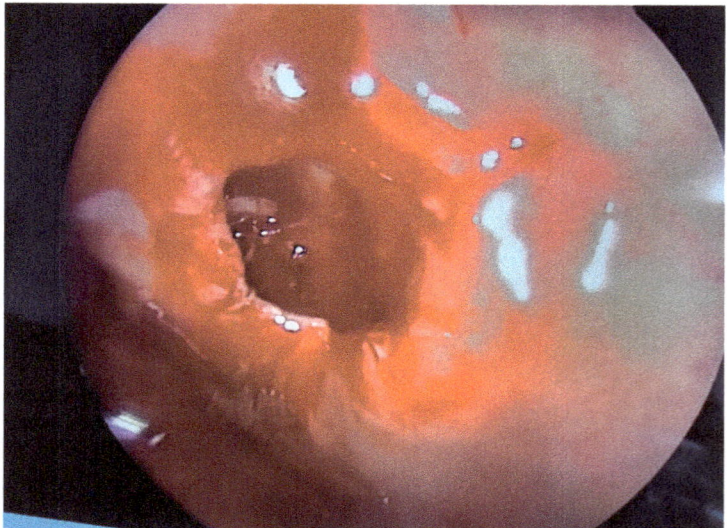

Figure 2. Intraoperative aspect—dissection of the mass within the left sphenoid sinus after tactical resection of the deviated nasal septum.

Histopathological examination and immunohistochemistry established the diagnosis of capillary hemangioma with desmoplastic stroma. The pathologist described, on hematoxylin–eosin (HE) staining, tumor proliferation composed of endothelial cells without atypia, forming delicate vascular structures without lumens. The aspect was of a benign vascular proliferation formed by endothelial cells that form fragile submucosal vascular structures; some vessels appeared slightly dilated and with intraluminal red blood cells (Figures 3 and 4). The pathologic assessment did not identify any ulcerations. Immunohistochemical analysis of the tumor showed that it was CD31- and CD34-positive, with Ki67 < 1%. Both immunohistochemical markers CD31 and CD34 are positive in endothelial cells, but CD31 is considered the most dependable endothelial marker [9].

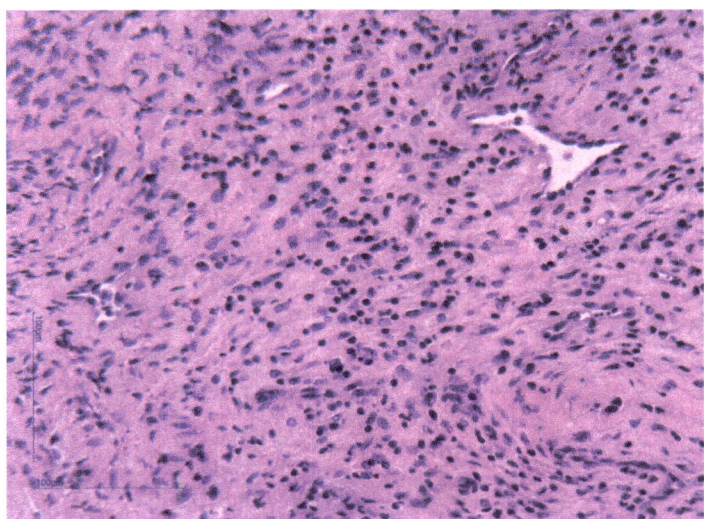

Figure 3. Solid area from a capillary hemangioma represented by a tumor proliferation composed of endothelial cells without atypia forming vascular structures without lumens. HE stain, ×400.

After surgery, clinical and endoscopic assessments were performed every month in the first three months, afterward the visits were scheduled for every three to six months. Flexible nasal endoscopy revealed patent nasal cavities and a patent left sphenoid sinus ostium (Figure 5). No signs of bleeding or abnormal nasal discharge were visible during any of the check-ups. Moreover, the patients' quality of life improved due to tactical removal of the deviated nasal septum and turbinoplasty. Postoperatively, the patient declared the absence of headaches and improved nasal breathing. Four months after resection, the patient received an enhanced brain (head) magnetic resonance imaging (MRI). The left sphenoid sinus was mass-free, without residual hemangioma (Figure 6).

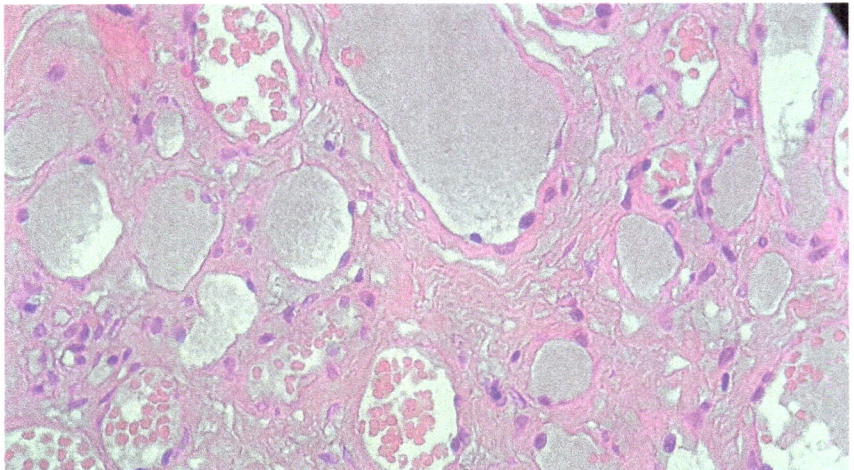

Figure 4. Classic appearance of a capillary hemangioma consisting of delicate vascular structures, some slightly dilated and with intraluminal red blood cells. HE stain, ×400.

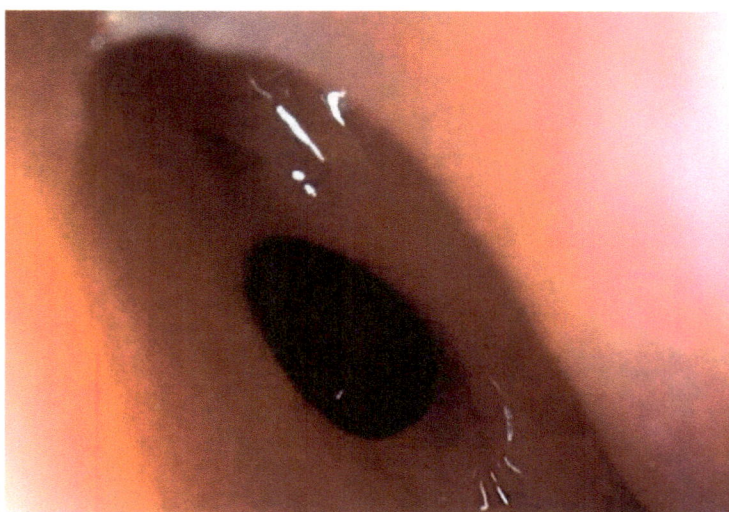

Figure 5. Postoperative aspect—enlarged left sphenoid sinus ostium with no signs of inflammation, no nasal or sinus discharge, and no bleeding.

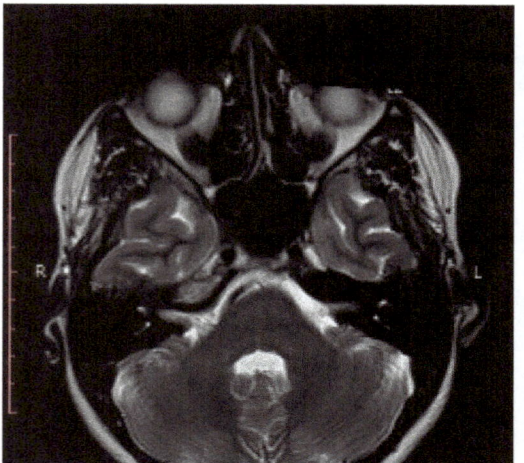 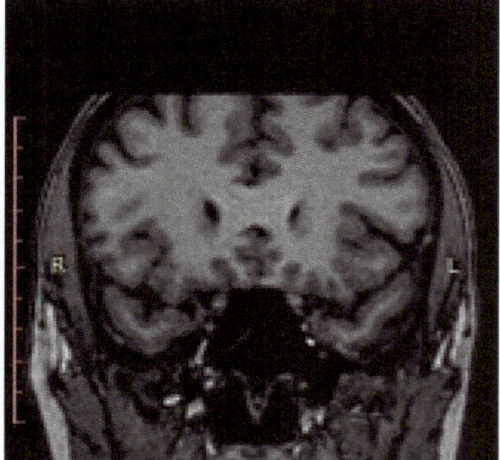

Figure 6. Enhanced brain MRI (axial and coronal plane)—no lesion detected within the left sphenoid sinus four months postoperatively.

3. Discussion

Hemangiomas are vascular tumors consisting of blood vessels and connective tissue that rarely affect the nose and paranasal sinuses and appear frequently on the skin in the head and neck region [9]. There are different types of classifications for hemangiomas depending on the moment of presentation and the pathologic and immunohistologic features. Hemangiomas can be congenital or infantile depending on the age of onset or presentation. From a histologic point of view, hemangiomas can be cavernous or capillary depending on the size of the blood vessels within the tumor [10]. Capillary hemangiomas have small-diameter vessels, while cavernous hemangiomas present large-diameter vessels [2,10]. Capillary hemangiomas have a characteristic pattern of vascular proliferation with a "trunk-and-branch" aspect, surrounded by pericytes, with a relative number of mitoses, fibromyoid stroma and well-represented inflammatory infiltrate [11]. Cavernous hemangiomas have large vascular spaces lined with endothelium [12]. Ulceration of the epithelium or atrophy can appear on microscopic examination of a capillary hemangioma [13]. In the nose and paranasal sinuses, capillary hemangiomas are more frequently encountered than cavernous hemangiomas [10]. A subtype of capillary hemangioma is lobular capillary hemangioma, also known as pyogenic granuloma. It appears on the skin and in oral and nasal mucosa (especially the anterior nasal septum, turbinates, nasal vestibule, or nasopharynx) [3,4]. The etiology of lobular capillary hemangioma is not completely understood, but some theories take into account hormonal implication (particularly pregnancy and contraceptive use), injury, trauma, and viral infections [3,13,14]. Lobular capillary hemangioma can be encountered during pregnancy and is defined by the term "granuloma gravidarum". It is located within the nasal cavities, and the main symptom is recurrent unilateral epistaxis. Managing nasal hemorrhage during pregnancy can be challenging for the ENT surgeon. The treatment should be efficient but as conservative as possible and care should be taken when prescribing certain drugs. Mohd Yusof J. et al. consider chemical cauterization with silver nitrate and anterior nasal packing to be first-line treatment for mild epistaxis during pregnancy [15]. In case of severe nose hemorrhage, surgical intervention with general anesthesia is necessary to control the epistaxis; all measures should be taken to minimize the risks of general anesthesia to the fetus [15]. Another classification of hemangiomas takes into account the presence or absence of a protein named endothelial cell glucose transporter 1 (GLUT1) [16]. In infantile hemangiomas, GLUT1 protein is expressed, whereas in congenital hemangiomas it is not [16]. A noteworthy aspect regarding hemangiomas of the nose and paranasal sinuses is their late presentation in adults (around 40 years), different from hemangiomas with other locations that appear at birth or soon afterward [10].

The symptoms can vary and depend on the location and size of the tumor, but unilateral nasal obstruction, recurrent unilateral epistaxis, and headache are among the commonest [14,17,18]. Hemangiomas are benign tumors with a slow growing rate. Usually, the patient is asymptomatic for a long period. When symptoms appear, the tumor has a considerable volume and exerts a mass effect on adjacent structures. Unilateral nasal obstruction develops progressively and advances slowly. In some cases, the nasal obstruction can be accompanied by rhinorrhea or mucopurulent nasal discharge if the drainage pathway of the affected sinus is blocked by the tumor. If the tumor is located in the anterior part of the nasal septum, unilateral recurrent anterior epistaxis is the dominant symptom. The severity of nasal hemorrhage is variable from mild to moderate and severe. In cases of mild and moderate epistaxis, local hemostatic maneuvers (nasal packing, chemical cauterization of site of bleeding) will control the bleeding. In cases of severe epistaxis, hospital admission is necessary, and emergency surgical maneuvers to control the nasal hemorrhage are imposed. A peculiarity of capillary hemangioma developing exclusively in the sinus cavity is the lack of nose bleeds in the clinical presentation of the patient. If the tumor is limited to a sinus cavity, then headache or facial pain represents the prevailing symptom. The unilaterality of the symptoms (and of the lesion) should raise suspicion of malignancy [10]. Another particular aspect of a lesion limited to the sinus cavity is the possibility of developing bony erosion through mass effect and locoregional extension without invasion into the surrounding structures. In advanced cases with orbital implication, ocular symptoms (proptosis, reduced eye mobility, impaired vision, ocular globe displacement) will accompany the nasal ones [19]. When intracranial involvement is also present, the neurologic symptoms are associated with the nasal manifestations [1]. A great range of neurologic symptoms can appear from diplopia to neurologic deficits and signs of increased intracranial pressure [8]. In the presented case, the patient had a history of chronic bilateral nasal obstruction and recurrent headaches. The intensity and particular features of the headache during the flight motivated the patient to seek medical attention. Although the symptoms were alleviated after the treatment prescribed by the general ENT specialist, the patient continued the medical investigations.

The imagistic assessment of choice is enhanced computed tomography, which allows identification of the site of the lesion, its characteristics, and its interaction with the surrounding structures. The relationship between the tumor and the base of the skull and orbit should be thoroughly checked. Binesh et al. reported two cases of ethmoid capillary hemangioma associated with bone erosion of the lamina papyracea in both adults and children; one case presented extensive bone erosion into the nasal septum and cribriform plate with extension into the anterior cranial fossa [19]. Pas M. et al. presented a case of left ethmoid and sphenoid sinus capillary hemangioma with involvement of the left cavernous sinus, extensive bone erosion, and intrasellar and parasellar extension [1].

The specific aspect of a capillary hemangioma on CT is a soft-tissue enhancing lesion associated (or not) with bone erosion located in the nose and/or paranasal sinuses [18]. According to some authors, the bone erosion is a result of the compression on the bony structures and is not an invasion of the surrounding bones [20]. Kim J.H. et al. described capillary hemangiomas from their series as well-defined, round–oval lesions, with significant enhancement at an early phase and diminished enhancement at the delayed phase on CT [12]. The same authors describe the appearance of a capillary hemangioma on MRI as low-signal masses on T1-weighted images with marked enhancement on contrast T1-weighted images and central masses surrounded by a hypo-intense peripheric rim on T2-weighted images [12].

Sometimes the histological diagnosis of capillary hemangioma can be difficult due to the endothelial proliferation pattern that resembles malignant lesions and ulceration that corresponds to granulation tissue [14]. Differential diagnosis can be made with nasal angiofibroma (when the patient is an adolescent male juvenile, angiofibroma can be taken into account), angiomatous polyp of the nose and sinuses, polypoid granulation tissue, inverted papilloma, lymphangioma, hemangiolymphangioma, glomangiopericytoma, or angiosarcoma [9,18,19,21]. Angiofibromas contain large-diameter blood vessels and stellate fibroblasts, which differ from the small-diameter vessels encountered in capillary hemangiomas [19]. Hemangiolymphangiomas are rare, lymph-containing vascular tumors characterized by multiple lymph vessels surrounded by loose fibrovascular stroma [2,21]. Glomangiopericytomas present more cells and less endothelial lining than capillary hemangiomas [19]. Angiosarcomas present malignant endothelial cells with extravascular extension and an infiltrative pattern, whilst capillary hemangiomas possess normal endothelial cells with no extravascular extension [11]. Histologic examination and immunohistochemistry establish the type of tumor. The aspect of the lesion on endoscopy and imagistic assessment can guide the surgeon, preoperatively, toward the correct diagnosis.

Surgical excision of the tumor is the preferred treatment method, and endoscopic trans-nasal surgery is most frequently used. Biopsies should be performed with care because of the high risk of bleeding due to the vascular nature of the tumor; any surgical maneuvers should be executed only after imagistic assessment [10]. Significant bleeding after biopsy should be expected when manipulating vascular tumors, and proper methods of hemostasis are imperative. Endoscopic trans-nasal removal of the tumor is considered safe and effective [22]. Furthermore, endoscopic sinus surgery is considered a minimally invasive approach for sinus hemangiomas with limited complications, reduced morbidity, and decreased hospitalization [10]. The excision can be made with electrocautery, laser, or even cryotherapy. Endoscopic surgery of intrasinusal lesions allows adequate visualization of the tumor and identification of the risk elements. Depending on the site and extension of the tumor, zero-degree or angled endoscopes can be used. Using both types (straight and angled) of endoscopes, the ENT surgeon can properly assess the sinus cavity and identify any residual tumor. Power instruments such as microdebriders should be carefully manipulated within sinus cavities, especially in the vicinity of surgical risk structures (orbit, skull base, internal carotid artery, optic nerve). Dissection with endoscopic forceps is recommended when bone erosion is identified on preoperative imagistic assessment. Preoperative CT is essential to understand the particularities of sphenoid sinus anatomy and its relation with the internal carotid artery and optic nerve—the two main risk structures in the area. Sphenoid sinus pneumatization is another factor that influences the effect on the internal carotid artery and the optic nerve. According to Fadda G.L.et al., the iatrogenic risk of injury of the aforementioned anatomic elements is higher when extensive pneumatization of the sphenoid sinus exists [23]. The presented case had significant asymmetry of the sphenoid sinus, with a small right sphenoid sinus and a wide left sphenoid sinus; this is a postsellar-type variation of pneumatization of the left sphenoid sinus. Due to the significant inequality of the sphenoid sinuses, both internal carotid arteries are in close proximity to the left sphenoid sinus. This makes them more susceptible to injury during sphenoid sinus approach. One study describes the postsellar variation as being less frequent in the studied population, but more commonly associated with protrusion of the internal carotid arteries and optic nerve within the sinus cavity [23]. Angiography with embolization may be performed before surgery, but there is no consensus among authors [6,14,20]. Preoperative embolization decreases the risk of significant bleeding during surgery and causes a regression of the tumor, allowing the ENT surgeon to manipulate the lesion and to properly dissect and ablate it. Due to the small number of reported cases and the lack of comprehensive studies, there are no available guidelines regarding the management of nasal and sinus capillary hemangiomas. Hasegawa et al. presented three cases of maxillary sinus hemangiomas that were embolized before surgery and limited perioperative bleeding was achieved (between 30 and 100 mL) [24]. Tzu-Hang C. et al. performed surgical excision of the tumor without prior embolization in all studied cases and reported no recurrence [20]. We performed endoscopic sinus surgery with no preoperative embolization in the presented case. Resection of the nasal septum and inferior turbinoplasty were necessary to create an adequate access pathway to the left sphenoid sinus and to improve nasal respiration. The particular features of the sphenoid sinus pneumatization in the presented case imposed a meticulous and prudent approach of the left sphenoid sinus cavity and its content. The choice of the adequate surgical technique and technology is adapted for every patient taking into account the effect of the technology on the healthy tissue surrounding the lesion and surgical risk elements in the vicinity [25].

The recurrence rate found in the literature varies from 0 to 42%; it depends on the study and follow-up period [20,26]. Bradshaw et al. consider that the recurrence rate depends on the technique and technology used for resection—8% recurrence rate for open excision and 40% recurrence rate for biopsy or electrocauterization—and advocate for complete resection of the tumor with a margin of healthy tissue to prevent recurrence [13]. The aforementioned authors also reported the possibility of spontaneously regression of the capillary hemangioma especially in adolescents, young adults, and pregnant women, but the regression process is not fully understood [13]. Smith et al. reported a 41.9% rate of recurrence for a mean follow-up interval of 58.6 months with a mean interval of 5.7 months between the surgery and the appearance of the recurrent tumor [26]. In their study, the presence of sinus capillary hemangiomas was limited: only one case of ethmoid lesion and no sphenoid sinus tumors. The same authors demonstrated a correlation between the age of the patient and recurrence; the mean age of the patients who developed recurrent capillary hemangioma of the nose and paranasal sinus was 50.1 years, whereas the mean age for non-recurrent tumor was 31.5 years [26]. Some authors state a 3.66% recurrence rate, but the follow-up period was relatively short (mean of 9 months) [27]. The management of recurrent capillary hemangioma is not standardized. Different approaches are available: surgical excision under general anesthesia, tumor ablation with local anesthesia, biopsy sampling, and electrocauterization. The study of Al-Ani et al., on 82 patients, demonstrated a left-side predilection of nasal capillary hemangiomas [27]. The case presented in this article was also a left-side tumor. In our case, at four months after surgery, both the endoscopic examination and brain MRI showed no residual tumor or recurrence. Taking into consideration the possibility of recurrence, we will continue follow up (clinic and endoscopic assessment every three to six months, and imagistic assessment after one year after surgery). An important aspect related to hemangioma recurrence is the lack of malignant transformation of the lesion [26].

The long-term prognosis of capillary hemangioma depends on the site of the lesion, the complete or incomplete removal of the tumor, and specific particularities of the patient (for example, pregnancy or other endocrinologic features) [8]. Given the complete removal of the tumor (assessed with enhanced head MRI four months after surgery), a favorable long-term prognosis is expected in this case. Nevertheless, the follow up will be realized as described above. The quality of life of the patient was improved after surgical resection of the tumor due to symptomatic relief. Improved nasal patency and absence of headaches were reported by the patient. The correct histologic diagnosis (histopathological examination and immunohistochemical analysis), according to the International Society for the Study of Vascular Anomalies, should be kept in mind when managing such cases [28,29].

4. Conclusions

Capillary hemangiomas are rare, benign vascular tumors encountered in the nose and paranasal sinuses. The clinical manifestations are not particular for this type of tumor, but the imagistic assessment can guide the surgeon to the correct diagnosis. The ENT specialist should have a high index of suspicion to diagnose capillary hemangioma within the nasal sinuses properly. Surgical resection of the tumor is the treatment of choice. Nowadays, endoscopic sinus surgery provides a good visualization of the surgical field and allows proper identification of the risk factors and correct assessment of the tumor. Complete resection of the tumor and the absence of malignant transformation (even for recurrences) are the two main features that advocate a favorable long-term prognosis for capillary hemangiomas.

Although this article represents a report of a single case of capillary hemangioma of the sphenoid sinus, the small number of cases reported in the literature make it relevant for the diagnosis and management of such tumors. Due to the lack of extensive studies of this diagnosis, there is no general consensus in its management nor in the postoperative rate of recurrence. The authors suggest that all encountered cases should undergo surveillance for a longer period of time in order to establish accurate statistical data.

Author Contributions: Conceptualization, R.H.; resources, A.V.D.; writing—original draft preparation, I.-G.I.; writing—review and editing, C.V., R.O.A.; visualization, C.D.S., C.A.P.; supervision, V.Z.; All authors have read and agreed to the published version of the manuscript.

Funding: This research received no external funding.

Institutional Review Board Statement: The study was conducted according to the guidelines of the Declaration of Helsinki in the current version and was approved by the local institutional ethics committee of "Prof. Dr. D. Hociota" Institute of Phonoaudiology and Functional ENT Surgery (protocol code 1764 and approved by 15 February).

Informed Consent Statement: Informed consent was obtained from all subjects involved in the study.

Data Availability Statement: Not applicable.

Conflicts of Interest: The authors declare no conflict of interest.

References

1. Pas, M.; Shimono, T.; Morisako, H.; Tsukamoto, T.; Kuramoto, R.; Horiuchi, D.; Tashiro, A.; Shigeki, S.; Miki, Y. Capillary hemangioma of the sphenoid sinus with intrasellar and parasellar extensions. *Radiol. Case Rep.* **2022**, *17*, 156–160. [CrossRef] [PubMed]
2. George, A.; Mani, V.; Noufal, A. Update on the classification of hemangioma. *J. Oral Maxillofac. Pathol.* **2014**, *18* (Suppl 1), S117–S120. [CrossRef] [PubMed]
3. Vukadinović, T.; Labus, M.; Spasić, S.; Đurđević, B.V.; Perić, A. Maxillary Sinus Lobular Capillary Hemangioma in a 15-Year-Old Boy. *Ear Nose Throat J.* **2021**, 0145561321993597. [CrossRef] [PubMed]
4. Kim, J.S.; Kwon, S.H. Sinonasal hemangioma: Diagnosis, treatment, and follow-up of 37 patients at a single center. *J. Oral Maxillofac. Surg.* **2017**, *75*, 1775–1783. [CrossRef]
5. Min, H.J.; Mun, S.K.; Lee, S.Y.; Kim, K.S. The Possible Role of Endoscopy in Diagnosis of Benign Tumors of the Nasal Cavity. *J. Craniofac. Surg.* **2017**, *28*, 973–975. [CrossRef]
6. Albesher, M.B.; Alharbi, M.H.; Alsumairi, M.B.; Hussein, N.M. Nasal lobular capillary hemangioma: Report of a case managed by endoscopic excision and pre-operative angio-embolization. *Int. J. Surg. Case Rep.* **2023**, *102*, 107866. [CrossRef]

7. Massman, L.J.; Conteh, F.; Cochran, E.J.; Zwagerman, N.T. Intracranial Capillary Hemangiomas: A Peripartum Presentation and Review of the Literature. *World Neurosurg.* **2021**, *145*, 220–228. [CrossRef]
8. Mehrizi, M.A.A.; Baharvahdat, H.; Saghebdoust, S. Recurrent posterior fossa intracranial capillary hemangioma in a pregnant woman: A case report and review of literature. *Ann. Med. Surgery.* **2022**, *84*, 104913. [CrossRef]
9. Tan, S.N.; Gendeh, H.S.; Gendeh, B.S.; Ramzisham, A.R. The Nasal Hemangioma. *Indian J. Otolaryngol. Head Neck Surg.* **2019**, *71* (Suppl 3), 1683–1686. [CrossRef]
10. Lightbody, K.A.; Wilkie, M.D.; Luff, D.A. Capillary haemangioma of the ethmoid sinus. *BMJ Case Rep.* **2013**, *2013*, bcr2013008695. [CrossRef]
11. Thompson, L.D.R.; Fanburg-Smith, J.C. Update on Select Benign Mesenchymal and Meningothelial Sinonasal Tract Lesions. *Head Neck Pathol.* **2016**, *10*, 95–108. [CrossRef]
12. Kim, J.H.; Park, S.W.; Kim, S.C.; Lim, M.K.; Jang, T.Y.; Kim, Y.J.; Kang, Y.H.; Lee, H.Y. Computed tomography and magnetic resonance imaging findings of nasal cavity hemangiomas according to histological type. *Korean J. Radiol.* **2015**, *16*, 566–574. [CrossRef]
13. Bradshaw, B.; Ulualp, S.O.; Rajaram, V.; Liu, C. Recurrent Epistaxis and Unilateral Intranasal Mass in A Teenager. *Am. J. Case Rep.* **2021**, *22*, e933075. [CrossRef]
14. Stubbs, D.; Poulios, A.; Khalil, H. Benign sinonasal capillary haemangioma. *BMJ Case Rep.* **2014**, *2014*, bcr2014207070. [CrossRef]
15. Mohd Yusof, J.; Abd Halim, A.; Wan Hamizan, A.K. Severe epistaxis in pregnancy due to nasal pyogenic granuloma: A case report. *J. Taibah Univ. Med. Sci.* **2020**, *15*, 334–337. [CrossRef]
16. Kollipara, R.; Dinneen, L.; Rentas, K.E.; Saettele, M.R.; Patel, S.A.; Rivard, D.C.; Lowe, L.H. Current Classification and Terminology of Pediatric Vascular Anomalies. *Am. J. Roentgenol.* **2013**, *201*, 1124–1135. [CrossRef]
17. Takaishi, S.; Asaka, D.; Nakayama, T.; Iimura, J.; Matsuwaki, Y.; Hirooka, S.; Takahashi, H.; Kojima, H.; Otori, N. Features of sinonasal hemangioma: A retrospective study of 31 cases. *Auris Nasus Larynx* **2017**, *44*, 719–723. [CrossRef]
18. Patil, P.; Singla, S.; Mane, R.; Jagdeesh, K.S. Nasal lobular capillary hemangioma. *J. Clin. Imaging Sci.* **2013**, *3*, 40. [CrossRef]
19. Binesh, F.; Khajehzadeh, F.; Kargar, Z.; Hakiminia, M.; Mirvakili, A. Lobular Capillary Hemangioma of the Ethmoid Sinus: A Report of Two Cases. *Indian J. Otolaryngol. Head Neck Surg.* **2019**, *71* (Suppl 3), 1668–1671. [CrossRef]
20. Chi, T.H.; Yuan, C.H.; Chien, S.T. Lobular capillary hemangioma of the nasal cavity: A retrospective study of 15 cases in Taiwan. *Balk. Med. J.* **2014**, *31*, 69–71. [CrossRef]
21. Vrînceanu, D.; Dorobăț, B.C.; Sajin, M.; Mogoantă, C.A.; Oprişcan, I.C.; Hîncu, M.C.; Georgescu, M.G. Cystic lymphangioma of nasopharynx in a 54-year-old man—Case report. A new histogenetic hypothesis. *Rom. J. Morphol. Embryol.* **2018**, *59*, 577–584. [PubMed]
22. Lim, H.R.; Lee, D.H.; Lim, S.C. Clinical Difference Between Capillary and Cavernous Hemangiomas of Nasal Cavity. *J. Craniofacial Surg.* **2021**, *32*, 1042–1044. [CrossRef] [PubMed]
23. Fadda, G.L.; Petrelli, A.; Urbanelli, A.; Castelnuovo, P.; Bignami, M.; Crosetti, E.; Succo, G.; Cavallo, G. Risky anatomical variations of sphenoid sinus and surrounding structures in endoscopic sinus surgery. *Head Face Med.* **2022**, *18*, 29. [CrossRef] [PubMed]
24. Hasegawa, H.; Matsuzaki, H.; Furusaka, T.; Oshima, T.; Masuda, S.; Unno, T.; Abe, O. Maxillary sinus hemangioma: Usefulness of embolization according to classification. *Braz. J. Otorhinolaryngol.* **2017**, *83*, 490–493. [CrossRef]
25. Gregorio, L.L.; Wu, C.L.; Busaba, N.Y. Lobular capillary hemangioma formation: An unusual complication of submucous resection with power instrumentation of the inferior turbinate. *Laryngoscope* **2015**, *125*, 2653–2655. [CrossRef]
26. Smith, S.C.; Patel, R.M.; Lucas, D.R.; McHugh, J.B. Sinonasal lobular capillary hemangioma: A clinicopathologic study of 34 cases characterizing potential for local recurrence. *Head Neck Pathol.* **2013**, *7*, 129–134. [CrossRef]
27. Al-Ani, R.M.; Bargas, O.M. Demographic and clinical criteria of intranasal lobular capillary hemangioma: As retrospective multicentric audit. *Egypt. J. Otolaryngol.* **2022**, *38*, 113. [CrossRef]
28. Kunimoto, K.; Yamamoto, Y.; Jinnin, M. ISSVA Classification of Vascular Anomalies and Molecular Biology. *Int. J. Mol. Sci* **2022**, *23*, 2358. [CrossRef]
29. Merrow, A.C.; Gupta, A.; Patel, M.N.; Adams, D.M. 2014 Revised Classification of Vascular Lesions from the International Society for the Study of Vascular Anomalies: Radiologic-Pathologic Update. *Radiographics* **2016**, *36*, 1494–1516. [CrossRef]

Disclaimer/Publisher's Note: The statements, opinions and data contained in all publications are solely those of the individual author(s) and contributor(s) and not of MDPI and/or the editor(s). MDPI and/or the editor(s) disclaim responsibility for any injury to people or property resulting from any ideas, methods, instructions or products referred to in the content.

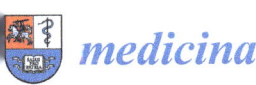

Review

Effect of Infraorbital and/or Infratrochlear Nerve Blocks on Postoperative Care in Patients with Septorhinoplasty: A Meta-Analysis

Do Hyun Kim [1,†], Jun-Beom Park [2,†], Sung Won Kim [1], Gulnaz Stybayeva [3] and Se Hwan Hwang [4,*]

1. Department of Otolaryngology-Head and Neck Surgery Seoul St. Mary's Hospital, College of Medicine, The Catholic University of Korea, Seoul 06591, Republic of Korea; dohyuni9292@naver.com (D.H.K.); kswcfs@ut.ac.kr (S.W.K.)
2. Department of Periodontics, College of Medicine, The Catholic University of Korea, Seoul 06591, Republic of Korea; jbassoon@catholic.ac.kr
3. Department of Physiology and Biomedical Engineering, Mayo Clinic, Rochester, MN 55905, USA; stybayeva.gulnaz@mayo.edu
4. Department of Otolaryngology-Head and Neck Surgery, Bucheon St. Mary's Hospital, College of Medicine, The Catholic University of Korea, Seoul 06591, Republic of Korea
* Correspondence: yellobird@catholic.ac.kr; Tel.: +82-32-340-7044; Fax: +82-32-340-2674
† These authors contributed equally to this work.

Abstract: *Background and Objectives*: Through a comprehensive meta-analysis of the pertinent literature, this study evaluated the utility and efficacy of perioperative infraorbital and/or infratrochlear nerve blocks in reducing postoperative pain and related morbidities in patients undergoing septorhinoplasty. *Materials and Methods*: We reviewed studies retrieved from the PubMed, SCOPUS, Embase, Web of Science, and Cochrane databases up to August 2023. The analysis included a selection of seven articles that compared a treatment group receiving perioperative infraorbital and/or infratrochlear nerve blocks with a control group that either received a placebo or no treatment. The evaluated outcomes covered parameters such as postoperative pain, the amount and frequency of analgesic medication administration, the incidence of postoperative nausea and vomiting, as well as the manifestation of emergence agitation. *Results*: The treatment group displayed a significant reduction in postoperative pain (mean difference = −1.7236 [−2.6825; −0.7646], I^2 = 98.8%), as well as a significant decrease in both the amount (standardized mean difference = −2.4629 [−3.8042; −1.1216], I^2 = 93.0%) and frequency (odds ratio = 0.3584 [0.1383; 0.9287], I^2 = 59.7%) of analgesic medication use compared to the control. The incidence of emergence agitation (odds ratio = 0.2040 [0.0907; 0.4590], I^2 = 0.0%) was notably lower in the treatment group. The incidence of postoperative nausea and vomiting (odds ratio = 0.5393 [0.1309; 2.2218], I^2 = 60.4%) showed a trend towards reduction, although it was not statistically significant. While no adverse effects reaching statistical significance were reported in the analyzed studies, hematoma (proportional rate = 0.2133 [0.0905; 0.4250], I^2 = 76.9%) and edema (proportional rate = 0.1935 [0.1048; 0.3296], I^2 = 57.2%) after blocks appeared at rates of approximately 20% *Conclusions*: Infraorbital and/or infratrochlear nerve blocks for septorhinoplasty effectively reduce postoperative pain and emergence agitation without notable adverse outcomes

Keywords: nerve block; nasal septum; rhinoplasty; pain; meta-analysis

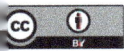

1. Introduction

Septorhinoplasty is a surgical procedure designed to improve the aesthetic features of the nasal region and correct any deformities. The postoperative phase can often involve significant discomfort, which arises from factors such as soft tissue trauma, irritation of periosteal tissues, and the effects of interventions on bones, including osteotomies [1,2]. Moreover, pain can be exacerbated by nasal packing after the surgery. Common postoperative complications include pain, edema, and periorbital ecchymosis [2,3]. There is a consensus that employing localized pain-management techniques postoperatively can lead to fewer complications and decreased overall costs [4]. The American Society of Anesthesiologists' guidelines for acute pain management during the perioperative stage recommend a multimodal analgesia approach, emphasizing the use of regional blockade techniques, where applicable [4]. While opioids are effective for managing postoperative pain, their use can lead to undesirable side effects such as sedation, respiratory depression, and episodes of nausea and vomiting [2,5]. Moreover, such potential adverse effects can hinder the patient's timely discharge from care [5]. This has led to an increasing emphasis on the application of peripheral nerve blocks during postoperative pain management. Some propositions even advocate for regional analgesia techniques to be the primary means of pain relief after plastic surgery [6]. Peripheral nerve blocks offer multiple advantages, such as reducing tissue edema, ensuring a more comprehensive range of anesthesia, and diminishing pain at the surgical site [7].

The infraorbital nerve, a branch of the maxillary division of the trigeminal nerve, plays a pivotal role in providing sensory innervation to the cutaneous areas around the nose and the nasal septum [7]. The infratrochlear nerve innervates the skin of the dorsum of the upper part and both sides of the nose. These two peripheral nerve blocks have been reported to facilitate pain management, reduce complications, and reduce anesthetic agent consumption after nasal procedures. Conducting a nerve block of this nerve has been shown to promote effective pain control, reduce complications, and decrease the requirement for anesthetic agents following nasal surgeries [8–14].

However, the effect of infraorbital and/or infratrochlear nerve blocks on the perinasal region remains a topic of debate [8,15]. We hypothesized that infraorbital and/or infratrochlear nerve blocks would be effective because septorhinoplasty is accompanied by significant postoperative pain. Therefore, we conducted a systematic review and meta-analysis to evaluate the influence of infraorbital and/or infratrochlear nerve blocks on postoperative care in patients undergoing septorhinoplasty.

2. Materials and Methods

This systematic review and meta-analysis was conducted in accordance with the guidelines set by the Preferred Reporting Items for Systematic Reviews and Meta-Analyses (PRISMA) [16]. The research protocol was proactively registered in the Open Science Framework (Charlottesville, VA, USA), accessible at the URL: https://osf.io/r3jve/ (accessed on 13 August 2023).

2.1. Search Strategy and Study Selection

The criteria, based on Population, Intervention, Comparison, Outcomes, and Study (PICOS), are as follows: (1) Population: patients who underwent septorhinoplasty; (2) Intervention: perioperative infraorbital and/or infratrochlear nerve blocks; (3) Comparison: either a placebo or no treatment; (4) Outcomes: grading of postoperative pain as reported by patients, quantity, and frequency of administered analgesic drugs, instances of postoperative nausea and vomiting and emergence agitation, and any events of adverse effects related to the infraorbital and/or infratrochlear nerve blocks; (5) Study design: not specified. Clinical studies up until August 2023 were sourced from PubMed, SCOPUS, Google Scholar, Embase, and the Cochrane Register of Controlled Trials. Key search terms employed included 'nerve block', 'rhinoplasty', 'septorhinoplasty', 'infraorbital nerve', 'infratrochlear nerve', 'pain', 'emergency agitation', 'nausea', and 'adverse effect.' Detailed search terms and queries are listed in Table S1. A librarian with more than a decade of experience facilitated the database searches, and the authors further examined references in the identified articles to ensure no omissions. Two independent reviewers (DHK and JP) meticulously assessed the titles and abstracts of potential studies, eliminating those considered irrelevant to perioperative infraorbital and/or infratrochlear nerve blocks. If abstracts did not provide enough information for a clear decision, the full texts of those studies were reviewed. Any disagreements between the two were settled by consulting a third reviewer (SHH).

To qualify for the review, studies had to meet specific criteria: they needed to involve patients undergoing septorhinoplasty and the application of an intraoperative infraorbital block. Studies focusing on additional procedures, such as sinus surgery, were excluded, ensuring the emphasis remained on septoplasty. Any research not offering clear, measurable data related to the outcomes of interest, or where extracting valuable information from the published results was impractical, was not considered. Figure 1 provides a visual representation of the search strategy used to pinpoint the studies included in this meta-analysis.

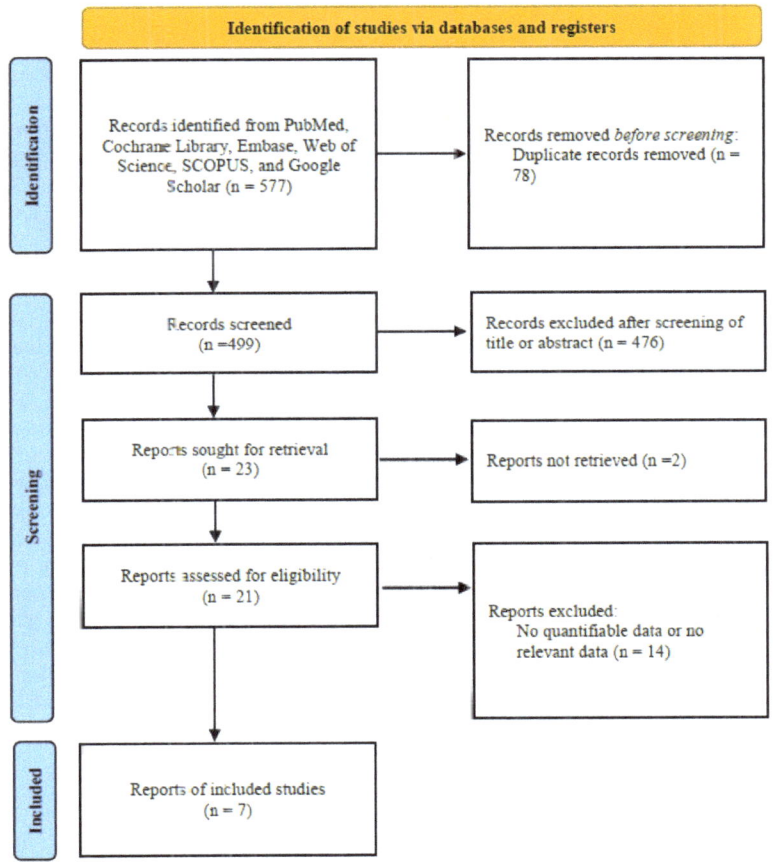

Figure 1. Diagram of study selection.

2.2. Data Extraction and Risk of Bias Assessment

Data from qualifying studies were extracted using standardized data collection forms [17–19]. The parameters assessed included the intensity of patient-reported postoperative pain, the amount and regularity of analgesic drug administration, the onset of postoperative nausea and vomiting, emergence agitation, and any reported adverse effects related to the infraorbital and/or infratrochlear nerve blocks. A comparison was made between the treatment group and the control group (those who received either no treatment or a saline injection) during the perioperative phase.

The data chosen for analysis encompassed patient demographics, pain intensity ratings given by patients, specifics regarding analgesic drug usage in terms of amount and regularity, rates of postoperative nausea and vomiting, events of emergence agitation, occurrences of side effects, and the stated *p*-values denoting the contrast between the treatment and control groups, as outlined in the chosen studies. This thorough data aggregation aimed to uncover the potential influence of the nerve block on postoperative complications and adverse effects.

2.3. Statistical Analyses

A statistical evaluation of the included studies was performed using the R-4.3.1 program developed by the R Software 4.3.1 Foundation based in Vienna, Austria. For quantitative variables, the meta-analysis was performed using either the standardized mean difference (SMD) or mean difference (MD). Employing SMD as a summary statistic allowed for the alignment of study outcomes onto a consistent scale, particularly when evaluations of similar outcomes were achieved using varied methods. This approach was chosen to gauge the quantity of administered analgesic medication, due to the lack of a universal scale across all studies. MD, indicating the average variance between the treatment and control groups, was calculated when the outcomes across studies were consistent and conveyed in similar units within the patient-reported pain grading scale. For metrics such as the regularity of analgesic medication administration, the incidence of postoperative nausea and vomiting, events of emergence agitation, and recorded side effects, the odds ratio (OR) was determined.

Heterogeneity was evaluated using the I^2 test, which describes the degree of variance across studies attributable to reasons beyond random chance, with values ranging from 0 (indicating no heterogeneity) to 100 (representing maximum heterogeneity). All reported findings were paired with a 95% confidence interval (CI), and *p*-values were cited for two-tailed tests. If significant heterogeneity in outcomes was detected, indicated by $I^2 > 50$, the random-effects model, following the DerSimonian–Laird method, was adopted. This model assumes different variances in true treatment effects among studies and anticipates a normal distribution of these. Where needed, subgroup analysis was also undertaken. Situations where heterogeneity was not significant, indicated by $I^2 < 50$, were examined using the fixed-effects model. This model, leveraging the inverse variance method, assumes a common source for all studies within the evaluated population.

To identify possible publication bias, both a funnel plot and Egger's test were utilized. The Duval and Tweedie's trim-and-fill method was also applied to adjust the combined effect size, accounting for any perceived publication bias. Moreover, sensitivity analyses were conducted to gauge the impact of individual studies on the overall meta-analysis results, which involved performing repeated meta-analyses, each time excluding one specific study.

3. Results

We evaluated a total of seven studies encompassing 414 participants. Detailed information about the individual studies is provided in Table 1, while the results of bias assessments can be found in Tables 2 and 3. Utilizing both Egger's test and Begg's funnel plot, specifically for assessing pain scores, we determined that there was no discernible publication bias among the incorporated studies ($p = 0.4912$). However, it is worth noting that an assessment of publication bias for other outcomes was not conducted due to the limited number of studies available, which made the creation of a funnel plot infeasible.

Table 1. Summary of studies included in the meta-analysis.

Study (Year)	Study Design	Number of Patients	Sex (Male/Female)	Age, Median (Range) or Mean (SD), y	Nation	Procedure	Medication	Anesthesia	Medication	Outcomes
Choi (2019) [8]	RCT	62	NA	21.97 ± 1.47	Korea	bilateral infraorbital and infratrochlear nerve blocks	0.5% ropivacaine	G/A	Isotonic saline	Postoperative pain score, used analgesic amount, frequency of used analgesic drug, incidence of postoperative nausea and vomiting, incidence of emergence agitation, incidence rate of edema and hematoma
Boselli (2016) [9]	RCT	36	13/23	38 ± 14	France	bilateral infraorbital and infratrochlear nerve blocks	10 mL of 0.25% levobupivacaine	G/A	Isotonic saline	Postoperative pain score, used analgesic amount, frequency of used analgesic drug, incidence of postoperative nausea and vomiting, incidence rate of edema and hematoma
Kacar (2020) [11]	RCT	52	24/28	27.38 ± 7.09	Turkey	bilateral infraorbital and infratrochlear nerve blocks	4 mL of 0.5% bupivacaine	G/A	G/A only	Postoperative pain score, used analgesic amount, frequency of used analgesic drug, incidence of emergence agitation
Elsayed (2020) [10]	Observational Study	40	26/14	26 (8)	Saudi Arabia	bilateral infraorbital and infratrochlear nerve blocks	5 mL of 0.25% levobupivacaine with 5 mL of diluted adrenaline 1:10,000	G/A	G/A only	Frequency of used analgesic drug
Yılmaz (2021) [12]	Observational Study	84	26/58	26.88 ± 5.45	Turkey	bilateral infraorbital and supraorbital nerve blocks	5 mg bupivacaine and 10 mg lidocaine for a total of 1.5 mL	G/A	G/A only	Postoperative pain score, used analgesic amount
Efe Atila (2022) [13]	Observational Study	60	27/33	30.5 ± 4	Turkey	bilateral infraorbital nerve blocks	15 mg bupivacaine hydrochloride to infraorbital foramen	G/A	G/A only	Postoperative pain score, frequency of used analgesic drug
Schumacher (2023) [14]	Observational Study	80	NA	27.6	USA	bilateral infraorbital nerve blocks	1.5 mL preoperative and postoperative bupivacaine	NA	NA	Incidence of postoperative nausea and vomiting

RCT, randomized controlled trials; G/A, general anesthesia; NA, not available.

Table 2. Quality of individual non-randomized controlled trial methodology.

Study	Selection [a]				Comparability [b]		Exposure [c]			Newcastle–Ottawa Scale Score
	1	2	3	4	5A	5B	6	7	8	
Elsayed (2020) [10]	Yes	No	Yes	Yes	No	No	Yes	Yes	Yes	6
Yılmaz (2021) [12]	Yes	No	No	Yes	Yes	Yes	Yes	Yes	Yes	7
Efe Atila (2022) [13]	Yes	No	Yes	Yes	No	No	Yes	Yes	Yes	6
Schumacher (2023) [14]	Yes	Yes	Yes	Yes	No	No	Yes	Yes	Yes	7

A star rating system was used to indicate the quality of a study, with a maximum rating of nine stars. A study could be awarded a maximum of one star for each numbered item within the selection and exposure categories. [a]: Selection (4 items): adequacy of case definition; representativeness of cases; selection of controls; and definition of controls. [b]: Comparability (1 item): comparability of cases and controls on the basis of design or analysis. [c]: Exposure (3 items): ascertainment of exposure; same method of ascertainment used for cases and controls; and non-response rate (same rate for both groups).

Table 3. Individual randomized controlled trial methodological quality.

Study	Random Sequence Generation	Allocation Concealment	Blinding of Participants and Personnel	Blinding of Outcome Assessment	Incomplete Outcome Data Addressed	Free of Selective Reporting	Risk of Bias of Randomized Studies
Choi (2019) [8]	Yes	Yes	Yes	Yes	Yes	Yes	Low
Boselli (2016) [9]	Yes	Yes	Yes	No	Yes	Yes	Low
Kacar (2020) [11]	Yes	Yes	Yes	No	Yes	Yes	High

3.1. Effect of Preoperative Infraorbital and/or Infratrochlear Nerve Blocks on Patient-Reported Pain Score and the Quantity and Frequency of Administered Analgesic Medication Compared to the Control Group

The postoperative pain score (MD = −1.7236 [−2.6825; −0.7646], I^2 = 98.8%), and quantity (SMD = −2.4629 [−3.8042; −1.1216], I^2 = 93.0%) and frequency (OR = 0.3584 [0.1383; 0.9287], I^2 = 59.7%) of administered analgesics, in the treatment group were markedly lower than the values in the control group, as shown in Figure 2. Notably, significant inter-study heterogeneity (I^2 > 50%) was observed in the mentioned outcomes.

The overall analysis did not differentiate based on who decided the quantity of analgesics administered (whether patient self-controlled or clinician-controlled), the interval after surgery when the pain score was assessed (within 2 h, 2–8 h, 8–24 h, or after 2 days), or the criteria for administering analgesics (a pain score > 3 or >7). This lack of differentiation likely contributed to the high heterogeneity (>50%) observed across all studies' results.

In a subgroup analysis that evaluated postoperative pain relative to the elapsed time, no significant variances were observed among the different time intervals (within 2 h: −1.5693 [−3.3455; 0.2068], I^2 = 98.9%; 2–8 h: 2.4546 [−5.0657; 0.1566], I^2 = 99.3%; 8–24 h: −1.6588 [−3.3991; 0.0815], I^2 = 98.6%; 2 days: −0.5000 [−0.8686; −0.1314], I^2 = NA) (p = 0.1895). These findings suggest that infraorbital and/or infratrochlear nerve blocks might maintain their efficacy up to 2 days postoperatively.

In a subgroup analysis that assessed the amount of analgesics administered based on the decision maker (patient vs. clinician), the quantity of analgesics self-administered by patients (−4.3254 [−5.1226; −3.5281], I^2 = NA) was significantly less than the amount decided by clinicians (−1.8263 [−2.6487; −1.0040], I^2 = 76.5%) (p < 0.0001). It is worth noting that postoperative pain intensity typically peaks within the first 24 h following surgery, with this pain often intensifying during the evening [13]. While only a single study utilized patient-controlled analgesics, the findings might indicate that nerve blocks can improve the patient's postoperative pain experience.

In a separate subgroup analysis that focused on the frequency of analgesic administration based on the criteria for administering them (either a pain score > 3 or >7), there were no significant differences between the two thresholds (pain score > 3: 0.4604 [0.1666; 1.2720], I^2 = 53.4%; >7: 0.2032 [0.0251; 1.6485], I^2 = 71.8%) (p = 0.4910). This suggests that nerve blocks might be equally effective for mitigating both moderate and severe postoperative pain.

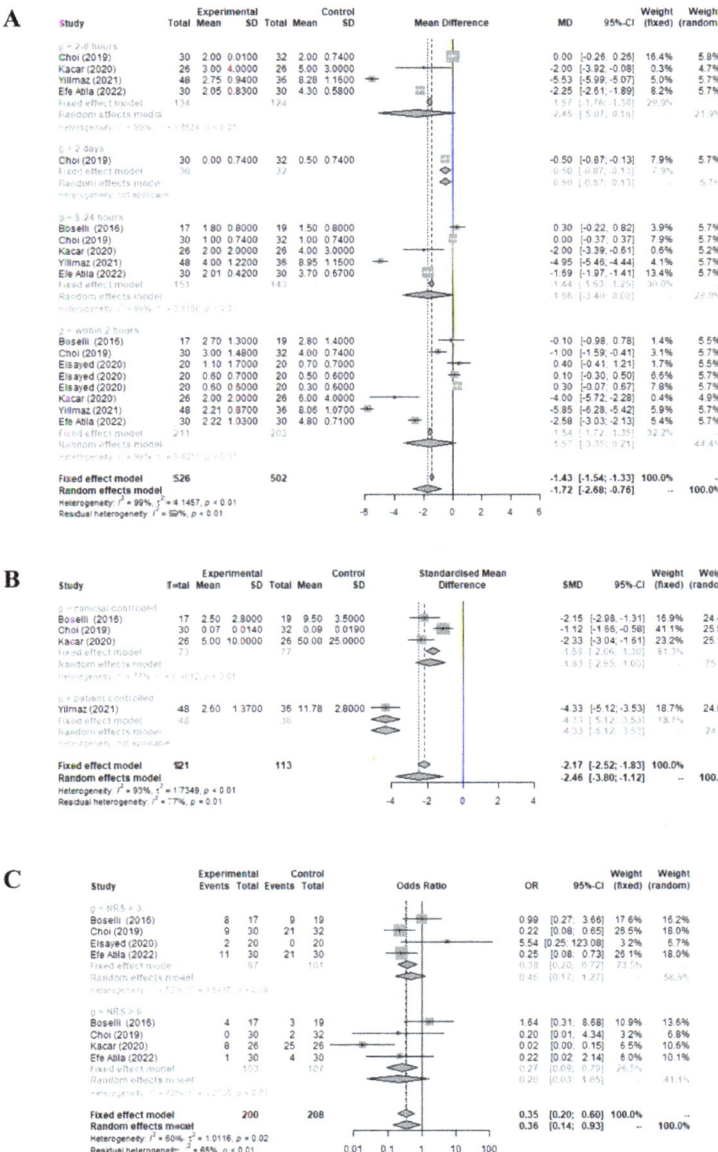

Figure 2. Comparison of preoperative infraorbital and/or infratrochlear nerve blocks versus placebo mean difference in postoperative pain score (**A**), standard mean difference in amount of analgesic used (**B**), and odds ratio for frequency of analgesic drug use (**C**) [8–13].

3.2. Effect of Preoperative Infraorbital and/or Infratrochlear Nerve Blocks on the Incidence of Postoperative Nausea and Vomiting, Emergence Agitation, and Occurrence of Side Effects Compared to the Control Group

The use of infraorbital and/or infratrochlear nerve blocks led to a significant reduction in the occurrence of emergence agitation (OR = 0.2040 [0.0907; 0.4590], I^2 = 0.0%) compared to the control group (Figure 3). Although the decrease in postoperative nausea and vomiting due to the infraorbital and/or infratrochlear nerve blocks did not achieve statistical significance, it is important to note a trend towards its reduction compared to the control group (OR = 0.5393 [0.1309; 2.2218], I^2 = 60.4%). Significant heterogeneity was evident among the analyzed studies ($I^2 > 50\%$) regarding the incidence of postoperative nausea and vomiting. This analysis did not differentiate the specific post-surgery time frames when assessing postoperative nausea and vomiting, such as during the immediate Post-Anesthesia Care Unit phase or within the 24 h that followed. This exclusion likely contributed to the notable heterogeneity (>50%) seen in the overall findings of the reviewed studies.

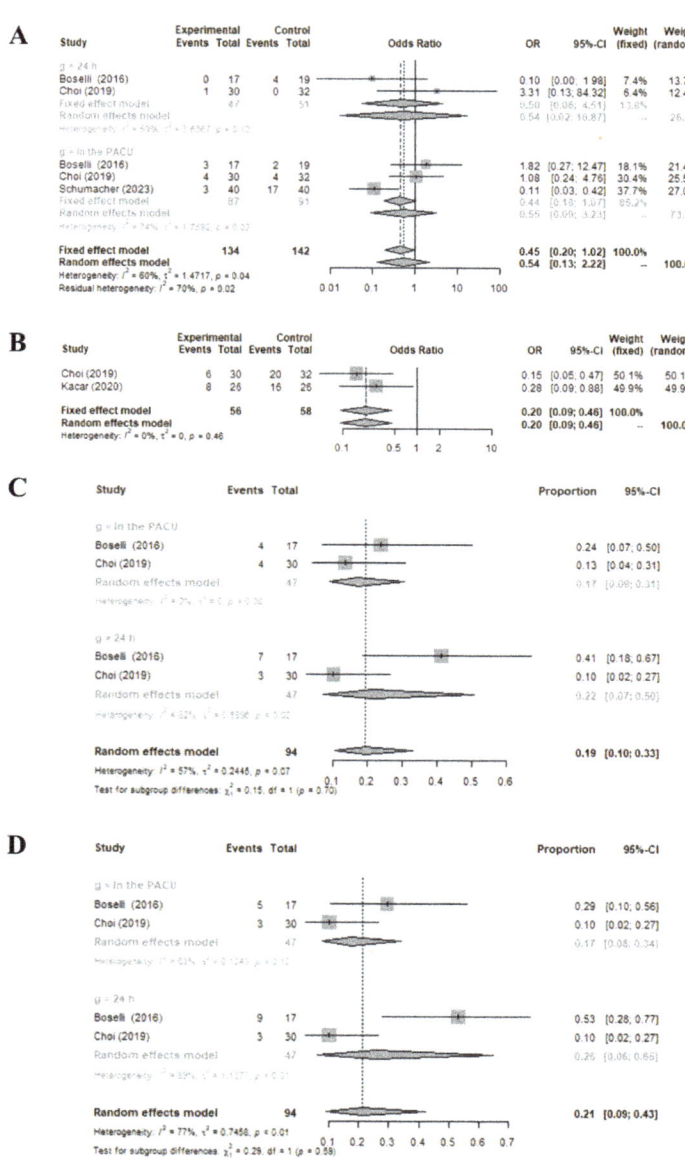

Figure 3. Comparison of preoperative infraorbital and/or infratrochlear nerve blocks versus placebo: odds ratio for incidence of postoperative nausea and vomiting (**A**) and emergence agitation (**B**), with incidence rates for edema (**C**) and hematoma (**D**) [8,9,11,14].

In a subgroup analysis that focused on the time of assessment (whether in the Post-Anesthesia Care Unit or within 24 h), no significant differences were identified (Post-Anesthesia Care Unit: 0.5397 [0.0173; 16.8663], $I^2 = 58.9\%$, 24 h: 0.5515 [0.0942; 3.2278], $I^2 = 73.9\%$) ($p = 0.9913$). This suggests that the beneficial effects of the infraorbital and/or infratrochlear nerve blocks in preventing postoperative complications persist up to 24 h after the operation.

Regarding side effects, no major adverse reactions, including neurological deficits, were highlighted in the studies included. However, incidences of hematoma (proportional rate = 0.2133 [0.0905; 0.4250], $I^2 = 76.9\%$) and edema (proportional rate = 0.1935 [0.1048; 0.3296], $I^2 = 57.2\%$) following nerve blocks were observed at a rate of ~20%

3.3. Sensitivity Analysis

An iterative sensitivity assessment was performed, wherein individual studies were consecutively excluded from the meta-analysis. No single study was found to significantly impact the overall trend.

4. Discussion

Our meta-analysis demonstrates that perioperative pain management utilizing infraorbital and/or infratrochlear nerve blocks effectively reduced postoperative pain and the usage of analgesic drugs. Moreover, there was a significant decline in the incidence of emergence agitation. Importantly, there were no notable adverse effects, including neurological deficits, reported.

Postoperative pain is characterized as acute inflammatory pain that originates with surgical trauma and typically resolves in tandem with tissue healing. When pain triggers a release of catecholamines, it can precipitate cardiovascular incidents, undesirable neuroendocrine or metabolic changes, thromboembolic events, pulmonary complications, and prolonged hospital stays [20]. It is crucial to efficiently address postoperative pain as it aids rapid mobilization, ensures adequate intake of fluids and nutrition, and accelerates the return to normal physical activities [21]. After surgical procedures, pain becomes a significant factor influencing patient well-being. Achieving comfort in the immediate postoperative stage plays a substantial role in enhancing patient contentment and overall satisfaction. Alongside conventional early analgesic approaches, the introduction of additional interventions that aim to reduce the need for analgesics and improve patient well-being is of utmost importance [22,23].

Emergence agitation is a postanesthetic phenomenon marked by psychomotor behaviors such as agitation, confusion, disorientation, and potential aggressive conduct that occurs during recovery from general anesthesia [24,25]. This state can pose significant challenges for patients, leading to complications such as injuries, bleeding, amplified pain sensations, accidental self-extubation, and the unintentional removal of catheters. Beyond the direct risks to patients, emergence agitation can also have negative ramifications for healthcare staff and may result in increased hospital costs [26]. Its occurrence has particularly been highlighted in relation to septorhinoplasty [8]. To counter this, adept pain management techniques have been proposed to reduce its incidence [8].

Nonetheless, achieving effective analgesic management remains a significant challenge. Postoperative pain affects a vast segment of the global population. The postoperative period inherently carries an increased likelihood of morbidity and mortality, with some cases potentially attributed to the use of analgesic agents [27–29]. Securing adequate analgesia through the use of regional nerve blocks, opioid analgesics, and nonsteroidal anti-inflammatory drugs has proven effective for both preventing and mitigating agitation, even for procedures traditionally considered to lack significant pain stimuli [30]. However, resorting to pharmacological preemptive measures can inadvertently lead to prolonged sedation and ensuing hemodynamic changes, which may include hypotension, hypertension, and bradycardia. These events can correlate with extended durations in the Post-Anesthesia Care Unit and a subsequent increase in overall hospital costs [8]. Furthermore, anesthetic variables play a crucial role in the onset of postoperative nausea and vomiting. These variables include the use of inhalational anesthetics, the length of anesthesia, the subsequent use of postoperative opioid analgesics, and the introduction of nitrous oxide [31]. A relationship between the administration of opioids during the postoperative period and an increased likelihood of postoperative nausea and vomiting has been suggested. This relationship appears to be dose-dependent [32].

Consequently, many patients often undergo treatment using a mix of non-opioid analgesic agents, a strategy known as multimodal analgesia [21]. The main goal of this approach is to achieve a synergistic or additive beneficial effect while reducing individual analgesic doses. This not only helps in preventing adverse effects but also reduces dependence on opioids and the associated range of opioid-related side effects [33,34]. Notable among the non-opioid drugs included in multimodal analgesic strategies are paracetamol, nonsteroidal anti-inflammatory drugs (NSAIDs), corticosteroids, ketamine, local anesthetics, and gabapentinoids [35]. Currently, various combinations of non-opioid analgesic drugs are employed in clinical settings [34]. In a forward-looking clinical study, a comparative evaluation assessed postoperative pain in patients undergoing specific otorhinolaryngologic surgeries with local anesthesia combined with sedation. Interestingly, the research revealed a significant difference, with patients who had septorhinoplasty experiencing significantly more pain compared to those who had septoplasty [36]. This observation aligns with another separate study where patients who had septoplasty showed little to no need for postoperative pain relief, maintaining effective pain management throughout the assessed postoperative phase [37]. Moreover, in the said study, patients who had undergone comprehensive nasal correction surgery displayed a steady improvement in pain scores, matching the levels seen in post-septoplasty patients just 6 days after the procedure. Taken together, these findings underscore the importance of a focused strategy to mitigate perioperative pain related to septorhinoplasty.

Peripheral nerve blocks involve the injection of a local anesthetic near the nerve that serves the surgical area. These anesthetics work by changing the sodium permeability of cell membranes, effectively halting nerve impulse transmission and leading to pain relief [38]. A distinctive feature of peripheral nerve blocks is their tendency to produce fewer side effects and complications, such as reduced swelling at the surgical site and lessened pain perception. When considering the sensory nerves relevant to septorhinoplasty surgery, the infraorbital and/or infratrochlear nerve blocks stand out in the facial region [39,40].

Our findings suggest that infraorbital and/or infratrochlear nerve blocks administered to patients undergoing septorhinoplasty provide effective pain control with minimal complications and reduce the reliance on perioperative opioids. Furthermore, the use of ultrasound guidance may increase the efficiency and safety of the procedure [41,42]. It is essential to highlight the significance of addressing agitation due to its potential detrimental effects on both the patient and the surgical site [43]. In addition, early post-surgical trauma can negatively influence the surgical results, which is particularly concerning in procedures such as rhinoplasty that involve modifications of intricate nasal bones. Consequently, adopting a cautious approach to minimize the risks posed by trauma induced by agitation is crucial, particularly for patients subjected to these surgeries [11]. While the precise efficiency of infraorbital and/or infratrochlear nerve blocks in countering agitation is still under investigation, previous studies, such as that by Choi et al. [8], indicate a strong link between pain and emergence agitation. Our observations echo this trend, with systemic magnesium administration being shown to reduce agitation during the recovery phase, which resonates with the known pharmacokinetics of magnesium. Moreover, the group that received nerve blocks experienced effective pain management throughout the postoperative phase.

Historically, efforts to alleviate emergence agitation have mainly centered on pharmacological solutions. Drugs such as ketamine, dexmedetomidine, and propofol have been found to be effective for managing emergence agitation in adults. However, it is worth noting that relying on pharmacological prevention can lead to prolonged sedation and hemodynamic changes, including hypotension, hypertension, and bradycardia. Such outcomes could result in extended durations in the Post-Anesthesia Care Unit, prompting considerations about cost-efficiency.

In the context of our research, we primarily concentrated on pain control using peripheral nerve blocks. As such, we champion the adoption of a multimodal pain management strategy, integrating systemic analgesics with peripheral nerve blocks, as the recommended method for septorhinoplasty when appropriate. Additionally, when performing septorhinoplasty, office-based local anesthesia can be facilitated by pain control caused by nerve blocks, and clinical data on this will also be needed.

However, this study is not without its limitations. Despite thorough subgroup analyses, fully addressing the heterogeneity regarding the effect of the perioperative nerve blocks on procedural morbidities was challenging. Several factors contribute to these challenges. First, the use of various local anesthetic agents in different studies, including levobupivacaine, ropivacaine, and bupivacaine, introduces variability. It is essential to note that the clinical characteristics of levobupivacaine and ropivacaine are similar to those of racemic bupivacaine, with differences mainly related to slight variation in anesthetic potency. Specifically, racemic bupivacaine displays higher potency compared to levobupivacaine and ropivacaine [44]. Second, we also included studies in which an infraorbital nerve block was performed but not an infratrochlear nerve block. This may contribute to the increased heterogeneity. It is critical to understand that the infraorbital nerve provides sensory innervation to the nasal skin and septum mobile nasi, whereas the infratrochlear nerve is responsible for the innervation of the nasal root [8]. In the future, additional clinical research will be needed on the effectiveness of individual nerve blocks for pain control after septorhinoplasty. The combined effect of varied anesthetic agents and the potential addition of an infratrochlear nerve block might be a primary source of the observed heterogeneity. Finally, another source of variability is the innate differences in peripheral nerve block techniques as executed by different clinicians. Each clinician's unique application approach can introduce variability, further adding to the heterogeneity noted in our findings.

5. Conclusions

This study underscores the efficacy of infraorbital and/or infratrochlear nerve blocks for septorhinoplasty in mitigating postoperative pain and emergence agitation. Furthermore, the application of this intervention did not present significant adverse outcomes, such as neurological deficits.

Supplementary Materials: The following supporting information can be downloaded at: https://www.mdpi.com/article/10.3390/medicina59091659/s1, Table S1. Search terms and queries.

Author Contributions: D.H.K., study conception and design, acquisition of data, analysis and interpretation of data, drafting the article and revisions, final approval of article; J.-B.P., study conception and design, analysis and interpretation of data, drafting the article and revisions, final approval of article; S.W.K., acquisition of data, analysis and interpretation of data, drafting the article and revisions, final approval of article; G.S., analysis and interpretation of data, drafting the article and revisions, final approval of article; S.H.H., study conception and design, acquisition of data, analysis and interpretation of data, drafting the article and revisions, final approval of article. All authors have read and agreed to the published version of the manuscript.

Funding: This work was supported by the National Research Foundation of Korea (NRF) grant funded by the Korea government (MSIT) (RS-2023-00209494, 2022R1F1A1066232), and the Korean Fund for Regenerative Medicine (KFRM) grant funded by the Korea government (23C0121L1). The sponsors had no role in the study design, data collection and analysis, decision to publish, or preparation of the manuscript.

Institutional Review Board Statement: An ethics statement is not applicable because this study is based exclusively on the published literature.

Informed Consent Statement: Informed consent was not required because this study is based exclusively on the published literature.

Data Availability Statement: The raw data of individual articles used in this meta-analysis are included in the main text or Supplementary Data.

Conflicts of Interest: The authors declare no conflict of interest.

References

1. Kim, D.H.; Kang, H.; Jin, H.J.; Hwang, S.H. Effect of piezoelectric osteotomy on postoperative oedema and ecchymosis after rhinoplasty. *Clin. Otolaryngol.* **2019**, *44*, 968–974. [CrossRef] [PubMed]
2. Wittekindt, D.; Wittekindt, C.; Schneider, G.; Meissner, W.; Guntinas-Lichius, O. Postoperative pain assessment after septorhinoplasty. *Eur. Arch. Otorhinolaryngol.* **2012**, *269*, 1613–1621. [CrossRef] [PubMed]
3. Gerbershagen, H.J.; Aduckathil, S.; van Wijck, A.J.; Peelen, L.M.; Kalkman, C.J.; Meissner, W. Pain intensity on the first day after surgery: A prospective cohort study comparing 179 surgical procedures. *Anesthesiology* **2013**, *118*, 934–944. [CrossRef] [PubMed]
4. Chou, R.; Gordon, D.B.; de Leon-Casasola, O.A.; Rosenberg, J.M.; Bickler, S.; Brennan, T.; Carter, T.; Cassidy, C.L.; Chittenden, E.H.; Degenhardt, E.; et al. Management of Postoperative Pain: A Clinical Practice Guideline from the American Pain Society, the American Society of Regional Anesthesia and Pain Medicine, and the American Society of Anesthesiologists' Committee on Regional Anesthesia, Executive Committee, and Administrative Council. *J. Pain* **2016**, *17*, 131–157.
5. Lam, D.M.H.; Choi, S.W.; Wong, S.S.C.; Irwin, M.G.; Cheung, C.W. Efficacy of Pregabalin in Acute Postoperative Pain Under Different Surgical Categories: A Meta-Analysis. *Medicine* **2015**, *94*, e1944. [CrossRef] [PubMed]
6. Joshi, G.P. Putting it all together: Recommendations for improving pain management in plastic surgical procedures. *Plast. Reconstr. Surg.* **2014**, *134*, 94s–100s. [CrossRef]
7. Cekic, B.; Geze, S.; Erturk, E.; Akdogan, A.; Eroglu, A. A comparison of levobupivacaine and levobupivacaine-tramadol combination in bilateral infraorbital nerve block for postoperative analgesia after nasal surgery. *Ann. Plast. Surg.* **2013**, *70*, 131–134. [CrossRef]
8. Choi, H.; Jung, S.H.; Hong, J.M.; Joo, Y.H.; Kim, Y.; Hong, S.H. Effects of Bilateral Infraorbital and Infratrochlear Nerve Block on Emergence Agitation after Septorhinoplasty: A Randomized Controlled Trial. *J. Clin. Med.* **2019**, *8*, 769. [CrossRef]
9. Boselli, E.; Bouvet, L.; Augris-Mathieu, C.; Bégou, G.; Diot-Junique, N.; Rahali, N.; Vertu-Ciolino, D.; Gérard, C.; Pivot, C.; Disant, F.; et al. Infraorbital and infratrochlear nerve blocks combined with general anaesthesia for outpatient rhinoseptoplasty: A prospective randomised, double-blind, placebo-controlled study. *Anaesth. Crit. Care Pain Med.* **2016**, *35*, 31–36. [CrossRef]
10. Elsayed, M.; Alosaimy, R.A.; Ali, N.Y.; Alshareef, M.A.; Althqafi, A.H.; Rajab, M.K.; Assalem, A.S.; Khiyami, A.J. Nerve Block for Septorhinoplasty: A Retrospective Observational Study of Postoperative Complications in 24 Hours. *Cureus* **2020**, *12*, e6961. [CrossRef]
11. Kaçar, C.K.; Uzundere, O.; Salık, F.; Akgündüz, M.; Bıçak, E.A.; Yektaş, A. Effects of Adding a Combined Infraorbital and Infratrochlear Nerve Block to General Anaesthesia in Septorhinoplasty. *J. Pain Res.* **2020**, *13*, 2599–2607. [CrossRef]
12. Yılmaz, R.; Arıcan, Ş.; Hacıbeyoğlu, G.; Tuncer Uzun, S. Effects of Bilateral Infraorbital-Supraorbital Nerve Block on Postoperative Pain Control and Drug Consumption in Rhinoplasty. *Eur. J. Ther.* **2021**, *27*, 235–240. [CrossRef]
13. Nihal, E.A.I. ATES Evaluation of Analgesic Effectivity of Infra Orbital Nerve Block in Open Septorhinoplasty Surgery: A Retrospective Study. *New Trend Med. Sci.* **2022**, *3*, 128–131.
14. Schumacher, J.K.; Cristel, R.T.; Talugula, S.; Shah, A.R. The Use of Adjunctive Perioperative Nerve Blocks in Rhinoplasty in the Immediate Postoperative Period. *Facial Plast. Surg. Aesthet. Med.* **2023**, *25*, 361–362. [CrossRef]
15. Wang, H.; Liu, G.; Fu, W.; Li, S.T. The effect of infraorbital nerve block on emergence agitation in children undergoing cleft lip surgery under general anesthesia with sevoflurane. *Paediatr. Anaesth.* **2015**, *25*, 906–910. [CrossRef] [PubMed]
16. Page, M.J.; McKenzie, J.E.; Bossuyt, P.M.; Boutron, I.; Hoffmann, T.C.; Mulrow, C.D.; Shamseer, L.; Tetzlaff, J.M.; Akl, E.A.; Brennan, S.E.; et al. The PRISMA 2020 statement: An updated guideline for reporting systematic reviews. *BMJ* **2021**, *372*, n71. [CrossRef]
17. Kim, D.H.; Kim, S.W.; Basurrah, M.A.; Hwang, S.H. Clinical and Laboratory Features of Various Criteria of Eosinophilic Chronic Rhinosinusitis: A Systematic Review and Meta-Analysis. *Clin. Exp. Otorhinolaryngol.* **2022**, *15*, 230–246. [CrossRef]
18. Hwang, S.H.; Kim, S.W.; Basurrah, M.A.; Kim, D.H. Efficacy of Steroid-Impregnated Spacers After Endoscopic Sinus Surgery in Chronic Rhinosinusitis: A Systematic Review and Meta-Analysis. *Clin. Exp. Otorhinolaryngol.* **2023**, *16*, 148–158. [CrossRef] [PubMed]
19. Kim, J.; Kim, D.H.; Hwang, S.H. Effectiveness of Dupilumab Treatment to Treat Chronic Rhinosinusitis with Nasal Polyposis: A Systematic Review and Meta-Analysis. *J. Rhinol.* **2023**, *30*, 62–68. [CrossRef]
20. Koputan, M.H.; Apan, A.; Oz, G.; Köse, E.A. The effects of tramadol and levobupivacaine infiltration on postoperative analgesia in functional endoscopic sinus surgery and septorhinoplasty. *Balkan Med. J.* **2012**, *29*, 391–394. [CrossRef] [PubMed]
21. Kehlet, H.; Dahl, J.B. Anaesthesia, surgery, and challenges in postoperative recovery. *Lancet* **2003**, *362*, 1921–1928. [CrossRef] [PubMed]
22. Vahabi, S.; Kazemi, A.H. Effects of clonidine as premedication on plasma renin activity, serum and urine electrolytes and body fluids in general anesthesia. A randomized double blind placebo controlled clinical trial. *Middle East J. Anaesthesiol.* **2011**, *21*, 71–76.

3. Vahabi, S.; Nadri, S.; Izadi, F. The effects of gabapentin on severity of post spinal anesthesia headache. *Pak. J. Pharm. Sci.* **2014**, *27*, 1203–1207. [PubMed]
4. Lepousé, C.; Lautner, C.A.; Liu, L.; Gomis, P.; Leon, A. Emergence delirium in adults in the post-anaesthesia care unit. *Br. J. Anaesth.* **2006**, *96*, 747–753. [CrossRef] [PubMed]
5. Vlajkovic, G.P.; Sindjelic, R.P. Emergence delirium in children: Many questions, few answers. *Anesth. Analg.* **2007**, *104*, 84–91. [CrossRef]
6. Hudek, K. Emergence delirium: A nursing perspective. *AORN J.* **2009**, *89*, 509–520. [CrossRef]
7. Aitkenhead, A.R. Injuries associated with anaesthesia. A global perspective. *Br. J. Anaesth.* **2005**, *95*, 95–109. [CrossRef]
8. Hansen, M.S.; Petersen, E.E.; Dahl, J.B.; Wetterslev, J. Post-operative serious adverse events in a mixed surgical population—A retrospective register study. *Acta Anaesthesiol. Scand.* **2016**, *60*, 1209–1221. [CrossRef]
9. Weiser, T.G.; Haynes, A.B.; Molina, G.; Lipsitz, S.R.; Esquivel, M.M.; Uribe-Leitz, T.; Fu, R.; Azad, T.; Chao, T.E.; Berry, W.R.; et al. Size and distribution of the global volume of surgery in 2012. *Bull. World Health Organ.* **2016**, *94*, 201–209f. [CrossRef]
10. Ibrahim, M.; Elnabtity, A.M.; Keera, A. Efficacy of external nasal nerve block following nasal surgery: A randomized, controlled trial. *Anaesthesist* **2018**, *67*, 188–197. [CrossRef]
11. Apfel, C.C.; Heidrich, F.M.; Jukar-Rao, S.; Jalota, L.; Hornuss, C.; Whelan, R.P.; Zhang, K.; Cakmakkaya, O.S. Evidence-based analysis of risk factors for postoperative nausea and vomiting. *Br. J. Anaesth.* **2012**, *109*, 742–753. [CrossRef] [PubMed]
12. Roberts, G.W.; Bekker, T.B.; Carlsen, H.H.; Moffatt, C.H.; Slattery, P.J.; McClure A.F. Postoperative nausea and vomiting are strongly influenced by postoperative opioid use in a dose-related manner. *Anesth. Analg.* **2005**, *101*, 1343–1348. [CrossRef] [PubMed]
13. Gritsenko, K.; Khelemsky, Y.; Kaye, A.D.; Vadivelu, N.; Urman, R.D. Multimodal therapy in perioperative analgesia. *Best Pract. Res. Clin. Anaesthesiol.* **2014**, *28*, 59–79. [CrossRef]
14. Ong, C.K.; Seymour, R.A.; Lirk, P.; Merry, A.F. Combining paracetamol (acetaminophen) with nonsteroidal antiinflammatory drugs: A qualitative systematic review of analgesic efficacy for acute postoperative pain. *Anesth. Analg.* **2010**, *110*, 1170–1179. [CrossRef] [PubMed]
15. Dahl, J.B.; Nielsen, R.V.; Wetterslev, J.; Nikolajsen, L.; Hamunen, K.; Kontinen, V.K.; Hansen, M.S.; Kjer, J.J.; Mathiesen, O. Post-operative analgesic effects of paracetamol, NSAIDs, glucocorticoids, gabapentinoids and their combinations: A topical review. *Acta Anaesthesiol. Scand.* **2014**, *58*, 1165–1181. [CrossRef] [PubMed]
16. Aydil, U.; Yilmaz, M.; Akyildiz, I.; Bayazit, Y.; Keseroglu, K.; Ceylan, A. Pain and safety in otorhinolaryngologic procedures under local anesthesia. *J. Otolaryngol. Head Neck Surg.* **2008**, *37*, 851–855. [PubMed]
17. Szychta, P.; Antoszewski, B. Assessment of early post-operative pain following septorhinoplasty. *J. Laryngol. Otol.* **2010**, *124*, 1194–1199. [CrossRef]
18. McCamant, K.L. Peripheral nerve blocks: Understanding the nurse's role. *J. Perianesth. Nurs.* **2006**, *21*, 16–26. [CrossRef]
19. Kanakaraj, M.; Shanmugasundaram, N.; Chandramohan, M.; Kannan, R.; Perumal, S.M.; Nagendran, J. Regional anesthesia in faciomaxillary and oral surgery. *J. Pharm. Bioallied Sci.* **2012**, *4*, S264–S269. [CrossRef]
20. Moskovitz, J.B.; Sabatino, F. Regional nerve blocks of the face. *Emerg. Med. Clin. N. Am.* **2013**, *31*, 517–527. [CrossRef]
21. Michalek, P.; Donaldson, W.; McAleavey, F.; Johnston, P.; Kiska, R. Ultrasound imaging of the infraorbital foramen and simulation of the ultrasound-guided infraorbital nerve block using a skull model. *Surg. Radiol. Anat.* **2013**, *35*, 319–322. [CrossRef] [PubMed]
22. Neagos, A.; Dumitru, M.; Vrinceanu, D.; Costache, A.; Marinescu, A.N.; Cergan, R. Ultrasonography used in the diagnosis of chronic rhinosinusitis: From experimental imaging to clinical practice. *Exp. Ther. Med.* **2021**, *21*, 611. [CrossRef] [PubMed]
23. Apan, A.; Aykac, E.; Kazkayasi, M.; Doganci, N.; Tahran, F.D. Magnesium sulphate infusion is not effective on discomfort or emergence phenomenon in paediatric adenoidectomy/tonsillectomy. *Int. J. Pediatr. Otorhinolaryngol.* **2010**, *74*, 1367–1371. [CrossRef] [PubMed]
24. Casati, A.; Putzu, M. Bupivacaine, levobupivacaine and ropivacaine: Are they clinically different? *Best Pract. Res. Clin. Anaesthesiol.* **2005**, *19*, 247–268. [CrossRef]

Disclaimer/Publisher's Note: The statements, opinions and data contained in all publications are solely those of the individual author(s) and contributor(s) and not of MDPI and/or the editor(s). MDPI and/or the editor(s) disclaim responsibility for any injury to people or property resulting from any ideas, methods, instructions or products referred to in the content.

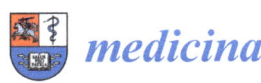 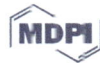

Systematic Review

Comparative Efficacy of Velopharyngeal Surgery Techniques for Obstructive Sleep Apnea: A Systematic Review

Ana Maria Vlad [1,2], Cristian Dragos Stefanescu [1,2,*], Iemima Stefan [2,3], Viorel Zainea [1,2] and Razvan Hainarosie [1,2]

[1] "Prof. Dr. Dorin Hociota" Institute of Phonoaudiology and Functional ENT Surgery, 21st Mihail Cioranu Street, 061344 Bucharest, Romania

[2] ENT Department, Faculty of Medicine, "Carol Davila" University of Medicine and Pharmacy, 030167 Bucharest, Romania

[3] Medical Center of Special Telecommunications Service, 060044 Bucharest, Romania

* Correspondence: dragos.stefanescu@umfcd.ro; Tel.: +40-730-047-455

Abstract: *Background*: In recent years, surgical interventions for obstructive sleep apnea (OSA) have evolved rapidly, with numerous techniques described in the literature. The approach to velopharyngeal surgery for obstructive sleep apnea has transformed over time, shifting from an aggressive removal of redundant excess soft tissue to less invasive reconstruction techniques that aim to preserve pharyngeal function while effectively managing sleep apnea. This review aims to evaluate and compare the efficacy of the surgical techniques utilized for OSA at the level of the palate and pharynx. It will cover both traditional and novel procedures. *Methods*: A comprehensive search of the major databases, such as PubMed/MEDLINE, Web of Science, and Scopus, was conducted to identify the relevant literature. We included articles written in English that analyzed the outcomes of adult patients who received velopharyngeal surgery for sleep apnea. Only comparative studies that examined at least two techniques were considered. *Results*: In all of the studies combined, the total number of patients who underwent velopharyngeal surgery was 614 in eight studies. All surgical procedures resulted in improvements in the apnea–hypopnea index (AHI). The highest success rates and best outcomes were achieved by barbed reposition pharyngoplasty (BRP) in most studies, ranging from 64.29% to 86.6%. BRP also demonstrated the most significant improvements in both objective and subjective parameters closely followed by ESP that obtained similar efficiency in some studies, especially when combined with anterior palatoplasty (AP), but with a higher incidence of complications. While LP showed moderate efficiency compared with BRP or ESP, the UPPP techniques exhibited greater outcome variability among studies, with a success rate ranging from 38.71% to 59.26%, and the best results observed in a multilevel context. *Conclusions*: In our review, BRP was the most preferred, effective, and safe among all velopharyngeal techniques, closely followed by ESP. However, older described techniques also showed good results in well-selected patients. Larger-scale studies, preferably prospective, that rigorously incorporate DISE-based strict inclusion criteria might be needed to assess the efficacy of different techniques and generalize the findings.

Keywords: obstructive sleep apnea; palatopharyngeal surgery; barbed reposition pharyngoplasty; expansion sphincter pharyngoplasty; uvulopalatopharyngoplasty

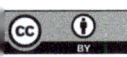

1. Introduction

It is estimated that worldwide, 936 million adults suffer from sleep apnea with important social and economic burdens secondary to the major complications it has on health [1].

Obstructive sleep apnea is characterized by recurrent upper airway collapse during sleep, leading to apnea/hypopnea with oxygen desaturation episodes. Various methods have been proposed for assessing upper airway (UA) obstruction. Drug-induced sleep endoscopy (DISE) is now widely regarded as the most effective approach for accurate localization of the collapse areas requiring targeted treatment planning [2]. Usually, multiple sites of obstruction are observed during DISE, with the most observed type of collapse at the palatal level [3]. CPAP remains the preferred initial treatment option with the strongest evidence of efficacy, as it can effectively open the upper airway at all levels. However, its limited compliance and acceptance rates make it necessary to explore alternative therapies [4].

For more than 40 years, since its first introduction in 1981 by Fujita et al. [5], UPPP remained one of the most common procedures performed for upper airway collapse, typically utilized as part of a multilevel approach due to inconsistent outcomes seen in single-level surgery [6]. The evaluation of a patient's suitability through several preoperative assessments to determine good patient selection might result in a more successful UPPP. However, despite careful patient selection and favorable outcomes in some cases, the procedure still carries a high risk of complications [7]. Anterior palatoplasty (AP) [8] and uvulopalatal flap (UPF) are other, similar procedures that address retropalatal obstruction, with favorable results in selected patients usually in mild to moderate sleep apnea [9].

With an increased understanding of palatopharyngeal anatomy, a move away from non-selective, resective procedures toward more refined and individualized treatment approaches has been adopted. Cahali et al. in 2004 were the first to show that addressing the lateral pharyngeal walls is necessary to achieve more positive surgical results [10]. Through his procedure, superior pharyngeal constrictor muscle is microdissected within the tonsillar fossa and cut, resulting in a laterally based flap of muscle that is attached to the palatoglossus muscle on the same side. However, dysphagia was an important issue, and a new technique was proposed a few years later. The expansion sphincter pharyngoplasty (ESP) technique isolates and rotates the palatopharyngeal muscle while leaving the superior pharyngeal constrictor muscle intact [11]. This determines the pulling of the muscle in a superoanterolateral direction with a less invasive approach. This proved to be an effective procedure, especially in patients with lateral wall collapse, determining fewer complications. In recent years, modified pharyngoplasties utilizing barbed sutures, also referred to as barbed pharyngoplasties (BPs), have been developed. The technique described by Vicini et al. in 2015 (barbed reposition pharyngoplasty) [12], involves repositioning the posterior pillar, specifically the palatopharyngeal muscle, to a more lateral and anterior location in order to increase the size of both the oropharyngeal inlet and the retropalatal space. Several studies reported excellent results with this technique, with minimal complications.

There has been a significant increase in the development of various procedures and modifications of surgical techniques to achieve the best possible results tailored to the individual characteristics of the upper airway. This systematic review aims to gather and explore all available evidence on the effectiveness and safety of different surgical techniques for treating obstructive sleep apnea in adults and provide insights into which technique may be the most effective and safe for patients. The analysis takes into account both objective parameters such as AHI and subjective parameters such as ESS. Success rates are reported for each technique, and trends in their usage are discussed.

2. Materials and Methods

2.1. General Study Design

This systematic review was carried out in compliance with The Preferred Items for Systematic Reviews and Meta-Analyses (PRISMA) guidelines [13].

2.2. Selection Criteria

The review was conducted using the PICOs protocol and encompassed studies that compared various techniques utilized in palatopharyngeal surgery, as follows:

(P): Population: Adult patients diagnosed with obstructive sleep apnea (OSA), undergoing palatopharyngeal surgery

(I): Intervention: Comparison of two or more surgical techniques used in palatopharyngeal surgery for OSA patients, such as, but not limited to, uvulopalatopharyngoplasty

(UPPP), barbed reposition pharyngoplasty (BRP), expansion sphincter pharyngoplasty (ESP), lateral pharyngoplasty (LP), or variations of these techniques.

(C): Comparison: Pre- and post-treatment outcomes of the different surgical techniques used.

(O): Outcome:

Primary outcomes: Assessment of treatment efficacy, including improvements in apnea–hypopnea index (AHI) and success rate,

Secondary outcomes Epworth Sleepiness Scale (ESS), complications.

(s): Study design: Both prospective and retrospective studies.

The exclusion criteria for the study were defined as follows:

1. Studies on the pediatric population.
2. Studies not in English.
3. Reviews, meta-analyses, editorial letters, technical notes.
4. Studies with insufficient or missing data.
5. Studies that did not analyze AHI.
6. Studies that did not compare at least two different palatopharyngeal surgical techniques or that compared variations of the same technique.
7. Studies that presented outcome variables (such as AHI) as an average rather than for each individual technique.

2.3. Search Strategy

Systematic electronic searches were performed by two different authors (A.M.V. and I.S) on PubMed/MEDLINE, Web of Science, and Scopus databases to identify relevant studies. The search strategies included different combinations of the following descriptors and/or medical subject headings (MeSH): ("palate surgery" OR "soft palate surgery" OR "uvula surgery" OR "Uvulopalatopharyngoplasty" OR UPPP) AND/OR "uvulopalatal flap" AND/OR ("lateral pharyngoplasty" OR "Cahali lateral pharyngoplasty") AND/OR ("Expansion sphincter pharyngoplasty" OR ESP) AND/OR ("Barbed reposition pharyngoplasty "OR barbed suture* OR BRP) AND ("sleep apnea" OR "obstructive sleep apnea" OR "OSA" OR "OSA surgery"). The search terms were adapted to the particular requirements of each database. Only studies that had been published within the last 5 years were considered for inclusion. The last search was conducted on 30 March 2023.

The search results obtained from each database were imported into the reference manager software Endnote, to manage and organize the articles. Duplicates were identified and subsequently removed.

2.4. Data Extraction

Initially, all articles underwent screening based on their titles and abstracts. Subsequently, the full-text versions of each publication were evaluated, and those considered unrelated to the scope of this review were excluded. The selected studies underwent independent evaluation by two investigators (A.M.V and I.S.), and necessary data were collected. The information extracted from the selected studies included: the name of the authors and the year of publication, study design, sample size, patients' profiles, surgical techniques compared, mean follow-up period, and objective or subjective outcomes (AHI, ESS). Any disagreement between the authors was discussed and resolved through consensus after consultation with the senior reviewer (C.D.S).

2.5. Statistical Analysis

Statistical analysis was conducted using the Jamovi software 2.3.26. The analysis was carried out using the mean difference as outcome measure to compare pre- and postoperative apnea–hypopnea index (AHI) and Epworth Sleepiness Scale (ESS) outcomes We adopted a random effects model to estimate effects measures by 95% confidence interval Forest plots for each outcome were provided. A total of 7 studies were included in the AHI analysis, and 6 studies were included in the ESS analysis. The Q-test and the I^2 statistic were calculated to assess the presence of data heterogeneity between studies. To compare the surgical techniques (UPP, ESP, and BRP), subgroup comparisons were performed. Binary variables were created to represent the utilization or non-utilization of each technique in the studies compared. For example, in the BRP vs. UPP comparison, a binary variable was assigned a value of 1 for sub-studies that performed the BRP technique and 0 for UPP studies. Similar binary variables were constructed for the other comparisons. These binary variables served as moderators in the analysis, enabling a direct comparison between the techniques while considering the specific technique employed in each study.

3. Results

3.1. Study Selection

The authors identified a total of 143 potentially suitable studies through the search strategy presented in the Methodology section. The studies' selection steps are summarized in Figure 1. After eliminating the duplicates through the Endnote reference manager, a total of 70 articles were analyzed regarding the title and abstract, applying the selection criteria to find the most appropriate studies for the review. All reviews, meta-analyses, editorial letters, and all studies that did not compare at least two surgical techniques were excluded, resulting in 23 full-text papers examined for eligibility. After removing the studies with incomplete or inappropriate information, eight studies were considered qualified for data extraction.

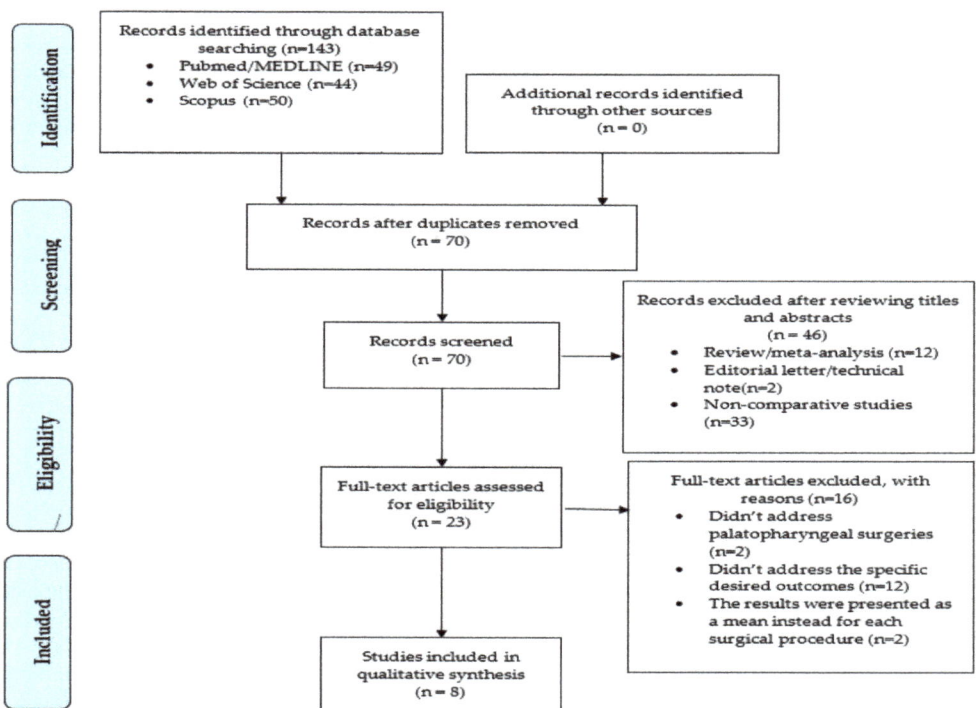

Figure 1. PRISMA flow diagram.

3.2. Study Characteristics and Patient Profiles

Table 1 provides a synthesis of the main features of the studies included (Table 1). The majority of included studies were retrospective [14–19], while two of them were prospective [20,21]. The sample size of each study exhibited variability, with the number of subjects ranging from 20 [14] to 122 [18]. The total count of patients who underwent velopharyngeal surgery across all studies was 614, for which uvulopalatopharyngoplasty (UPP) and variations in the technique (m-UPP, RF-UPP) were described and performed in four studies (209 patients), anterior palatoplasty (AP) in two studies (52 patients), uvulopalatoflap placement in one study (23 patients), and lateral pharyngoplasty (LP/CLP) in two studies (41 patients). BRP and ESP were performed in five (166 patients) and four studies, respectively.

Table 1. Main characteristics of the included studies.

Author (Year)	Study Design	Patient Number	Mono-/Multilevel	Follow-up	Mean Age	Sex (M:F)	BMI	Snoring/OSA	DISE
Lorusso et al., 2022 [14] Italy	Retrospective study	MESP = 10 MBRP = 10	Monolevel	12 months	48.4 ± 4.8 41.6 ± 11.77	20M:0F	28.4 ± 3.06 28.7 ± 3.02	Mild to moderate OSA	Yes
Lombo et al., 2022 [15] Portugal	Retrospective study	UPP=36 RF-UPP=31 BRP=25	Monolevel	12 months	49.36 ± 9.6	85M:7F	29.14 ± 2.94	OSA + snorers	Yes
Tsou et al., 2021 [16] China	Retrospective study	UPPP = 31 BRP = 31	Multilevel + TORSBTR	6 months	39.61 ± 11.63 37.51 ± 9.42	24M:7F 26M:5F	28.20 ± 3.62 28.22 ± 3.19	Moderate to severe OSA	Yes
Martinez et al., 2020 [17] Spain	Retrospective study	UPP = 31 LP = 11 ESP = 17 BRP = 23	Monolevel	4 months	42.0 ± 19.78	70M:12F	27.63 ± 3.7	Moderate to severe OSA	Yes
A. Minni et al., 2021 [18] Italy	Retrospective study	UPPP = 80 BRP = 42	Mono/ multilevel (±HS)	18 months	43 (37–47) 42 (38–47)	51M:29F 20M:22F	25 (24–26) 27 (25–28)	Moderate to severe OSA	No
Babademez et al., 2020 [19] Turkey	Retrospective study	BRP= 45 ESPwAP = 53	Monolevel	18.8 months (median)	37.3 ± 8.9 41.6 ± 9.4	31M:14F 41M:12F	29.3 ± 3.1 28.8 ± 4.2	Mild to severe OSA	Yes
Karakok et al., 2018 [20] Turkey	Prospective study	AP = 30 LP = 30 ESP = 33	Monolevel	5.90 ± 6.23 months	40.7 ± 9.59	27M:3F 30M:0F 32M:1F	27.67 ± 2.96	OSA + snorers	No
Haytogiu et al., 2018 [21] Turkey	Prospective study	AP = 22 UFP = 23	Monolevel	6 months	39.2 41.3	12M:10F 14M:9F	28.0 ± 1.6 27.3 ± 1.8	Mild to moderate OSA	No

UPP—classical uvulopalatoplasty, UPPP—modified uvulopalatoplasty, LP—lateral pharyngoplasty, ESP—expansion sphincter pharyngoplasty, MESP—modified ESP, BRP—barbed reposition pharyngoplasty, MBRP—modified BRP, AP—anterior palatoplasty, UFP—uvulopalatal flap placement, HS—hyoid suspension, TORSBTR—transoral robotic base of tongue reduction, BMI—body mass index, DISE—Drug Induced Sleep Endoscopy.

3.3. Outcomes

Table 2 provides a summary of the outcomes from all the studies that were reviewed.

Table 2. Included studies outcomes.

Author (Year)	Surgical Techniques	Pre-op AHI	Post-op AHI	Pre-op ESS	Post-op ESS	Success Criteria	Success Rate
Lorusso et al., 2022 [14] Italy	MESP vs. MBRP	23.9 ± 6.62 vs. 22.03 ± 5.05	11 ± 3.3 a vs. 12.47 ± 5.03 a	10.4 ± 3.1 vs. 9.1 ± 2.07	5.1 ± 3.17 a vs. 4.5 ± 2.5 a	Sher criteria AHI reduction > 50 and AHI value < 20	90% vs. 80%
Lombo et al., 2022 [15] Portugal	UPP (classical) vs. RF-UPP vs. BRP	29.88 ± 19.40 vs. 23.19 ± 10.34 vs. 23.53 ± 9.68	23.78 ± 18.46 a vs. 20.43 ± 14.88 a vs. 14.06 ± 10.23 a	nd	nd	Sher criteria AHI reduction > 50 and AHI value < 20	57% vs. 54% vs. 66%

Table 2. Cont.

Author (Year)	Surgical Techniques	Pre-op AHI	Post-op AHI	Pre-op ESS	Post-op ESS	Success Criteria	Success Rate
Tsou et al., 2021 [16] Chins	UPPP (modified) vs. BRP	45.13 ± 19.31 vs. 46.21 ± 22.03	28.75 ± 23.09 a vs. 21.60 ± 21.54 a	11.01 ± 4.52 vs. 9.03 ± 4.52	7.82 ± 3.45 a vs. 6.60 ± 3.82 a	Sher criteria AHI reduction > 50 and AHI value < 20	38.71% vs. 67.74%
Martinez et al., 2020 [17] Spain	UPP (classical) vs. LP vs. ESP vs. BRP	48.91 ± 22.32 vs. 46.3 ± 34.02 vs. 28.29 ± 13.32 vs. 43.74 ± 27.17	20.55 ± 22.9 a vs. 17.84 ± 13 a vs. 13.19 ± 16.8 a vs. 8.79 ± 10.85 a	9.6 ± 4.95 vs. 9.78 ± 4.21 vs. 7.12 ± 5.43 vs. 8.33 ± 4.7	6.89 ± 4.1 a vs. 6.4 ± 3.2 vs. 4.54 ± 3.33 vs. 5.19 ± 3.3 a	Sher criteria AHI reduction > 50 and AHI value < 20	58.06% vs. 54.55% vs. 64.71% vs. 78.26%
Minni et al., 2021 [18] Italy	UPPP (modified) vs. UPPP + HS vs. BRP vs. BRP + HS	27 (24–29) vs. 27 (24–29) vs. 29 (28–31) vs. 28 (26–30)	16 (14–17) a vs. 11 (10–11) a vs. 10 (9–11) a vs. 10 (9–11) a	12 (12–13) vs. 13 (12–13) vs. 13 (12–13) vs. 13 (12–13)	12 (11–12) vs. 11 (11–12) vs. 10 (10–11) vs. 11 (10–12)	AHI < 20, ESS < 10, both reduced > 50%	nd
Babademez et al., 2020 [19] Turkey	BP vs. ESPwAP	25.9 ± 13.6 vs. 28.5 ± 16.8	7.4 ± 5.5 a vs. 9.1 ± 6.9 a	11.2 ± 3.7 vs. 12.6 ± 4.9	3.4 ± 1.5 a vs. 4.1 ± 1.8 a	Sher criteria AHI reduction > 50 and AHI value < 20	86.6% vs. 84.9%
Karakok et al., 2018 [20] Turkey	AP vs. LP vs. ESP	16.90 ± 10.26 vs. 17.69 ± 12.47 vs. 26.83 ± 21.68	14.27 ± 15.43 vs. 12.05 ± 15.23 a vs. 9.08 ± 10.35 a	9.35 ± 4.67 vs. 13.21 ± 4.89 vs. 11.06 ± 5.21	6.80 ± 4.59 vs. 8.28 ± 4.84 a vs. 4.25 ± 3.19 a	Modified Sher criteria AHI reduction > 50 and AHI value < 15	45% vs. 64% vs. 74%
Haytogiu et al., 2018 Turkey [21]	AP vs. UFP	17.5 ± 8.2 vs. 18.5 ± 7.9	8.1 ± 7.3 a vs. 8.6 ± 6.9 a	13.6 ± 3.3 vs. 10.8 ± 3.3	6.4 ± 3.3 a vs. 5.4 ± 4.8 a	Sher criteria AHI reduction > 50 and AHI value < 20	81.8% vs. 82.6%

UPP—classical uvulopalatoplasty, UPPP—modified uvulopalatoplasty, LP—lateral pharyngoplasty, ESP—expansion sphincter pharyngoplasty, MESP- modified ESP, BRP—barbed reposition pharyngoplasty, MBRP—modified BRP, AP—anterior palatoplasty, UFP—uvulopalatal flap placement, HS—hyoid suspension, a—of statistical significance as reported by authors, nd—not determined, AHI—apnea–hypopnea index, ESS—Epworth sleep scale.

3.3.1. AHI Outcomes

All studies provided pre- and post-operative data regarding AHI. However, just seven studies were taken into account for meta-analysis since one of the studies expressed the results as median and quartile intervals instead of mean and standard deviation. The analysis was carried out using the standardized mean difference of AHI as the outcome measure.

A comprehensive database was created by subdividing each study based on the techniques and the corresponding outcomes. The random-effects model was fitted to the data, incorporating 18 sub-studies in the analysis. The observed standardized mean differences ranged from 0.1981 to 2.3633, with most estimates being positive (100%). The estimated average standardized mean difference based on the random-effects model was 1.0416 (95% CI: 0.7825 to 1.3007). Therefore, the average outcome differed significantly from zero ($z = 7.8794$, $p < 0.0001$), indicating a meaningful effect of the velopharyngeal techniques on the AHI.

According to the Q-test, the true outcomes appeared to be heterogeneous ($Q(17) = 61.9697$, $p < 0.0001$, $tau^2 = 0.2152$, $I^2 = 71.5731\%$). However, despite this heterogeneity, the studies generally supported the estimated average outcome. An examination of the studentized residuals revealed that none of the studies had a value larger than ±2.9913, and hence, there was no indication of outliers in the context of this model. Additionally, none of the studies could be considered to be overly influential.

A forest plot was generated to visually display the mean differences between the velopharyngeal techniques in the included studies. The forest plot provides a clear overview of the effect sizes and their confidence intervals for each technique, allowing for easy comparison and interpretation (Figure 2).

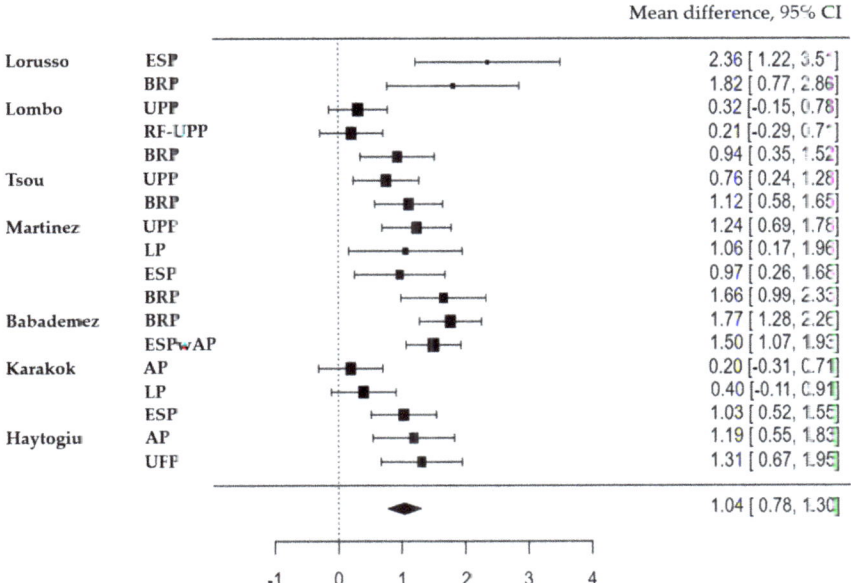

Figure 2. Forest plot AHI-Comprison between pre- and postoperative results.

3.3.2. Subgroup Analysis

In the subgroup analysis, a random-effects model was applied to the UPP, BRP, and ESP techniques (Figure 3). These techniques were selected because they had sufficient studies available for analysis. However, it was not possible to perform a subgroup analysis for the other techniques due to limited data availability. Only one or two studies were available for those techniques, which did not provide enough data to conduct a meaningful comparison. Nevertheless, the results and trends of the other techniques were described and discussed based on the available studies.

Uvulopalatoplasty

The uvulopalatopharyngoplasty (UPPP) procedure was examined in four studies, and all studies showed a statistically significant reduction in the apnea–hypopnea index (AHI). In two studies [15–17], the performed technique was the classical one, described by Fujita et al. [5], and in the other two [16–18], the modified version according to Fairbanks et al. was used [22]. The analysis using the random-effects model for the UPP approach showed a mean difference of 1.24 (95% CI: 0.1694 to 1.0714) with an overall effect Z score = 2.6962 ($p = 0.0070$). Based on the Q-test results (Q(3) = 9.3795, $p = 0.0246$), it appeared that the outcomes observed in the studies were not consistently similar. The I^2 value of 63.67% indicated a moderate level of heterogeneity.

Subgroup/Study	Pre-op AHI			Post-op AHI			
UPP	Mean	SD	Total	Mean	SD	Total	Mean difference
Lombo et al. UPP	29.88	23.78	36	23.78	18.46	36	0.32 [−0.15, 0.76]
Lombo et. al. RF-UPP	23.19	10.34	31	20.43	14.88	31	0.21 [−0.29, 0.71]
Tsou et al.	45.13	19.31	31	28.75	23.09	31	0.76 [0.24, 1.28]
Martinez et al.	48.91	22.32	31	20.55	22.90	31	1.24 [0.69, 1.78]
Subtotal (CI 95%)			129			129	
Overall effect: Z=2.70 (p=0.0007)							
Heterogeneity: Q (3) =9.37 (P=0.025), I²=68.68%							

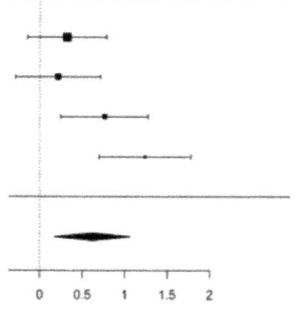

BRP	Mean	SD	Total	Mean	SD	Total	Mean difference
Lorusso et al.	22.03	5.05	10	12.47	5.03	10	1.82 [0.77, 2.86]
Lombo et al.	23.53	9.68	25	14.06	10.23	25	0.94 [0.35, 1.52]
Tsou et al.	46.21	22.03	31	21.60	21.54	31	1.12 [0.58, 1.65]
Martinez et al.	43.74	27.17	23	8.79	10.85	23	1.66 [0.99, 2.33]
Babademez et al.	25.90	13.60	45	7.40	5.50	45	1.77 [1.28, 2.26]
Subtotal (CI 95%)			134			134	1.44 [1.05, 1.79]
Overall effect: Z= 7.50 (p<0.001)							
Heterogeneity: Q (3) = 6.89 (p= 0.142), I²=43.42%							

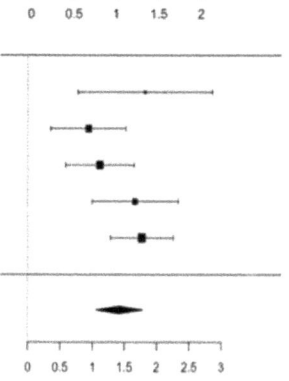

ESP	Mean	SD	Total	Mean	SD	Total	Mean difference
Lorusso et al.	23.90	6.61	10	11.00	3.31	10	2.36 [1.22, 3.51]
Martinez et al.	28.29	13.32	17	13.19	16.80	17	0.97 [0.26, 1.68]
Babademez et al.	28.50	16.80	53	9.10	6.90	53	1.50 [1.07, 1.93]
Karakok et al.	26.83	21.68	33	9.08	10.35	33	1.03 [0.52, 1.55]
Subtotal (CI 95%)			113			113	1.33 [0.93, 1.73]
Overall effect: Z= 6.46 (p<0.001)							
Heterogeneity: Q (3) =5.99 (p=0.112), I²=40.3%							

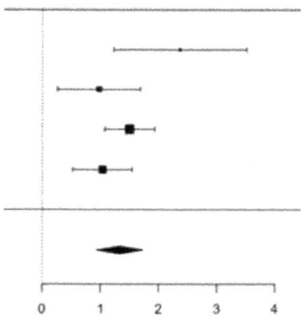

Figure 3. Subgroup analyses of AHI outcomes using random-effects model.

Barbed Reposition Pharyngoplasty

In all six studies in which it was evaluated, the BRP technique obtained a statistically significant improvement in AHI. The analysis of five studies suggested that the BRP procedure led to a significant improvement in AHI based on the average difference observed across the included studies (z-value = 7.4986, $p < 0.0001$). The 95% confidence interval (CI) for this estimate ranged from 1.0466 to 1.7874, suggesting a high level of confidence in the results The analysis did not find significant variation in the true outcomes, as indicated by the Q-test (Q(4) = 6.8923, $p = 0.1417$, $I^2 = 43.4237\%$). This suggests that, overall, the studies showed similar results in terms of the effect of BRP on AHI improvement.

Expansion Sphincter Pharyngoplasty

ESP was addressed in four studies, with a statistically significant improvement of AHI in all of them. The estimated average standardized mean difference based on the random-effects model was 1.3308 (95% CI: 0.9272 to 1.7344), indicating a significant difference from zero ($z = 6.4625$, $p < 0.0001$). Regarding heterogeneity, the Q-test showed no significant amount of heterogeneity in the true outcomes ($Q(3) = 5.9937$, $p = 0.1119$, $I^2 = 40.3042\%$). This suggests that the true outcomes across the studies were generally consistent with the estimated average outcome, although some heterogeneity may have existed.

Comparisons between UPP, ESP, and BRP

Using moderator variables allowed us to assess whether the effect sizes (mean differences) varied depending on the technique used. When comparing the UPP and BRP techniques, the mixed-effects model analysis showed a significant difference in the mean AHI reduction (coefficient = 0.802, se = 0.295, $Z = 2.723$, $p = 0.006$, 95% CI: 0.225 to 1.380). Specifically, the BRP technique, used as moderator, was associated with a larger mean difference in AHI compared to the UPP technique. Similar results were observed for the ESP technique, which was associated with a larger mean difference in the outcome compared to the UPP technique (coefficient = 0.726, se = 0.324, $Z = 2.241$, $p = 0.025$, 95% CI: 0.091 to 1.362).

The positive coefficients suggested that the BRP and ESP techniques may be more effective in achieving the desired outcome compared to UPP. However, the use of BRP as a moderator did not significantly affect the AHI outcome when compared to ESP (coefficient = 0.216, se = 0.288, $Z = 0.752$, $p = 0.452$, 95% CI: −0.347 to 0.780). This suggests that there was no significant difference between the BRP and ESP techniques in terms of their impact on reducing AHI using the data from the studies.

The Other Techniques

Two studies evaluated lateral pharyngoplasty (LP) in comparison to other palatopharyngeal techniques [17,20]. Both studies reported a significant reduction in AHI (17.84 ± 13 from 46.3 ± 34.02 and 12.05 ± 15.23 from 17.69 ± 12.47). Anterior palatoplasty (AP) was described in two studies. The decrease in AHI value was statistically significant only in the Haytagiu et al. study (8.1 ± 7.3a from 17.5 ± 8.2) compared to in the Karakok et al. study (14.27 ± 15.43 from 16.90 ± 10.26). The UFP technique, mentioned in one study, was responsible for a great reduction in AHI (18.5 ± 7 9 to 8.6 ± 6.9).

3.3.3. ESS Outcomes

The subjective outcomes for the techniques were measured in seven of eight studies using the Epworth Sleepiness Scale (ESS). Six studies had the necessary data to analyze the results. The estimated average standardized mean difference based on the random-effects model was 1.2631, with a 95% CI= 0.8877–1.6385 and a z-value= 6.5943 (p-value < 0.0001). This implies that surgery had a significant positive effect on the ESS subjective parameters. According to the Q-test, the true outcomes appeared to be heterogeneous ($Q(14) = 83.3390$, $p < 0.0001$, $tau^2 = 0.4385$, $I^2 = 82.2159\%$). Hence, although the average outcome was estimated to be positive, in some studies the true outcome may in fact have been negative. A forest plot was generated to visually display the mean differences in ESS between the velopharyngeal techniques in the included studies (Figure 4).

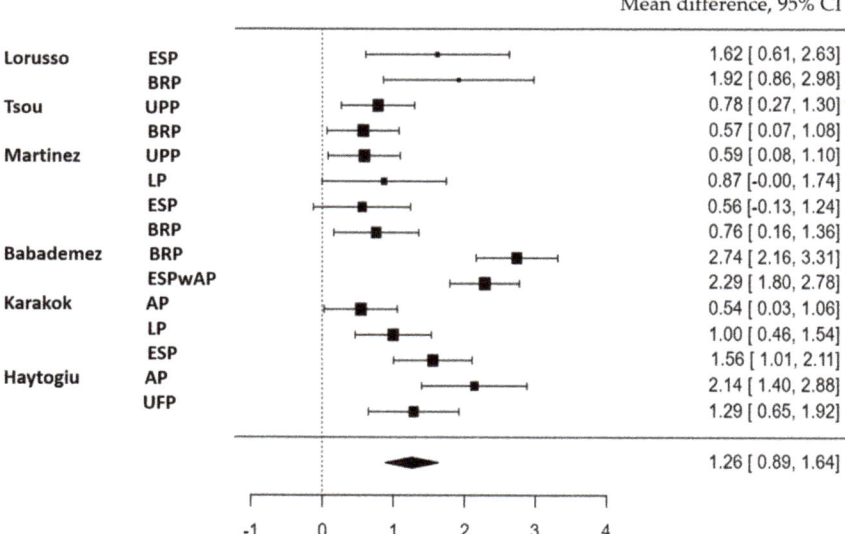

Figure 4. Forest plot ESS—Comparison between pre- and postoperative results.

3.3.4. Success Rate

The success rate was determined in seven studies. The majority of studies used the Sher criteria of success rate (AHI reduction > 50 and AHI value < 20). For the BRP technique, the surgical success rate ranged between 66% and 86.6%, with the best outcomes in the majority of studies. However, it achieved similar outcomes compared with the modified ESP described by Lorusso et al. (80% vs. 90%) [14] and with ESPwAP analyzed by Babademez et al. (86.6% vs. 84.9%) [19]. The success rate of the ESP technique ranged from 64.81% to 90%. For the UPP technique, the surgical success rate was found to vary significantly among the studies, with the lowest success rate of 38.71% and the highest of 58.06%. Regarding AP, results differed considerably between studies, with Haytogiu et al. [21] reporting a success rate of 81.8%, and Karakok et al. [20] reporting a success rate of only 45%. LP obtained a success rate of 54.55% [17] and 64% [20], respectively. Being described in just one study [21] in comparison to AP, uvulopalatoflap placement obtained a favorable outcome with an overall procedural success rate of 82.6%.

3.4. Factors That Might Influence the Results

Having only the mean age available and not individual participant BMI limited our ability to conduct a moderation analysis using age as a separate predictor. The same was available for the BMI variable. However, we performed a mixed-effects model analysis using severity of disease as a moderator, categorizing it into two levels: mild to moderate (coded as 1) and moderate to severe (coded as 2). The intercept estimate was 1.810, while the moderator estimate was −0.349, suggesting a negative association between the severity of the disease (specifically moderate to severe) and the outcome variable (AHI mean difference). Nevertheless, this association was not statistically significant ($p = 0.142$).

3.5. Complications

Complications were addressed in seven studies. Table 3 provides a summary of the number of patients who experienced complications in each study, along with their corresponding citations. Lorusso et al. [14] described a persistent feeling of a foreign body in the throat, both in MESP and MBRP, that disappeared after a few months, and suggested the pain was more prolonged in the MESP group. Additionally, two cases of early bleeding were described. A lasting sensation of a foreign body was the most frequently observed complication of UPPP in the Lombo study [15] compared to BRP, which had the highest incidence of early bleeding. Tsou et al. [16] found not significantly statistically notable variations in the incidence of bleeding, dysgeusia, and globus among the two groups

Table 3. Postoperative complications for different techniques.

Complications	Techniques						
	UPPP	RF-UPP	BRP	ESP	LP	AP	LFF
Foreign Body Sensation/Globus	8 [15] 3 [16]	5 [15]	2 [14] 2 [15] 7 [16]	2 [14]	-	1 [21]	8 [21]
Nose regurgitation	-	-	-	-	2 [20]	2 [20] 1 [21]	-
Velopharyngeal insufficiency	-	-	-	-	1 [20]	1 [20]	-
Prolonged pain	3 [15]	1 [15]	1 [15]	-	-	-	-
Early bleeding	2 [15] 2 [16]	-	4 [15] 1 [16]	2 [14] 4 [20]	2 [20]	-	-
Suture dehiscence	1 [15]	-	2 [15]	-	-	-	-
Dysphagia	6 [16]	-	5 [16]	7 [20]	9 [20]	3 [20]	-
Dysgeusia	1 [16]	-	1 [16]	-	-	-	-

However, globus was more prevalent in the BRP group compared to the UPP group (22.58% vs. 9.67%). Martinez et al. [17] did not observe any particular complications other than minor bleeding. Postoperative pain was lower with the BRP technique compared to ESPwAP, as suggested by Babademez et al. [19] In the Karakok study [20], difficulty in swallowing and nasal regurgitation were present in all three groups, while velopharyngeal insufficiency was found only in the AP and LP groups. However, nasal regurgitation and nasal velopharyngeal insufficiency resolved within 1 month postoperatively. Postoperative bleeding was also described after the LP and ESP procedures, with two patients from the ESP group requiring reintervention. Haytogiu et al. [21] reported that postoperative pain at rest and during swallowing was significantly lower after AP compared to UPF. However, the foreign body sensation persisted for 6 months after UPF in seven patients compared to only one patient in the AP group.

4. Discussion

A meta-analysis published by Pang et al. in 2018 on palatal surgery for sleep apnea demonstrated a significant change in the utilization of the UPPP technique over a 17-year period, with its decreased usage in comparison to other techniques. The UPPP procedures performed during the 2011–2018 period encompassed 12.6% of all techniques used on 2715 patients compared to 25.6% during the 2001–2010 period [23]. This pattern was observable in several of the studies that we included, particularly those that gathered data retrospectively over an extended timeframe. Lombo et al. (2022) analyzed surgical techniques for sleep apnea performed in their institution between 2001 and 2020, and Martinez et al. between 2006 and 2018. In both studies, a shift away from traditional UPPP over the years and toward more focused and less invasive procedures was suggested (LP, ESP). Both authors adopted the BRP technique after 2015, as proposed by Viccini et al. [12].

The observed trend may be attributed to an improved understanding of the underlying anatomical and pathological mechanisms involved in sleep apnea, which has been facilitated by the rising utilization of drug-induced sleep endoscopy (DISE). This technique is believed to mimic natural sleep conditions more closely than alternative diagnostic methods, which may have contributed to its increasing popularity and adoption in recent years. A study by one author included in our analysis [20] also mentioned that at the beginning of his prospective study in 2011, DISE was not widely recognized or promoted at the time and, thus, he opted for alternative diagnostic procedures to visualize the obstructed site, such as the Mueller maneuver during awake nasal endoscopy. At the same time, this situation was encountered also by Lombo et al. [15] and Martinez et al. [17], who performed DISE only on some of the patients included. The majority of authors conducted a video fibroscopic examination, with or without the Mueller maneuver prior to surgery. Nevertheless, research indicates that in around 50% of patients with OSA, DISE leads to changes in surgical treatment plans when compared to awake evaluations [24]. Despite the increasing use and recognition of DISE, as well as the publication of the European position paper on DISE in 2014 and its subsequent update in 2017, there is still no wide agreement on a specific protocol for interpreting the procedure, especially regarding upper airway classification [2]. A recent review concluded that the VOTE classification was the preferred scoring system among different studies [25]. Two studies in our review used VOTE classification during DISE in assessing surgical plans and operative indications [16,19], and one study used NOHL grading [14], while the others did not mention any DISE criteria for patient selection. Nevertheless, only Lorusso et al. [14] conducted a post-surgical DISE to assess the impact of palatopharyngeal surgery on the upper airway space and confirm the appropriate selection of patients [14]. The results indicated a significant transverse reduction in oropharyngeal obstruction after both MESP and MBRP, as well as a slight decrease in hypopharyngeal obstruction, which was slightly more pronounced in the MESP group. Establishing a validated model that connects the results of DISE classification with surgical treatment plans and outcomes would provide a reliable basis for making well-informed decisions about surgical options.

Even though the UPP significantly decreased AHI in all included studies, the success rates varied highly, ranging from 38.71% to 59.26%. This can be attributed to variances in the selection criteria adopted by various studies, as well as subtle distinctions in the techniques performed. Our observations were similar to those obtained in a large systematic review published by Stock et al. that reported success/response rates between 35% and 95.2% after UPPP [26]. However, performing UPPP along with hyoid suspension significantly increases its efficacy compared to single-level surgery, through the effect it has on latero-lateral diameters of hypopharynx, widening the transverse oropharyngeal space, as Minni. et al. observed in their study [18]. The success rate rose from 40.74% to 59.26% with this combination of techniques. This finding is based on the study published in 2021 by Tessel et al. [27] that achieved noteworthy results for UPPP practiced in conjunction with HS in patients with moderate to severe OSA, with a success rate of 76.9%. Nonetheless, UPPP could have favorable outcomes as a single-level surgery in well-selected patients, as a recent meta-analysis suggests [28]. Predominantly velopharyngeal obstruction and Friedman stage 1 are predictors of success, while low hyoid position can negatively impact the surgical outcome.

The anterior palatoplasty outcomes were contradictory in the studies included in the review, as Haytogiu et al. [21] reported a success rate of 81.8% compared with only 45% obtained by Karakok et al. [20]. This was unexpected, as both authors had comparable inclusion criteria (small tonsils, retropalatal obstruction), and tonsillectomy was not performed in either of the studies. However, Karakok reported a lack of postoperative PSG for 10 patients in the AP group, which might have influenced the results. In Haytogiu's study, the uvulopalatal flap (UPF) technique exhibited outcomes comparable to those with AP, with success rates of 82.6% and 81.8%, respectively. These findings were in line with the results obtained in another study that reported success rates of 84% and 86% for UPF and AP, respectively [29]. Notably, both studies demonstrated that patients who underwent UPF experienced higher levels of pain. This may suggest that AP could be the preferred treatment option for patients with similar characteristics.

Barbed reposition pharyngoplasty has widely grown in popularity since the first mention of the technique in 2015 by Viccini et al. [12]. A systematic review published in 2022, including all relevant articles regarding the procedure, found that barbed reposition pharyngoplasty is a simple, fast, and secure procedure for treating palatopharyngeal issues that can be used on its own or as part of a more complex surgical approach [30]. This was also reflected in our review, as BRP obtained the best results in the majority of studies in both objective and subjective parameters and mono- and multi-level procedures in patients with mild to severe disease. Moreover, as Minni et al. observed in their study, an association of hyoid suspension did not lead to an improvement in outcomes compared to UPPP (64.29% vs. 65.52%, respectively) [18]. Thus, it can be assumed that a satisfactory enlargement of the retropalatal area can be achieved without requiring the need for HS in the case of BRP, as the authors suggested. However, similar favorable results were observed in the modified version of the expansion sphincter pharyngoplasty (MESP) technique developed by Lorusso et al. [14] that demonstrated a surgical success rate of 90%, comparable with that of MRP (80%) [14,19,31]. The combination of AP with ESP in the Babademez study [19] proved to be beneficial, with a success rate of 84.9%, as it approaches both antero-posterior and latero-lateral collapse in the retropalatal space. Moreover, a randomized control trial published by Ciger et al. concluded that ESP combined with AP can effectively address various types of pharyngeal obstruction (antero-posterior, latero-lateral and concentrical) [32]. According to a 2019 multicenter study on palate surgery complications by Pang et al [7], foreign body sensation was found to be the most prevalent complication, particularly in the UPP group. Our study corroborates this finding. Interestingly, our study revealed that many patients in the BRP group also experienced foreign body sensations. This could be attributed to the fact that most of the patients in this group with this symptom underwent a multilevel approach (BRP plus base of tongue reduction). In the LP group in our study, the most prevalent symptom was dysphagia, which aligns with Pang et al.'s statement and decision to shift toward non-invasive procedures such as ESP, initially introduced by Pang. For the BRP and ESP techniques, early bleeding was the complication most mentioned in the studies. However, this could also be the result of tonsillectomy that was performed in the same operative time. Nonetheless, a notable reduction in postoperative pain was observed with the BRP technique compared with ESP in the Lorusso and Babademez studies [14,19]. Additionally, it was noted that the operation time was shorter. A recent meta-analysis also reported that both techniques have comparable effectiveness in terms of AHI, ODI, LOS, and ESS, but BRP is faster to execute [31].

Study Limitations

Consistent with other recently published reviews [33], we observed a lack of prospective studies directly comparing the velopharyngeal surgical techniques. Most of the studies included in this review were retrospective, which might imply an inferior level of evidence, being prone to selection bias. However, the inclusion of longitudinal studies helped us to obtain an overview of how surgical approaches changed over the years, from an aggressive approach to more reconstructive and more focused procedures. The attempt to better understand the anatomy and physiology of the upper airway in obstructive sleep apnea also determined a change in diagnostic procedures, with extended usage of DISE in the preoperative plan, which might have had an impact on surgical results in some studies. The longitudinal nature of the studies and the accumulation of experience in performing DISE over time allowed for the refinement of patient selection for surgery, which may have had an impact on the surgical outcomes.

5. Conclusions

A trend toward adopting the BRP surgical technique has emerged due to its excellent outcomes with minimal complications and a relatively short operation time. Our results show that BRP achieved the most favorable objective and subjective outcomes among the studies reviewed, with consistent results in both single and multilevel settings. Although ESP closely follows BRP in terms of efficiency, it comes with a higher risk of complications such as postoperative prolonged pain and shows better results when combined with techniques such as AP that target antero-posterior collapse. However, other, older techniques, such as UPPP, UPF, AP, or LP in mono- or multilevel settings, also have good results when performed in well-selected patients. The heterogeneity observed in the studies, both in terms of surgical outcomes and patient selection criteria, led us to conclude that more prospective studies with standardized selection criteria for each group of patients are needed to generalize the outcomes. Despite the well-established role of DISE worldwide, there is still a lack of specific consensual criteria regarding the upper airway classification of obstruction patterns. The introduction of such criteria may assist surgeons in selecting the appropriate therapeutic strategy for each patient and researchers in obtaining more accurate and generalizable results.

Author Contributions: A.M.V. had equal contribution with C.D.S. in designing the research, data acquisition, analysis and interpretation of data and wrote the manuscript. V.Z. and R.H. performed data acquisition, analysis and interpretation of data and manuscript drafting. A.M.V., I.S. and C.D.S. contributed to statistical analysis, critical revision of the manuscript for important intellectual content. All authors have read and agreed to the published version of the manuscript.

Funding: This research received no external funding.

Institutional Review Board Statement: Not applicable.

Informed Consent Statement: Not applicable.

Data Availability Statement: Not applicable.

Conflicts of Interest: The authors declare no conflict of interest.

References

1. Benjafield, A.V.; Ayas, N.T.; Eastwood, P.R.; Heinzer, R.; Ip, M.S.M.; Morrell, M.J.; Nunez, C.M.; Patel, S.R.; Penzel, T.; Pépin, J.L.D.; et al. Estimation of the global prevalence and burden of obstructive sleep apnoea: A literature-based analysis. *Lancet. Respir. Med.* **2019**, *7*, 687. [CrossRef] [PubMed]
2. De Vito, A.; Llatas, M.C.; Ravesloot, M.J.; Kotecha, B.; De Vries, N.; Hamans, E.; Maurer, J.; Bosi, M.; Blumen, M.; Heiser, C.; et al. European position paper on drug-induced sleep endoscopy: 2017 Update. *Clin. Otolaryngol. Off. J. ENT-UK Off. J. Neth. Soc. Oto-Rhino-Laryngol. Cervico-Facial Surg.* **2018**, *43*, 1541–1552. [CrossRef]
3. Vroegop, A.V.; Vanderveken, O.M.; Boudewyns, A.N.; Scholman, J.; Saldien, V.; Wouters, K.; Braem, M.J.; Van De Heyning, P.H.; Hamans, E. Drug-induced sleep endoscopy in sleep-disordered breathing: Report on 1249 cases. *Laryngoscope* **2014**, *124*, 797–802. [CrossRef] [PubMed]
4. Soose, R.J. Novel Surgical Approaches for the Treatment of Obstructive Sleep Apnea. *Sleep Med. Clin.* **2016**, *11*, 189–202. [CrossRef]
5. Fujita, S.; Conway, W.; Zorick, F.; Roth, T. Surgical correction of anatomic azbnormalities in obstructive sleep apnea syndrome: Uvulopalatopharyngoplasty. *Otolaryngol.-Head Neck Surg. Off. J. Am. Acad. Otolaryngol.-Head Neck Surg.* **1981**, *89*, 923–934. [CrossRef] [PubMed]
6. Ja, P. Lessons from 50 Years of Uvulopalatopharyngoplasty. *J. Sleep Disord. Ther.* **2016**, *5*, 3–5. [CrossRef]
7. Pang, K.P.; Vicini, C.; Montevecchi, F.; Piccin, O.; Chandra, S.; Yang, H.C.; Agrawal, V.; Chung, J.C.K.; Chan, Y.H.; Pang, S.B.; et al. Long-term Complications of Palate Surgery: A Multicenter Study of 217 Patients. *Laryngoscope* **2020**, *130*, 2281–2284. [CrossRef]
8. Pang, K.P.; Tan, R.; Puraviappan, P.; Terris, D.J. Anterior palatoplasty for the treatment of OSA: Three-year results. *Otolaryngol.-Head Neck Surg. Off. J. Am. Acad. Otolaryngol.-Head Neck Surg.* **2009**, *141*, 253–256. [CrossRef]
9. Alcaraz, M.; Bosco, G.; Pérez-Martín, N.; Morato, M.; Navarro, A.; Plaza, G. Advanced Palate Surgery: What Works? *Curr. Otorhinolaryngol. Rep.* **2021**, *9*, 271–284. [CrossRef]
10. Cahali, M.B. Lateral pharyngoplasty: A new treatment for obstructive sleep apnea hypopnea syndrome. *Laryngoscope* **2003**, *113*, 1961–1968. [CrossRef]
11. Pang, K.P. Expansion sphincter pharyngoplasty: A new technique for the treatment of obstructive sleep apnea. *Otolaryngol.-Head Neck Surg. Off. J. Am. Acad. Otolaryngol.-Head Neck Surg.* **2007**, *137*, 110–114. [CrossRef] [PubMed]
12. Vicini, C.; Hendawy, E.; Campanini, A.; Eesa, M.; Bahgat, A.; AlGhamdi, S.; Meccariello, G.; DeVito, A.; Montevecchi, F.; Mantovani, M. Barbed reposition pharyngoplasty (BRP) for OSAHS: A feasibility, safety, efficacy and teachability pilot study. "We are on the giant's shoulders". *Eur. Arch. Oto-Rhino-Laryngol. Off. J. Eur. Fed. Oto-Rhino-Laryngol. Soc. (EUFOS) Affil. Ger. Soc. Oto-Rhino-Laryngol.-Head Neck Surg.* **2015**, *272*, 3065–3070. [CrossRef] [PubMed]
13. Moher, D.; Liberati, A.; Tetzlaff, J.; Altman, D.G.; Altman, D.; Antes, G.; Atkins, D.; Barbour, V.; Barrowman, N.; Berlin, J.A.; et al. Preferred reporting items for systematic reviews and meta-analyses: The PRISMA statement. *PLoS Med.* **2009**, *6*, e1000097. [CrossRef] [PubMed]

14. Lorusso, F.; Dispenza, F.; Sireci, F.; Immordino, A.; Immordino, P.; Gallina, S. Management of pharyngeal collapse in patients affected by moderate obstructive sleep apnoea syndrome. *Acta Otorhinolaringol. Ital. Organo Uff. Soc. Ital. Otorinolaringol. Chir. Cervico-Facciale* **2022**, *42*, 273–280. [CrossRef]
15. Lombo, C.; Costa, R.; Martins, M.; Matos, C.; Fonseca, R. Pharyngoplasty for obstructive sleep apnea: The influence of surgical technique. *Acta Otorrinolaringol. Esp* **2022**, *73*, 362–369. [CrossRef]
16. Tsou, Y.A.; Hsu, C.C.; Shih, L.C.; Lin, T.C.; Chiu, C.J.; Tien, V.H.C.; Tsai, M.H.; Chang, W.D. Combined Transoral Robotic Tongue Base Surgery and Palate Surgery in Obstructive Sleep Apnea Syndrome: Modified Uvulopalatopharyngoplasty versus Barbed Reposition Pharyngoplasty. *J. Clin. Med.* **2021**, *10*, 3169. [CrossRef]
17. Martínez Ruiz de Apodaca, P.P.M.R.; Llatas, M.C.; Gras, M.V.; Galofre, J.D. Improving surgical results in velopharyngeal surgery: Our experience in the last decade. *Acta Otorrinolaringol. Esp.* **2020**, *71*, 197–203. [CrossRef]
18. Minni, A.; Cialente, F.; Ralli, M.; Colizza, A.; Lai, Q.; Placentino, A.; Franco, M.; Rossetti, V.; De Vincentiis, M. Uvulopalatopharyngoplasty and barbed reposition pharyngoplasty with and without hyoid suspension for obstructive sleep apnea hypopnea syndrome: A comparison of long-term functional results. *Bosn. J. Basic Med. Sci.* **2021**, *21*, 364–369. [CrossRef]
19. Babademez, M.A.; Gul, F.; Teleke, Y.C. Barbed palatoplasty vs. expansion sphincter pharyngoplasty with anterior palatoplasty. *Laryngoscope* **2020**, *130*, E275–E279. [CrossRef]
20. Karakoc, O.; Binar, M.; Aydin, U.; Genc, H.; Akcam, T.; Gerek, M. A tertiary center experience with velopharyngeal surgical techniques for treatment of snoring and obstructive sleep apnea. *Auris Nasus Larynx* **2018**, *45*, 492–498. [CrossRef]
21. Haytoğlu, S.; Arikan, O.K.; Muluk, N.B.; Tuhanioğlu, B.; Çörtük, M. Comparison of anterior palatoplasty and uvulopalatal flap placement for treating mild and moderate obstructive sleep apnea. *Ear Nose Throat J.* **2018**, *97*, 69–78. [CrossRef] [PubMed]
22. Fairbanks, D.N.F. Operative Techniques of Uvulopalatopharyngoplasty. *Ear Nose Throat J.* **1999**, *78*, 846–850. [CrossRef] [PubMed]
23. Pang, K.P.; Plaza, G.; Baptista, P.M.; Reina, C.O.; Chan, Y.H.; Pang, K.A.; Pang, E.B.; Wang, C.M.Z.; Rotenberg, B. Palate surgery for obstructive sleep apnea: A 17-year meta-analysis. *Eur. Arch. Oto-Rhino-Laryngol. Off. J. Eur. Fed. Oto-Rhino-Laryngol. Soc. (EUFOS) Affil. Ger. Soc. Oto-Rhino-Laryngol.-Head Neck Surg.* **2018**, *275*, 1697–1707. [CrossRef]
24. Certal, V.F.; Pratas, R.; Guimarães, L.; Lugo, R.; Tsou, Y.; Camacho, M.; Capasso, R. Awake examination versus DISE for surgical decision making in patients with OSA: A systematic review. *Laryngoscope* **2016**, *126*, 768–774. [CrossRef] [PubMed]
25. Amos, J.M.; Durr, M.L.; Nardone, H.C.; Baldassari, C.M.; Duggins, A.; Ishman, S.L. Systematic Review of Drug-Induced Sleep Endoscopy Scoring Systems. *Otolaryngol.-Head Neck Surg.* **2018**, *158*, 240–248. [CrossRef]
26. Stuck, B.A.; Ravesloot, M.J.L.; Eschenhagen, T.; de Vet, H.C.W.; Sommer, J.U. Uvulopalatopharyngoplasty with or without tonsillectomy in the treatment of adult obstructive sleep apnea-A systematic review. *Sleep Med.* **2018**, *50*, 152–165. [CrossRef]
27. Van Tassel, J.; Chio, E.; Silverman, D.; Nord, R.S.; Platter, D.; Abidin, M.R. Hyoid Suspension with UPPP for the Treatment of Obstructive Sleep Apnea. *Ear Nose Throat J.* **2021**, *102*, NP212–NP219. [CrossRef]
28. Cho, J.H.; Choi, J.H.; Cho, S.H.; Kim, S.N.; Suh, J.D. Predicting Outcomes after Uvulopalatopharyngoplasty for Adult Obstructive Sleep Apnea: A Meta-analysis. *Otolaryngol.-Head Neck Surg. Off. J. Am. Acad. Otolaryngol.-Head Neck Surg.* **2016**, *155*, 904–913. [CrossRef]
29. Marzetti, A.; Tedaldi, M.; Passali, F.M. Preliminary findings from our experience in anterior palatoplasty for the treatment of obstructive sleep apnea. *Clin. Exp. Otorhinolaryngol.* **2013**, *6*, 18–22. [CrossRef]
30. Iannella, G.; Lechien, J.R.; Perrone, T.; Meccariello, G.; Cammaroto, G.; Cannavicci, A.; Burgio, L.; Maniaci, A.; Cocuzza, S.; Di Luca, M.; et al. Barbed reposition pharyngoplasty (BRP) in obstructive sleep apnea treatment: State of the art. *Am. J. Otolaryngol.* **2022**, *43*, 103197. [CrossRef]
31. Neruntarat, C.; Khuancharee, K.; Saengthong, P. Barbed Reposition Pharyngoplasty versus Expansion Sphincter Pharyngoplasty: A Meta-Analysis. *Laryngoscope* **2021**, *131*, 1420–1428. [CrossRef] [PubMed]
32. Ciğer, E.; İşlek, A. Anterior Palatoplasty with Expansion Sphincter Pharyngoplasty for All Type of Pharyngeal Collapse. *Laryngoscope* **2022**, *132*, 1313–1319. [CrossRef] [PubMed]
33. Maniaci, A.; Di Luca, M.; Lechien, J.R.; Iannella, G.; Grillo, C.; Grillo, C.M.; Merlino, F.; Calvo-Henriquez, C.; De Vito, A.; Magliulo, G.; et al. Lateral pharyngoplasty vs. traditional uvulopalatopharyngoplasty for patients with OSA: Systematic review and meta-analysis. *Sleep Breath.* **2022**, *26*, 1539–1550. [CrossRef] [PubMed]

Disclaimer/Publisher's Note: The statements, opinions and data contained in all publications are solely those of the individual author(s) and contributor(s) and not of MDPI and/or the editor(s). MDPI and/or the editor(s) disclaim responsibility for any injury to people or property resulting from any ideas, methods, instructions or products referred to in the content.

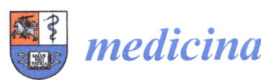

Case Report

Olfactory Neuroblastoma—A Challenging Fine Line between Metastasis and Hematology

Trandafir Cornelia Marina [1], Balica Nicolae Constantin [1,2,*], Baderca Flavia [3], Sarau Oana Silvana [4], Poenaru Marioara [1] and Cristian Andrei Sarau [5]

1. ENT Department, Spitalul Clinic Municipal de Urgenta, Victor Babeş University of Medicine and Pharmacy, Bulevardul. Revoluției No. 6, 300054 Timisoara, Romania
2. ENT Department, Victor Babeş University of Medicine and Pharmacy, 300041 Timişoara, Romania
3. Department of Microscopic Morphology, Victor Babeş University of Medicine and Pharmacy, 300041 Timişoara, Romania
4. Department of Hematology, Victor Babeş University of Medicine and Pharmacy, 300041 Timişoara, Romania
5. Department of Medical Semiology I, Victor Babeş University of Medicine and Pharmacy, 300041 Timişoara, Romania
* Correspondence: balica@umft.ro

Abstract: Developing in a limited space, rare tumors located at the nose and paranasal sinuses are sometimes difficult to diagnose due to their modest clinical presentation, which is uncorrelated with anatomopathological diversity. This limits the preoperative diagnosis without added immune histochemical study; for that reason, we present our experience with these tumors with the intention of raising awareness. The patient included in our study was investigated by our department through clinical and endoscopic examination, imaging investigations, and an anatomic-pathological study. The selected patient gave consent for participation and inclusion in this research study in compliance with the 1964 Declaration of Helsinki.

Keywords: olfactory neuroblastoma; rare sinonasal tumors; endoscopic surgery; management strategy; myeloma

1. Introduction

Tumors in the nose and paranasal sinuses are rare lesions, affecting <1 in 100,000 people per year [1]. These tumors may have monomorphic, nonspecific symptomatology, but they require a prompt and accurate diagnosis due to their poor prognosis and evolution.

While new discoveries are made worldwide, especially to assess new methods of prevention, diagnosis, or specialized treatment, the rarity of these cases remains an obstacle in choosing the management option.

Olfactory neuroblastoma, also referred to as esthesioneuroblastoma, represents an oncological entity of neuroectodermal origin arising in the upper part of the nasal cavity. Its incidence represents 2–3% of all nasal neoplasms [2].

The etiology and risk factors are still unknown. As with most sinonasal tumors, the symptoms are nonspecific, most commonly epistaxis, nasal obstruction, and hyposmia. A biopsy is essential for diagnosis, while CT scans and MRI images are used for the staging system.

These tumors are locally aggressive, with the propensity to spread into the anterior skull base as well as to metastasize to the cervical lymph nodes, thorax, and bones [3].

Cervical metastases are described in 5–8% of cases at diagnosis and in 15–25% of patients as recurrence [4,5]. The management of the neck in olfactory neuroblastoma is still controversial.

In our day, three separate staging systems exist. Kadish et al. [6] proposed in 1976 a staging of olfactory neuroblastoma in three groups based on the extension of the disease,

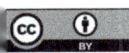

which is still widely used (group A—tumor limited to the nasal fossa; group B—extension to the paranasal sinuses; group C—extension beyond the paranasal sinuses). The staging has evolved, and a modified Kadish system was proposed with an additional group D describing tumors with the locoregional or distant presence of metastases. Some institutions apply the TNM staging system by the American Joint Committee on Cancer (AJCC) based on the Dulguerov modified version of staging [6,7] (Table 1).

Table 1. Staging systems for olfactory neuroblastoma.

Kadish System (1976)		Kadish Modified System		TNM Staging System for Olfactory Neuroblastoma from the Dulguerov Modified Version	
Group A	Tumor confined to nasal cavity	Group A	Tumor confined to nasal cavity	T1	Tumor involving the nasal cavity and/or paranasal sinuses (excluding sphenoid), sparing the most superior ethmoidal cells
Group B	Tumor involved nasal cavity and paranasal sinuses	Group B	Tumor involved nasal cavity and paranasal sinuses	T2	Tumor involving the nasal cavity and/or paranasal sinuses (including the sphenoid) with extension to or erosion of the cribriform plate
Group C	Tumor spread beyond the nasal cavity and paranasal sinuses	Group C	Tumor extent beyond nasal cavity and paranasal sinuses, including involvement of the cribriform plate, base of the skull, orbit or intracranial cavity	T3	Tumor extending into the orbit or protruding into the anterior cranial fossa, without dural invasion
		Group D	Tumor with metastasis to cervical lymph nodes or distant sites	T4	Tumor involving the brain
				N0	No cervical lymph-node metastasis
				N1	Any form of cervical lymph-node metastasis
				M0	No metastases
				M1	Distant metastasis

There is no agreed-upon standard treatment for olfactory neuroblastoma. Surgical treatment and radiotherapy represent the most frequently used approaches. Chemotherapy treatment modalities can be used in selected cases. Open surgical approaches, such as extracranial and anterior craniofacial resection, are preferred in the treatment of ONB. The development of an endoscopic approach over the past few decades has gained popularity and offered many advantages (better cosmetic outcome and better visualization of some deep areas within the sinonasal region), representing a valid treatment for olfactory neuroblastoma [4,8].

Multimodal treatment associating surgery with radiation therapy has been demonstrated to have the best survival rates; however, the infrequency of olfactory neuroblastoma and its heterogeneous clinical biology limit the possibility of creating specific protocols of treatment [3,9–11].

Recurrence may be encountered years after treatment; therefore, long-term follow-up is recommended [9].

Multiple myeloma currently affects 250,000 people globally [12]. According to the 2022 Canadian data, the incidence is 10.1 per 100,000 men and 6.4 per 100,000 women, with an average age of diagnosis in the 6thdecade for both [13].

The diagnosis is made based on the evidence of one or more of the CRAB criteria (C—hypercalcemia, R—renal insufficiency, A—anemia, and B—bone lesions), with biopsy confirmation of bone marrow infiltration by 10% clonal plasma cells or detection of a plasmacytoma. The laboratory diagnosis includes a variety of biochemical examinations (serum protein electrophoresis, urine protein electrophoresis, urine immunofixation, serum free light chains, and total protein) associated with the monitoring of end-organ damage [14,15].

2. Case Report

A 45-year-old patient was admitted to our department with epistaxis from the right nasal fossa. He received conservative treatment using an anterior nasal tampon (Merocel) for 2 days, and he returned a few days later with recurrent symptomatology. The patient underwent an endoscopic examination, where he presented a solitary, smooth mass in the right nasal fossa.

The patient underwent CT and MRI of the head and neck prior to surgical resection; the CT scan identified a heterogeneous, natively hyperdense tissue mass, located at the level of the right nasal cavity, which it filled for the most part. The mass-produced remodeling and bone erosion, with partial visualization of the right inferior nasal turbinates. The native CT appearance was nonspecific in the differential diagnosis, including an inverted papilloma, sinonasal polyp, or adenocarcinoma. The right maxillary sinus was filled with mixed, parafluid, and tissue densities (Figure 1).

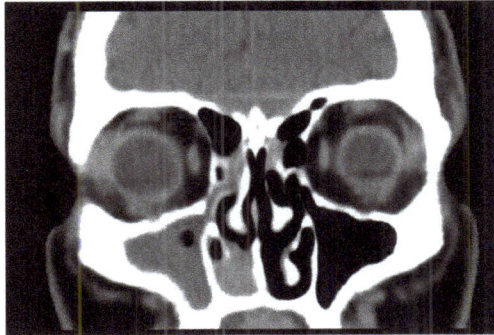

Figure 1. Preoperative CT scan showing a nonspecific opacification of the right nasal fossa (inferior meatus) with partial erosion of the inferior turbinate. There was no evidence of invasion into the skull base, cribriform plate, or olfactory cleft. The CT scan demonstrated density and mucosal thickening of the maxillary sinus.

The patient underwent a chest and abdominal CT scan and MRI, and there was no proof of distant metastasis. The patient was staged according to the Kadish system.

The tumor was located in the nasal fossa, without intracranial extension or erosion of the cribriform plate. An endoscopic approach was performed. The tumor was successfully removed with negative margins; a right maxillary antrostomy was performed. A Merocel was placed in the nasal fossa and removed after 48 h. In order to avoid the risk of infection, for all endoscopic surgeries, we use an antibioprophylaxis for 48–72 h, initiated on the day of the surgery.

The patient had no complications (no CSF leak, no neurologic symptoms), and no epistaxis was found after the postoperative Merocel removal. The patient stayed in the hospital for less than a week.

Tissue fragments were immunohistologically studied; the fragments were initially fixed in formalin. Positive and negative controls were performed.

The tumor consisted of a polypoid thickened respiratory mucosa through a pseudolobular tumor proliferation that develops exclusively in the lamina propria, respecting the structure of the covering epithelium. Tumor cells were relatively monomorphic, small in size, weakly basophilic or weakly acidophilic, with a nucleus with irregularly or finely dispersed chromatin and inconstant nucleoli; some cells have a central nucleus, and in other cells, the position of the nucleus is eccentric, rare mitoses (1–2 cp × 40), with solid and trabecular growth architecture in a fibrous stroma and the formation of pseudorosettes (Homer Wright rosettes), and frequently in perivascular position, encasing small and medium vessels. Positive and negative controls were performed.

Immunohistochemical reactions are performed on the paraffin block. The negative immunoreactions in tumor cells were identified (CD45, AE1/AE3, CD34, SMA, desmina, and CD99). BCL-2 was positive, and PGP9.5 was positive.

Correlating the histological aspects (Figure 2) with immunohistochemical staining, the diagnosis of neuroectodermal tumor was established, with the subtype of olfactory neuroblastoma (BCL2-positive and PGP9.5-positive) determined at G2 differentiation (Figure 3).

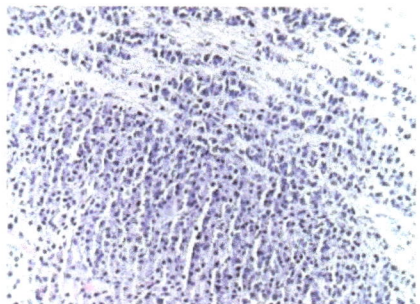

Figure 2. Olfactory neuroblastoma (HE stain, 40×) showing a solid and trabecular growth pattern composed of round, small cells that are relatively uniform with scanty cytoplasm and scattered chromatin pattern.

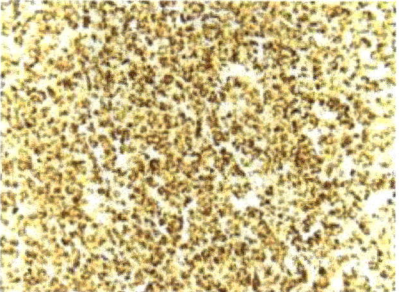

Figure 3. Immunohistochemical stain (PGP 9.5, ob 40×) showing intense cytoplasmic positive reaction of PGP 9.5 in all tumor cells.

After the surgical endoscopic removal of the tumor and the confirmation of the diagnosis by the anatomopathological exam, the patient was referred for radiotherapy. He underwent 33 sessions of radiotherapy treatment (DT = 50 Gy/fr/38 days) on the right nasal fossa. Radiotherapy was well tolerated.

Follow-up was conducted by the oncology and radiotherapy departments, where postoperative imaging of the head and neck was performed. No recurrence was identified. The ENT follow-up was scheduled every 3 months during the first year for nasal endoscopy, every 6 months during the second and third years, and annually thereafter without recurrence or symptoms.

In the fifth year after the primary diagnosis, the patient complained of lumbosacral and humeral bone pain.

He underwent a CT scan and an MRI, which indicated osteolytic lesions of the vertebral bodies C6, C7, C8. T7 (16 mm), and T11, as well as the costal arches and bone basin (11 cm at the level of the right iliac wing with the extension to the right iliac muscle and a 10 mm lesion at the left iliac wing). The CT scan identified an important circumferential thickening of the mucosa of the right maxillary sinus that almost completely occupied it, with otherwise normally aerated paranasal sinuses.

The lesions raised suspicion of multiple myeloma or long-distance metastasis. A biopsy of the sinus mucosa was performed with local anesthesia; the patient was referred to a hematologist and scheduled for a whole-body positron emission computer tomography (PET-CT) and a bone biopsy. The sinus biopsy revealed hypertrophic mucosa and the absence of tumoral cells.

The whole-body PET-CT showed the activated metabolism of a mass in the right iliac wing measuring 10 to 7.5 cm, which invaded the neighboring endo- and exopelvic structures. The mass showed an inhomogeneous uptake of FDG. Other similarly moderate FDG-capturing osteolytic lesions could be distinguished in the right posterior fourth costal arch (invasive and dimensional progression compared to the CT scan performed 1 week before), the right fourth anterior costal arch, the left sixth lateral costal arch, the sternal manubrium, the medial angle of the left scapula, C7 (with a major risk of subsidence), T7, and T9 vertebral bodies, the right lateral clavicular extremity, the right humeral head, apex of the right temporal bone, the right parietal bone, and the left sciatic tuberosity [Figures 4 and 5].

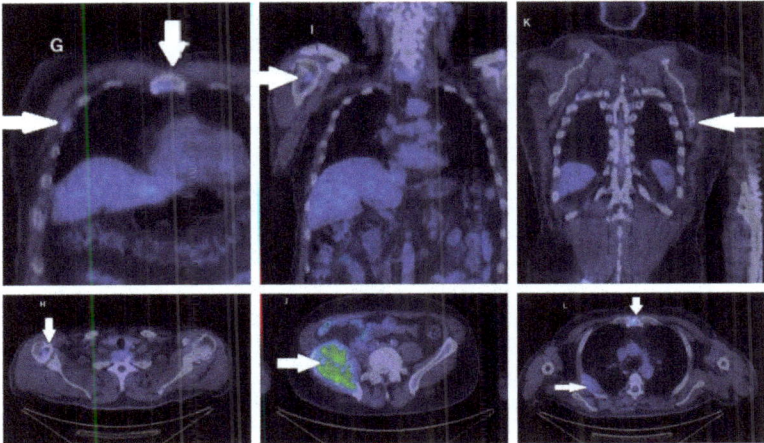

Figure 4. PET-CT showed an activated metabolism (arrow) of a mass in the right iliac wing of 10/7.5 cm that invaded the neighboring endo- and exopelvic structures. The mass showed an inhomogeneous uptake of FDG. Other similarly moderate FDG-capturing osteolytic lesions could be distinguished in the right posterior fourth costal arch (invasive and dimensional progression compared to the CT scan performed 1 week before), the right fourth anterior costal arch, the left sixth lateral costal arch, the sternal manubrium, the medial angle of the scapula on the left, the C7 (with a major risk of subsidence), the T7 and T9 vertebral bodies, the right lateral clavicular extremity, the right humeral head, the apex, the right temporal bone, right parietal bone, and the left sciatic tuberosity.

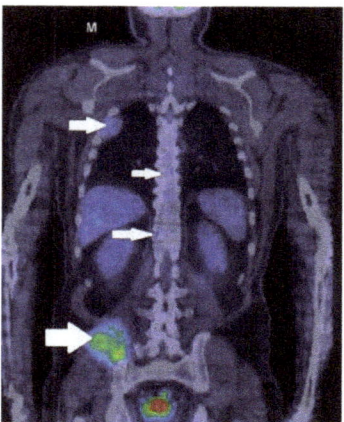

Figure 5. The whole-body PET-CT showed (arrow) the activated metabolism of a 10 to 7.5 cm mass in the right iliac wing that invaded the neighboring endo- and exopelvic structures. The mass showed an inhomogeneous uptake of FDG. Other similarly moderate FDG-capturing osteolytic lesions could be distinguished in T7 and T9 vertebral bodies, the right lateral clavicular extremity, and the right humeral head.

The bone marrow biopsy concluded medullary iron blockage with moderate hyperplasia of the plasmacyte, affecting 4.5% of nucleated cells.

Based on the complete blood cell counts, the protein electrophoresis, the serum electrophoresis, the immunoquantification, and the bone marrow biopsy, the diagnosis of monoclonal gammopathy of unspecified etiology of type IgG with lambda chains was established.

A bone biopsy was taken from the iliac lesion, demonstrating the diagnosis of multiple myeloma type IgG with kappa chains (CD-138 positive; kappa chains weakly intensify CD79a-positive, CD56-positive, and CD20-negative for lambda chains). The Ki37 cell proliferation index was 40%. The disease was classified as stage III according to the International Staging System (R2-ISS) for overall survival in multiple myeloma.

The patient underwent hematological treatment with daratumumab, bortezomib, thalidomide, dexamethasone, and bisphosphonate. The symptoms of bone pain were relieved. The patient is still in the follow-up stage.

3. Discussion

As a rare malignant tumor of the nasal cavity with a frequency of only 0.4 million per year, olfactory neuroblastoma was described for the first time in 1924 [16].

The tumor can affect both children and adults; in adults, the disease generally occurs between the fifth and sixth decades of life. Its origin is still unknown. No lifestyle risk, environmental, or geographic factors are linked to its apparition. The symptoms may vary from unilateral nasal obstruction (70%) to epistaxis (46%; see [7,9]). The gold standard of diagnosis for olfactory neuroblastoma is a biopsy and an anatomopathological examination.

Having neuroectodermal and epithelial origins, olfactory neuroblastoma presents itself as a unilateral, polypoid tumor formation of low consistency with a nonspecific clinical presentation. The olfactory epithelium can be identified in the mucosa of the superior and middle turbinates and also in the mucosa of the nasal septum [17].

The immunohistochemical examination is based on positive markers for S100, BCL2 [17], and PGP9.5 and negative markers for keratin, muscle, melanoma, and lymphoma.

Olfactory neuroblastoma poses a high risk of local invasion, recurrence, and distant metastasis [18]. Dulguerov et al. found in their meta-analysis that cervical lymph node metastasis is the most important prognostic factor in olfactory neuroblastoma that negatively affects survival [9].

Castelnuovo et al. reported, in a total of 10 patients treated with endoscopic surgery, the presence of cervical metastasis 21 months after surgery. The patients underwent a bilateral modified neck dissection plus radiotherapy [19]. Some studies recommend cervical neck dissection for metastases occurring 6 months or more after treatment of the primary site. Naples et al. found in a meta-analysis that elective supra-omohyoid neck dissection is a reasonable option for patients with Kadish stage B and TNM stage N0 [4,5].

Based on our experience, we think that the endonasal approach achieves a complete resection for small, localized lesions when no reconstruction is needed, and all the lesions can be resected with negative margins. Our patient was, at the time of the diagnosis, N0M0, so we did not perform a neck dissection. The endonasal excision allows rapid recovery and returns to daily activities for the patients, improving their quality of life.

The infrequency of these tumors has limited the possibility of categorizing the prognostic factors and specific protocols of treatment. Several staging systems have been proposed. The most commonly used was proposed by Kadish et al. in 1976 and modified in 1993. Nowadays, some institutions apply the TNM staging system by the AJCC based on the Dulguerov modified version of staging [9,20,21] (Table 1).

A meta-analysis compared the outcomes of the Kadish and Dulguerov staging systems, finding that both systems correlated with prognostic factors in terms of disease-free and overall survival, with the Dulguerov system having a superior performance [21].

CT and MRI images are essential for correct staging. PET-CT can identify local recurrences and metastases. The anatomopathological examination is the gold standard for diagnosis.

The typical recommended treatment for olfactory neuroblastoma consists of endoscopic surgery resection associated with radiochemotherapy. Endonasal endoscopic surgery is preferred due to its efficient local control and lower morbidity [22]. In our center, we consider and use the open approach when there is an extensive tumor with intracranial involvement or when a pericranial flap for reconstruction is needed [23].

However, in this particular case, the imaging suggests no involvement of the cribriform plate, base of the skull, orbit, or intracranial cavity. As described in the literature, endoscopic resection allows the total excision of small lesions. Due to its location in the right nasal fossa and the fact that it had not spread into the adjacent structures, we performed an endoscopic approach.

In a retrospective study by Gallia et al., eight patients with olfactory neuroblastoma treated by endonasal endoscopic surgery were identified. They had a complete resection and negative intraoperative margins, with no evidence of disease over a mean follow-up of over 27 months [3].

Newer radiotherapy techniques have been added, reducing cerebral and ocular toxicity over time [24]. Neoadjuvant chemotherapy for tumor reduction can improve surgical management by reducing the size of the tumor and its complications [25–27].

Due to the delayed regional recurrences associated with olfactory neuroblastoma, prolonged surveillance is recommended. We highlight in our report the aggressiveness of this tumor and the importance of including PET-CT in the monitoring follow-up protocol for olfactory neuroblastoma while also considering that distant metastases (approximately 10%) can occur irrespective of the grade of the tumor [28].

In our report, osteolytic lesions raised the suspicion of distant metastases of the olfactory neuroblastoma and multiple myeloma. Distant recurrences of olfactory neuroblastoma are described in the literature. In an article by Loy et al., 34% of patients developed recurrent disease, and the most distant metastases were osseous (humerus, lumbar spine, and diffuse bone metastases) [29]. The symptomatology of the patient correlated with their history of olfactory neuroblastoma, raising the suspicion of a distant recurrence of the disease. However, the clinical ENT exam and negative biopsy of the sinus confirmed a hematological malignancy.

In multiple myeloma, malignant plasma cells proliferate in the bone marrow, displacing normal blood cells and leading to disease and symptom manifestations such as generalized weakness, weight loss, bone pain, hypercalcemia, and anemia [30].

Although our patient was diagnosed with a hematological disease and there is no correlation between multiple myeloma and olfactory neuroblastoma, it should be noted that long-term follow-up of an olfactory neuroblastoma patient is mandatory. The presence of a multidisciplinary team around the patient can identify and treat relapses, long-distance metastases, or even a hematological disease.

4. Conclusions

Rare sinonasal tumors present similar symptomatology, originating in a relatively small anatomical space. The patients often have a long history before their initial presentation. The treatment modalities have changed over time with the evolution of endoscopic surgery, and a multidisciplinary approach may improve the survival rate and the patient's quality of life. Lifelong follow-up is crucial, combined with imaging surveillance, given the possibility of distant metastases occurring many years after treatment of the primary tumor or, as in our case, an early diagnosis of hematological disease.

Author Contributions: Conceptualization and methodology, P.M.; software, C.A.S.; validation: B.N.C.; formal analysis and investigation: B.F. and S.O.S.; writing—original draft preparation, T.C.M.; writing—review and editing, T.C.M.; visualization: All authors have read and agreed to the published version of the manuscript.

Funding: This research received no external funding.

Institutional Review Board Statement: Thisstudy was conducted in accordance with the Declaration of Helsinki andapproved by the ethical committee of the institution (CECS No 30/2015/rev 2022).

Informed Consent Statement: Written informed consent was obtained from the patient to publish this paper.

Conflicts of Interest: The authors declare no conflict of interest.

References

1. Lund, V.J.; Clarke, P.M.; Swift, A.C.; McGarry, G.W.; Kerawala, C.; Carnell, D. Nose and paranasal sinus tumours: United Kingdom National Multidisciplinary Guidelines. *J. Laryngol. Otol.* **2016**, *130* (Suppl. S2), S111–S118. [CrossRef]
2. Faragalla, H.; Weinreb, I. Olfactory neuroblastoma: A review and update. *Adv. Anat. Pathol.* **2009**, *16*, 322–331. [CrossRef]
3. Gallia, G.L.; Reh, D.D.; Salmasi, V.; Blitz, A.M.; Koch, W.; Ishii, M. Endonasal endoscopic resection of esthesioneuroblastoma: The Johns Hopkins Hospital experience and review of the literature. *Neurosurg. Rev.* **2011**, *34*, 465–475. [CrossRef] [PubMed]
4. Naples, J.G.; Spiro, J.; Tessema, B.; Kuwada, C.; Kuo, C.L.; Brown, S.M. Neck recurrence and mortality in esthesioneuroblastoma: Implications for management of the N0 neck. *Laryngoscope* **2016**, *126*, 1373–1379. [CrossRef] [PubMed]
5. Zanation, A.M.; Ferlito, A.; Rinaldo, A.; Gore, M.R.; Lund, V.J.; McKinney, K.A.; Suárez, C.; Takes, R.P.; Devaiah, A.K. When, how and why to treat the neck in patients with esthesioneuroblastoma: A review. *Eur. Arch. Otorhinolaryngol.* **2010**, *267*, 1667–1671. [CrossRef] [PubMed]
6. Kadish, S.; Goodman, M.; Wang, C.C. Olfactory neuroblastoma. A clinical analysis of 17 cases. *Cancer* **1976**, *37*, 1571–1576. [CrossRef] [PubMed]
7. Dulguerov, P.; Calcaterra, T. Esthesioneuroblastom February a: The UCLA experience 1970–1990. *Laryngoscope* **1992**, *102*, 843–849. [CrossRef]
8. Abdelmeguid, A.S.; Bell, D.; Roberts, D.; Ferrarotto, R.; Phan, J.; Su, S.Y.; Kupferman, M.; Raza, S.; DeMonte, F.; Hanna, E. Long-Term Outcomes of Olfactory Neuroblastoma: MD Anderson Cancer Center Experience and Review of the Literature. *Laryngoscope* **2022**, *132*, 290–297. [CrossRef]
9. Dulguerov, P.; Allal, A.S.; Calcaterra, T.C. Esthesioneuroblastoma: A meta-analysis and review. *Lancet Oncol.* **2001**, *2*, 683–690. [CrossRef]
10. Jethanamest, D.; Morris, L.G.; Sikora, A.G.; Kutler, D.I. Esthesioneuroblastoma: A population-based analysis of survival and prognostic factors. *Arch. Otolaryngol. Head Neck Surg.* **2007**, *133*, 276–280. [CrossRef]
11. Ozsahin, M.; Gruber, G.; Olszyk, O.; Karakoyun-Celik, O.; Pehlivan, B.; Azria, D.; Roelandts, M.; Kaanders, J.H.; Cengiz, M.; Krengli, M.; et al. Outcome and prognostic factors in olfactory neuroblastoma: A rare cancer network study. *Int. J. Radiat. Oncol. Biol. Phys.* **2010**, *78*, 992–997. [CrossRef] [PubMed]

12. Fitzmaurice, C.; Allen, C.; Barber, R.M.; Barregard, L.; Bhutta, Z.A.; Brenner, H.; Dicker, D.J.; Chimed-Orchir, O.; Dandona, R.; Satpathy, M.; et al. Global Burden of Disease Cancer Collaboration. Global, Regional, and National Cancer Incidence, Mortality, Years of Life Lost, Years Lived with Disability, and Disability-Adjusted Life-years for 32 Cancer Groups, 1990 to 2015: A Systematic Analysis for the Global Burden of Disease Study. *JAMA Oncol.* **2017**, *3*, 524–548, Erratum in *JAMA Oncol.* **2017**, *3*, 418. [PubMed]
13. Myeloma Canada. Available online: https://myelomacanada.ca/en/about-multiple-myeloma/what-is-myeloma/statistics (accessed on 23 February 2023).
14. Kosmala, A.; Bley, T.; Petritsch, B. Imaging of Multiple Myeloma. *Rofo* **2019**, *191*, 805–816. [CrossRef] [PubMed]
15. Wallington-Beddoe, C.T.; Mynott, R.L. Prognostic and predictive biomarker developments in multiple myeloma. *J. Hematol. Oncol.* **2021**, *14*, 151. [CrossRef] [PubMed]
16. Czapiewski, P.; Kunc, M.; Haybaeck, J. Genetic and molecular alterations in olfactory neuroblastoma: Implications for pathogenesis, prognosis and treatment. *Oncotarget* **2016**, *7*, 52584–52596. [CrossRef]
17. Kim, J.W.; Kong, G.; Lee, C.H.; Kim, D.Y.; Rhee, C.S.; Min, Y.G.; Kim, C.W.; Chung, J.H. Expression of Bcl-2 in olfactory neuroblastoma and its association with chemotherapy and survival. *Otolaryngol. Head Neck Surg.* **2008**, *139*, 708–712.
18. Castelnuovo, P.; Turri-Zanoni, M.; Battaglia, P.; Antognoni, P.; Bossi, P.; Locatelli, D. Sinonasal Malignancies of Anterior Skull Base: Histology-driven Treatment Strategies. *Otolaryngol. Clin. N. Am.* **2016**, *49*, 183–200. [CrossRef]
19. Castelnuovo, P.; Bignami, M.; Delù, G.; Battaglia, P.; Bignardi, M.; Dallan, I. Endonasal endoscopic resection and radiotherapy in olfactory neuroblastoma: Our experience. *Head Neck* **2007**, *29*, 845–850. [CrossRef]
20. Morita, A.; Ebersold, M.J.; Olsen, K.D.; Foote, R.L.; Lewis, J.E.; Quast, L.M. Esthesioneuroblastoma: Prognosis and management. *Neurosurgery* **1993**, *32*, 706–714, discussion 714–715. [CrossRef]
21. Arnold, M.A.; Farnoosh, S.; Gore, M.R. Comparing Kadish and Modified Dulguerov Staging Systems for Olfactory Neuroblastoma: An Individual Participant Data Meta-analysis. *Otolaryngol. Head Neck Surg.* **2020**, *163*, 418–427. [CrossRef]
22. Montava, M.; Verillaud, B.; Kania, R.; Sauvaget, E.; Bresson, D.; Mancini, J.; Froelich, S.; Herman, P. Critical analysis of recurrences of esthesioneuroblastomas: Can we prevent them? *Eur. Arch. Oto-Rhino-Laryngol.* **2014**, *271*, 3215–3222. [CrossRef] [PubMed]
23. Balica, N.; Cotulbea, S.; Poenaru, M.; Marin, A.H.; Doros, C.; Lupescu, S.; Boia, E.R.; Stefanescu, H. Olfactory neuroblastoma-Case report. *Front. ORLQ. Mag. Med. Cl.* **2014**, *V*, 20–24.
24. Abdelmeguid, A.S. Olfactory Neuroblastoma. *Curr. Oncol. Rep.* **2018**, *20*, 7. [CrossRef] [PubMed]
25. Bartel, R.; Gonzalez-Compta, X.; Cisa, E.; Cruellas, F.; Torres, A.; Rovira, A.; Manos, M. Importance of neoadjuvant chemotherapy in olfactory neuroblastoma treatment: Series report and literature review. *Acta Otorrinolaringol. Esp.* **2018**, *69*, 208–213. [CrossRef] [PubMed]
26. Modesto, A.; Blanchard, P.; Tao, Y.G.; Rives, M.; Janot, F.; Serrano, E.; Benlyazid, A.; Guigay, J.; Ferrand, F.R.; Delord, J.P.; et al. Multimodal treatment and long-term outcome of patients with esthesioneuroblastoma. *Oral. Oncol.* **2013**, *49*, 830–834. [CrossRef] [PubMed]
27. Su, S.Y.; Bell, D.; Ferrarotto, R.; Phan, J.; Roberts, D.; Kupferman, M.E.; Frank, S.J.; Fuller, C.D.; Gunn, G.B.; Kies, M.S.; et al. Outcomes for olfactory neuroblastoma treated with induction chemotherapy. *Head Neck* **2017**, *39*, 1671–1679. [CrossRef]
28. Thompson, L.D. Olfactory neuroblastoma. *Head Neck Pathol.* **2009**, *3*, 252–259. [CrossRef]
29. Loy, A.H.; Reibel, J.F.; Read, P.W.; Thomas, C.Y.; Newman, S.A.; Jane, J.A.; Levine, P.A. Esthesioneuroblastoma: Continued follow-up of a single institution's experience. *Arch. Otolaryngol. Head Neck Surg.* **2006**, *132*, 134–138. [CrossRef] [PubMed]
30. Morrison, T.; Booth, R.A.; Hauff, K.; Berardi, P.; Visram, A. Laboratory assessment of multiple myeloma. *Adv. Clin. Chem.* **2019**, *89*, 1–58. [CrossRef]

Disclaimer/Publisher's Note: The statements, opinions and data contained in all publications are solely those of the individual author(s) and contributor(s) and not of MDPI and/or the editor(s). MDPI and/or the editor(s) disclaim responsibility for any injury to people or property resulting from any ideas, methods, instructions or products referred to in the content.

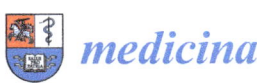

Case Report

The Role of Inverted Papilloma Surgical Removal for Sleep Apnea Treatment Success—A Case Report

Ana Maria Vlad [1,2], Cristian Dragos Stefanescu [1,2,*], Catalina Voiosu [1,2] and Razvan Hainarosie [1,2]

1. Institute of Phonoaudiology and Functional ENT Surgery, 21st Mihail Cioranu Street, 050751 Bucharest, Romania
2. Faculty of Medicine, "Carol Davila" University of Medicine and Pharmacy, 37th Dionisie Lupu Street, 020022 Bucharest, Romania
* Correspondence: dragos.stefanescu@umfcd.ro; Tel.: +40-730047455

Abstract: In recent years, increased attention has been directed to sleep apnea syndrome due to its high prevalence and preventable severe health consequences. Besides enhancing the risk of cardiovascular, cerebrovascular, and metabolic disorders, it determines increased daytime somnolence, cognitive impairment, and delayed reaction time. These symptoms, determined by sleep fragmentation and chronic hypoxemia, can result in a decrease in professional performance and, moreover, could have tragic implications, especially in patients with high-risk professions. We present the case of a 58-year-old male truck driver, known to suffer from uncontrolled OSA and chronic obstructive pulmonary disease, who presented to our ENT department for incapacitating daytime somnolence and severe nasal obstruction. These symptoms were caused by a voluminous sinonasal inverted papilloma, occupying the entire left cavity with extension in the nasopharynx. Following nose permeabilization, the patients' APAP compliance grew substantially, with a dramatic decrease in daytime sleepiness and improvement in polysomnographic parameters. Due to the overlap syndrome of OSA and COPD, an oxygen supplementation was added to PAP therapy by a pulmonologist, improving pulse-oximetry parameters and resulting in the best outcome for the patient. Through this case report, we aim to emphasize the importance of multimodal, personalized treatment of sleep apnea with a focus on nasal surgical permeabilization. At the same time, we sustain a multidisciplinary approach, especially in patients with sleep apnea and associated pathologies, to obtain therapeutic success. We propose increased attention to the early recognition and proper treatment of sleep apnea in patients with high-risk professions as it prevents catastrophes.

Keywords: sleep apnea; nasal surgery; inverted papilloma; CPAP; multimodal treatment; CCPD

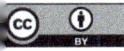

1. Introduction

Sleep apnea is a multifactorial disease that determines the partial or total obstruction of the upper airway during sleep. Left untreated, it results in important health consequences such as cardiovascular, cerebrovascular, and metabolic disorders. Through micro awakenings and oxygen desaturation characterizing the pathology, it leads to daytime sleepiness, cognitive impairment, psychological problems, and a significant reduction in quality of life. Secondary to the patients' delayed reaction time, especially in those suffering from frequent desaturations during sleep, OSA can result in tragic traffic road accidents [1]. Inverted papilloma is a rare benign sinonasal tumor characterized by a strong potential for local destruction, a high rate of recurrence, and a risk of malignant transformation. Nasal obstruction can be the main symptom, especially in voluminous tumors. The treatment of choice nowadays is surgical excision via an endoscopic nasosinusal approach with a favorable outcome [2].

In recent years, a multimodality approach has been studied and applied in the integrative management of obstructive sleep apnea. The role of nasal breathing during the night in healthy individuals is well-established. The implications of nasal obstruction on sleep apnea have been addressed in several studies. The switch to mouth breathing secondary to nasal blockage is associated with increased OSA severity and worse oximetric variables [3]. However, isolated nose surgery for sleep apnea improvement is controversial. Still, nasal surgery significantly improves subjective symptoms of daytime somnolence and is considered to have an important role in CPAP compliance and efficiency [4]. This is of great importance in enhancing the quality of life and results in an indirect reduction of health consequences through correct CPAP utilization. In some cases, in the same patient, sleep apnea and chronic obstructive pulmonary disease (CPOD) can coexist, resulting in so-called overlap syndrome, which brings some particularities in diagnosis and treatment [5].

In this paper, we present the case of a patient known to have sleep apnea and COPD who presented at the hospital with severe daytime sleepiness and nasal obstruction determined by a voluminous inverted papilloma. This is a representative case of individualized care requirements for sleep apnea. Through our case report, we demonstrate that a multimodal, multidisciplinary approach results in successful OSA outcomes and a significant increase in patients' quality of life.

2. Case Report

A 58-year-old patient, known to have sleep apnea and COPD, was referred to our ENT department for a 2-year history of persistent left nasal obstruction, mouth breathing, snoring, daytime somnolence, and gradually worsening sleep apnea episodes. His past medical history consists of an inverted papilloma diagnosed ten years anteriorly, for which he underwent surgery. No recurrences were observed after the end of the treatment.

The patient experienced significant daytime sleepiness that interfered with their daily life. They scored 24 on the Epworth Sleepiness Scale, and reported instances of falling asleep while driving as a truck driver. Hospital admission was sought for further evaluation and management. The flexible nasopharyngoscopic examination revealed the obstruction site. A voluminous papillomatous, yellowish tumor entirely blocked the left nasal fossa extending toward the ipsi- and contralateral choana. (Figure 1). An anterior left nasal deviation was also noted. Mucopurulent secretions were visualized in both nasal fossae.

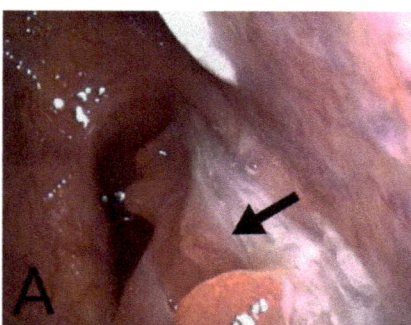 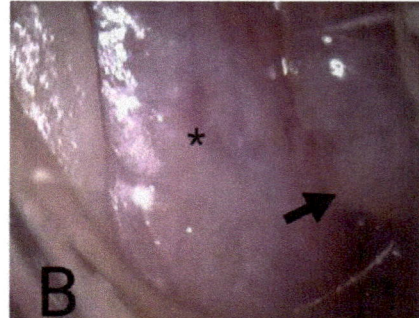

Figure 1. Endoscopic view of the nasal tumor (**A**) right choanal extension of the tumor (black arrow) (**B**) tumor occupying the entire left nasal fossa (black arrow), anterior nasal deviation (*).

A computed tomographic scanning of the head and paranasal sinuses was performed, showing extensive parafluid-solid densities completely occupying the left maxillar, ethmoidal, sphenoidal sinuses and the entire left nasal cavity, expanding in the nasopharynx through the left choana. (Figure 2).

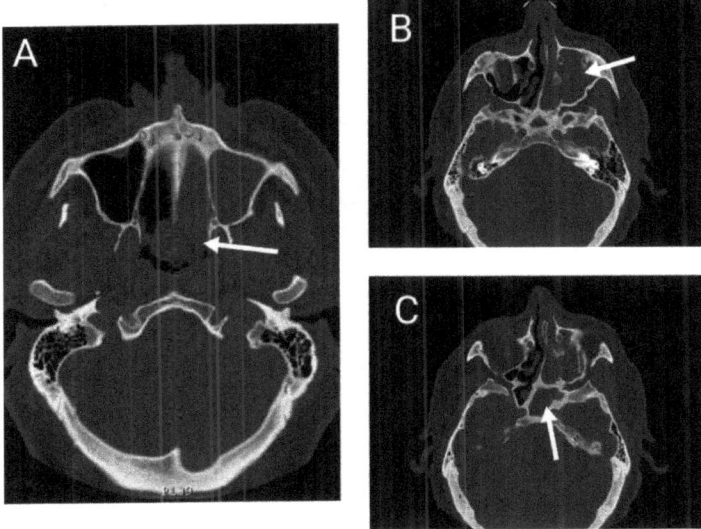

Figure 2. CT scan of the head and paranasal sinuses showing tumor extension in the (**A**) nasal cavity, nasopharynx, and contralateral choana, (**B**) maxillary sinus, (**C**) sphenoidal sinus.

A polysomnographic study showed severe obstructive sleep apnea syndrome (AHI = 67.8) with the most prolonged apnea episode duration of 1 min and 55 s (Table 1). Most episodes were represented by obstructive apneas (oA = 73%), while central and mixed apneas represented 1% and 12%, respectively. The rest of the 13% were hypopneas (Chart).

Table 1. Polysomnographic respiratory parameters at presentation.

Respiratory Evaluation	Findings
AHI (Desat.Cor.) [Per hour]	67.8 (54.9)
RDI (Desat.-Cor.) [Per hour]	67.8 (54.9)
Apnea Index HI (Desat.-Cor.) [Per hour]	58.9 (46.3)
Hypopnea Index HI (Desat.-Cor.) [Per hour]	9.0 (8.6)
No. of Apnea [n]	309
Of them Central: [n]	3
Mean duration of apneas [Sec]	27
No. of Hypopnea [n]	47
Total Apnea/Hypopnea time (RDT) [Hrs]	2:31:45
Apnea/Hypopnea time per hour [Min Per hour]	28:55
Longest Apnea [Min] (t = 22:01:32)	1:55
Longest Hypopnea [Min] (t = 23:25:10)	1:18

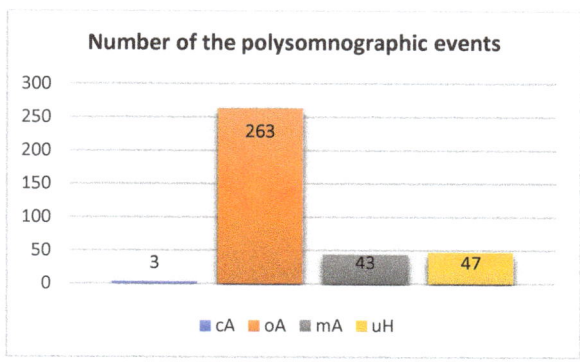

Chart 1. Overview of the polysomnographic events.

These frequent and prolonged apnea episodes influenced pulsoxymetric parameters (Chart 2), determining a desaturation index of 90.0, with a mean O2 saturation of 74% and a minimum saturation of 50% during sleep (Table 2), (Chart 3). The SpO2 reading on the pulse oximeter was 86% during the day, with a pulse range of 65 to 111.

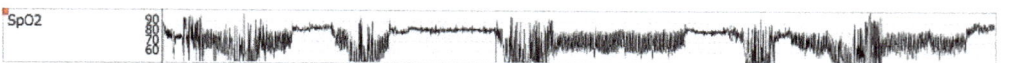

Chart 2. SpO2 variations during examination time.

Table 2. Polysomnographic SpO2 and pulse parameters at presentation.

Evaluation of SpO2/Pulse	Findings
Desaturation-Index DI [per hour]	90.0
No. of desaturations [n]	597
No. of desaturations < 90% [n]	597
Total time [Hrs]	3:24:05
Time per hour [Min Per hour]	30:45
Lowest Desaturation [%] (04:29:38)	50
Longest Desaturation [Sec] (29:39:00)	55
Mean Duration [sec]	20
Mean Desaturation [%]	67
Mean. Saturation [%] (04:48:11)	74
Max. Saturation [%] (22:54:09)	100
Min. Saturation [%] (22:54:09)	50
T90 [%]	98.5
Min. Pulse (01:15:37) [1/min]	65
Max. Pulse (04:40:01) [1/min]	111
Mean Pulse [1/min]	89

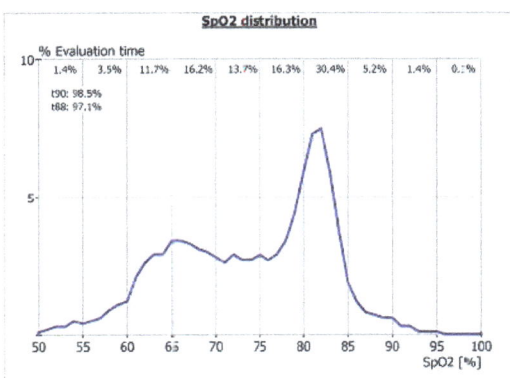

Chart 3. Overview of the polysomnographic SpO2 variations during examination time.

Blood tests were performed, revealing modified complete blood count parameters: hemoglobin 17.9 g/dL (N = 13.1–17), hematocrit 56.2%(N = 39–50%), MCV 103.5 fL (N = 81–101), and RDW 15.7% (N = 11.5–14.5%).

With the patient's informed consent, surgical intervention was proposed. Under general anesthesia with orotracheal intubation, sinonasal videoendoscopic surgery was performed. It consisted of the excision of the tumoral mass from the nasal cavity and nasopharynx with subsequently left maxillary sinus antrostomy, anterior ethmoidectomy, and sphenoidotomy. (Figure 3) Bioptic fragments from the significant sites of tumor extension were sent to the anatomopathological laboratory for histopathological examination.

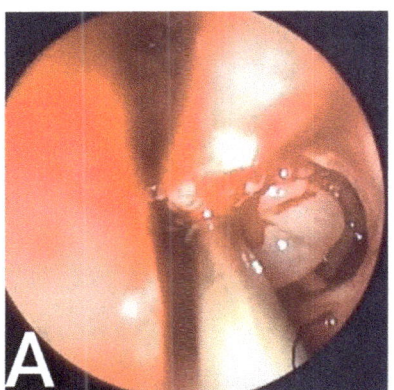
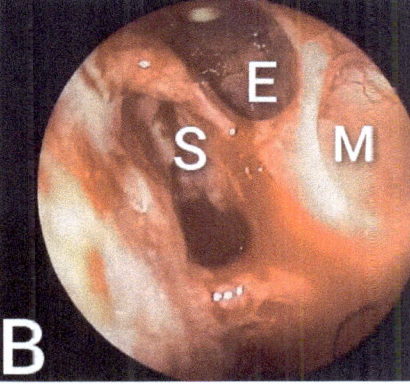

Figure 3. Intraoperative view: (**A**) part of tumor occupying left maxilar sinus (**B**) sphenoical (S), posterior ethmoidal (E) and maxillary (M) sinuses free of tumor.

The postoperative care consisted of intravenous antibiotics, hemostatic agents, and analgesics for pain management. The patient had a favorable result without postoperative complications. The histopathological result was suggestive of inverted papilloma.

Postoperatively, the symptoms of nasal obstruction and daytime somnolence diminished substantially. Even if the leading cause of the patient's complaints had been eliminated, further steps were made to manage the case better. Considering that the patient had multi-level obstruction determining sleep apnea (anteroposterior diminished pharyngeal diameter, elongated uvula, increased neck circumference), an APAP mask was recommended

The polysomnography showed a residual AHI of only 5.4/h in the first month after surgery and PAP therapy prescription. However, even if considerably reduced, pulse oximetry parameters did not reach the levels of desired therapeutic success. APAP treatment was completed with oxygen supplementation during sleep to better manage desaturation episodes. This measure resulted in a very favorable outcome with a ODI of only 18.6 (vs. 90 at first presentation), mean O2 saturation of 91%, and a minimum saturation of 76% (Table 3).

Table 3. Polysomnographic SpO2 and pulse parameters after surgery and PAP implementation.

Evaluation of SpO2/Pulse	Findings	
	APAP without Oxygen Supplementation	APAP with Oxygen Supplementation
Desaturation-Index DI [per hour]	41.8	18.6
No. of desaturations [n]	195	130
No. of desaturations < 90% [n]	193	90
Total time [Hrs]	1:05:12	1:03:39
Time per hour [Min Per hour]	13:58	9:06
Lowest Desaturation [%] (04:29:38)	50	76
Longest Desaturation [Sec] (29:39:00)	1:19	1:58
Mean Duration [sec]	20	29
Mean Desaturation [%]	78	88
Mean. Saturation [%] (04:48:11)	84	91
Max. Saturation [%] (22:54:09)	100	100
Min. Saturation [%] (22:54:09)	50	76
T90 [%]	83.7	18.4
Min. Pulse (01:15:37) [1/min]	32	55
Max. Pulse (04:40:01) [1/min]	171	92
Mean Pulse [1/min]	68	66

Daytime SaO2 increased from 84% before surgery to 93% ten days after surgery. (Figure 4) Secondary to nocturnal oxygen supplementation, the daytime SaO2 reached 96%.

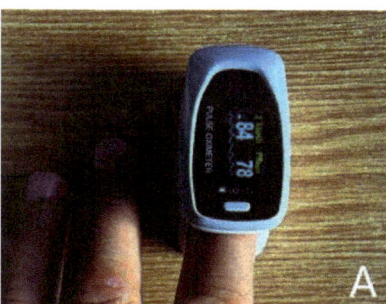 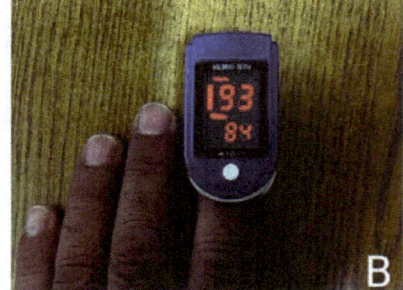

Figure 4. Daytime SaO2 before surgery (**A**) and two weeks after surgery and APAP therapy (**B**).

Secondary polycythemia, highlighted by increased hemoglobin and hematocrit, has been rectified after treatment implementation. Following three months under therapeutic measures, hematocrit decreased by almost 10% (from 56.2 to 47.2%) and hemoglobin by approximately 2 g/d (from 17.9 to 16 g/dL).

A videoendoscopic examination of the nasal cavity was repeated three months after the surgical intervention. The nose was permeable, with no recurrence of nasal tumor observed (Figure 5).

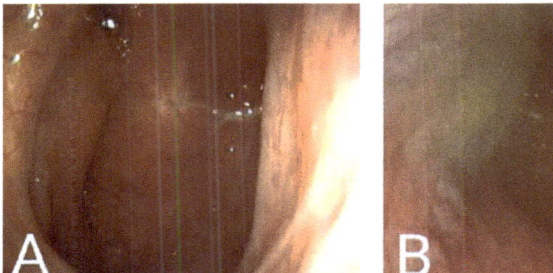

Figure 5. Videoendoscopic examination showing (**A**) right and (**B**) left permeable choana.

The patient completed the Epworth daytime sleepiness scale revealing a score of 0 points, compared to a score of 24 before the treatment. He described that his quality of life improved significantly.

3. Discussion

Obstructive sleep apnea (OSA) is a pathology characterized by recurrent episodes of airway collapse, determining upper airway obstruction during sleep. This leads to subsequent oxygen desaturation, chronic intermittent hypoxia, and repetitive micro awakening, resulting in daytime sleepiness and a wide range of health problems.

The prompt treatment of sleep apnea in the particular case of our patient had a special significance considering his profession. As a truck driver, he represented a real risk for the population. It has been demonstrated that sleep fragmentation and intermittent hypoxemia, characterizing sleep apnea episodes, leads to excessive daytime sleepiness, cognitive processing, and reaction time delays. The most recent and most extensive study on this subject, conducted in Denmark, including all citizens diagnosed with OSA from 1995 to 2015, concluded that sleep apnea patients are not only at an increased risk for road traffic accidents, but also tend to be involved in more severe accidents [1].

We can state that the nasal obstruction determined by the nasal tumor and subsequent severe daytime sleepiness were the main factors that motivated the patient to come to the hospital. Even though he was diagnosed with sleep apnea ten years anteriorly, he chose not to follow any treatment because he did not have such disturbing symptoms as those produced by the tumor. At the same time, he decided not to use APAP therapy even after the onset of the symptoms because of the discomfort created by the high nose resistance.

Nasal breathing is the preferred breathing route during sleep, and various pathophysiological mechanisms could explain the implication of nose obstruction on sleep-disordered breathing and OSA. Firstly, conforming to the Starling resistor model, increased nasal resistance might amplify the collapsibility of oropharyngeal soft tissue due to negative pressure downstream. At the same time, a blocked nose might determine a compensatory switch to mouth breathing that is unfavorable during sleep due to the narrowing of the pharyngeal space, secondary to the base of tongue collapse. Additionally, in the absence of nasal airflow, the receptors for nasal respiratory reflex are not activated, resulting in decreased muscle tone and ventilation. Moreover, a significant quantity of NO is produced in the nose; bypassing it, reduced NO is transferred to the lungs, with subsequent poor blood oxygenation [6–9].

Several studies approached the effect of isolated nasal surgery on sleep apnea improvement. However, in most articles, there was no statistically relevant improvement in the objective parameters quantifiable by polysomnography. The most recently published systematic review (Schoustra et al. 2022) concluded that the apnea-hypopnea index (AHI) did not improve substantially after isolated nasal surgery in most studies. Yet, it had an impressive effect on daytime sleepiness and overall quality of life [10]. Nonetheless, the authors observed a slight decrease in AHI in the patients followed for more than three months postoperatively and suggested that future research papers should focus more on the extended follow-up to quantify the changes in polysomnographic indices better.

In our case, it is hard to measure the exact impact of surgery on daytime sleepiness due to the patient using CPAP immediately after tumor removal. However, the combination of nasal surgery and CPAP use led to a significant improvement in the patient's Epworth Sleeping Scale score, reducing it from 24 to 0. There is limited re-search on the relationship between inverted papilloma and sleep apnea, but several studies have explored the connection between other causes of nasal obstruction and OSA. A clinical trial published in 2019 [11]. concluded that endoscopic sinus surgery for nasal polyps improves sleep efficiency by dramatically decreasing the arousal index on polysomnography following nasal permeabilization. Through this mechanism, a significant reduction of daytime somnolence resulted.

It is interesting to note the discordance between the subjective and objective parameters change following nasal surgery. Iwata et al. 2020 came up with an intriguing explanation for this phenomenon [12]. They assume that besides lowering daytime sleepiness, the comfortable and profound sleep following nasal permeabilization determines greater collapsibility of pharyngeal structures. Thus, the two processes cancel each other out, resulting in an unchanged AHI.

In agreement with previous studies, a review published in 2022 regarding the holistic care of patients with sleep apnea concluded that restoring nasal breathing is indispensable in optimizing OSA treatment outcomes [4]. This statement is sustained by our case, too. We used a personalized, multimodal treatment for our patient, with great success in improving both subjective and objective quantifiable parameters of OSA. After endoscopic nasal surgery for tumor removal, an APAP mask was recommended. The patient was very compliant to night-time ventilation therapy, with a mean usage time of 87% three months after the surgery. This high compliance is consistent with various studies in the literature sustaining the importance of nasal surgery for CPAP adherence. Brimioulle et al., 2022, reviewed the literature to emphasize the bidirectional link between nose and CPAP use. Even if CPAP's effects on the nose remain uncertain, all studies reported a correlation between lower nasal resistance and higher CPAP compliance [13].

The overlap syndrome describes the coexistence of obstructive sleep apnea in patients with chronic obstructive pulmonary disease (COPD) [14]. It has been shown that overlap patients are particularly prone to oxygen desaturation during sleep, making the overnight oxygen desaturation frequency (ODI) the most crucial variable to evaluate in this category of patients [5]. Our patient's polysomnographic indices show extremely frequent desaturations (ODI = 90), supporting the data in the literature. PAP remains the standard treatment for OSA and is also accepted for overlap syndrome. However, in some cases, CPAP alone may not be sufficient for hypoxemia correction, and supplemental oxygen might be needed [15]. Even though the CPAP therapy reduced the oxygen desaturation index by more than half, it was not sufficient for therapeutic success in our case. With 4 L of supplemental oxygen, the measured parameters improved substantially, resulting in an ODI of only 18.6 and a mean oxygen saturation of 91%. These therapeutic measures positively impacted blood test results resolving secondary polycythemia. Hemoglobin and hematocrit reached normal values three months after treatment implementation. Considering the known association between elevated hematocrit levels and increased cardiovascular and all-cause mortality [16], the reduction of almost 10% in our case (from 56.2% to 47.2%) may translate into potentially favorable clinical outcomes.

4. Conclusions

Daytime somnolence determined by sleep apnea can result in cognitive function deterioration followed by a decline in professional performance and, in the case of high-risk professions (driver, locomotive mechanic, pilot, etc.), can lead to major transportation disasters.

Nasal surgery facilitates non-invasive pressure support because the patients require lower pressures for similar effects. This implies an improvement in PAP therapy compliance with consequent benefits for the patient, for society (by reducing accidents), and for the health system (by reducing the costs associated with chronic preventable conditions).

The interdisciplinary (ENT, pneumology) and multimodal (nasal surgery, non-invasive ventilation) approaches represent an adequate therapeutic solution for patients suffering from sleep apnea with multiple comorbidities.

Author Contributions: A.M.V. had equal contribution with C.D.S. in designing the research, data acquisition, analysis and interpretation of data, and wrote the manuscript. C.V. and R.H. performed the experiments, data acquisition, analysis and interpretation of data and manuscript drafting. A.M.V., C.D.S. and R.H. contributed to statistical analysis, critical revision of the manuscript for important intellectual content. All authors have read and agreed to the published version of the manuscript.

Funding: This research received no external funding.

Institutional Review Board Statement: The study was conducted according to the guidelines of the Declaration of Helsinki, and approved by the Ethics Committee) of Institute of Phonoaudiology and Functional ENT Surgery.

Informed Consent Statement: Written informed consent was obtained from the patient for the publication of the data; the privacy data regulation was followed.

Data Availability Statement: Not applicable.

Conflicts of Interest: The authors declare no conflict of interest.

References

1. Udholm, N.; Rex, C.E.; Fuglsang, M.; Lundbye-Christensen, S.; Bille, J.; Udholm, S. Obstructive sleep apnea and road traffic accidents: A Danish nationwide cohort study. *Sleep Med.* **2022**, *96*, 64–69. [CrossRef] [PubMed]
2. Lisan, Q.; Laccourreye, O.; Bonfils, P. Sinonasal inverted papilloma: From diagnosis to treatment. *Eur. Ann. Otorhinolaryngol. Head Neck Dis.* **2016**, *133*, 337–341. [CrossRef] [PubMed]
3. Hsu, Y.; Lan, M.Y.; Huang, Y.C.; Kao M.C.; Lan, M.C. Association between Breathing Route, Oxygen Desaturation, and Upper Airway Morphology. *Laryngoscope* **2021**, *131*, E659–E664. [CrossRef] [PubMed]
4. Tsai, M.S.; Chen, H.C.; Liu, S.Y.C.; Lee, L.A.; Lin, C.Y.; Chang, G.H.; Tsai, Y.; Lee, Y.C.; Hsu, C.M.; Li, H.Y. Holistic care for obstructive sleep apnea (OSA) with an emphasis on restoring nasal breathing: A review and perspective. *J. Chin. Med Assoc. JCMA* **2022**, *85*, 672–678. [CrossRef] [PubMed]
5. McNicholas, W.T. COPD-OSA Overlap Syndrome: Evolving Evidence Regarding Epidemiology, Clinical Consequences, and Management. *Chest* **2017**, *152*, 1318–1326. [CrossRef] [PubMed]
6. De Sousa Michels, D.; da Mota Silveira Rodrigues, A.; Nakanishi, M.; Sampaio, A.L.L.; Venosa, A.R. Nasal Involvement in Obstructive Sleep Apnea Syndrome. *Int. J. Otolaryngol.* **2014**, *2014*, 717419. [CrossRef]
7. Ishii, L.; Roxbury, C.; Godoy, A.; Ishman, S.; Ishii, M. Does Nasal Surgery Improve OSA in Patients with Nasal Obstruction and OSA? A Meta-analysis. *Otolaryngol. Head Neck Surg.* **2015**, *153*, 326–333. [CrossRef] [PubMed]
8. Awad, M.I. Nasal Obstruction Considerations in Sleep Apnea. *Otolaryngol. Clin. N. Am.* **2018**, *51*, 1003–1009. [CrossRef] [PubMed]
9. Torre, C.; Capasso, R.; Zaghi, S.; Williams, R.; Liu, S.Y.-C. High incidence of posterior nasal cavity obstruction in obstructive sleep apnea patients. *Sleep Sci. Pract.* **2017**, *1*, 286. [CrossRef]
10. Schoustra, E.; van Maanen, P.; den Haan, C.; Ravesloot, M.J.L.; de Vries, N. The Role of Isolated Nasal Surgery in Obstructive Sleep Apnea Therapy—A Systematic Review. *Brain Sci.* **2022**, *12*, 1446. [CrossRef] [PubMed]
11. Nourizadeh, N.; Rasoulian, B.; Majidi, M.R.; Ardani, A.R.; Rezaeitalab, F.; Asadpour, H. Sleep quality after endoscopic sinus surgery in patients with sinonasal polyposis. *Auris Nasus Larynx* **2019**, *46*, 866–870. [CrossRef] [PubMed]
12. Iwata, N.; Nakata, S.; Inada, H.; Kimura, A.; Hirata, M.; Yasuma, F. Clinical indication of nasal surgery for the CPAP intolerance in obstructive sleep apnea with nasal obstruction. *Auris Nasus Larynx* **2020**, *47*, 1018–1022. [CrossRef] [PubMed]
13. Brimioulle, M. Nasal function and CPAP use in patients with obstructive sleep apnoea: A systematic review. *Sleep Breath. = Schlaf Atm.* **2022**, *26*, 1321–1332. [CrossRef] [PubMed]
14. Singh, S.; Kaur, H.; Singh, S.; Khawaja, I. The Overlap Syndrome. *Cureus* **2018**, *10*, e3453. [CrossRef] [PubMed]
15. Owens, R.L. Sleep-Disordered Breathing and COPD: The Overlap Syndrome. *Respir. Care* **2010**, *55*, 1333. [PubMed]
16. Martelli, V.; Carelli, E.; Tomlinson, G.A.; Orchanian-Cheff, A.; Kuo, K.H.M.; Lyons, O.D.; Ryan, C.M. Prevalence of elevated hemoglobin and hematocrit levels in patients with obstructive sleep apnea and the impact of treatment with continuous positive airway pressure: A meta-analysis. *Hematology* **2022**, *27*, 889–901. [CrossRef] [PubMed]

Disclaimer/Publisher's Note: The statements, opinions and data contained in all publications are solely those of the individual author(s) and contributor(s) and not of MDPI and/or the editor(s). MDPI and/or the editor(s) disclaim responsibility for any injury to people or property resulting from any ideas, methods, instructions or products referred to in the content.

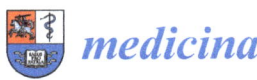

Article

Efficacy of Continuous Suctioning in Adenoidectomy Haemostasis—Clinical Study

Veronica Epure [1,2,*], Razvan Hainarosie [1,3,*] and Dan Cristian Gheorghe [1,2]

1. ENT Department, Carol Davila University of Medicine and Pharmacy, 020021 Bucharest, Romania
2. ENT Department, "Marie Curie" Children Hospital, Bd. C. Brâncoveanu 20, 041451 Bucharest, Romania
3. I.F.A.C.F.-ORL Prof Dr. D. Hociota, M. Cioranu 21, 061344 Bucharest, Romania
* Correspondence: veronica_epure@yahoo.co.uk (V.E.); razvan.hainarosie@umfcd.ro (R.H.)
Tel.: +40-214604260 (V.E.); +40-214102170 (R.H.)

Abstract: *Introduction*: Adenoidectomy is often the first major surgical challenge for the child's haemostatic system, and controlling intraoperative bleeding can be a challenge for the surgeon. Different methods have been used intraoperatively by surgeons in order to enhance haemostasis. The cold air effect (continuous suctioning) has been used by some surgeons during adenoidectomy; however, no documentation of its haemostatic effect has been made. *Objectives*: Our prospective randomised controlled study enrolled a sample of 140 children undergoing adenoidectomy, and we studied the effect of continuous suctioning on the duration of haemostasis in paediatric adenoidectomy. *Materials and Methods*: We evaluated the effect of using continuous suctioning during haemostasis at the end of adenoidectomy procedures, comparing variables such as total surgery time, total haemostasis time, and intraoperative blood loss, between two groups: 70 adenoidectomy procedures where no continuous suctioning was used to enhance haemostasis versus the other 70 patients where continuous suctioning was the haemostatic method employed. RESULTS: After statistical analysis of the recorded data, we found that the total duration of adenoidectomy, the duration of haemostasis in adenoidectomy, and the intraoperative blood loss were significantly lower in patients in whom cold air was used for haemostasis. Intraoperative haemostasis failure (and consequent use of electrocautery for haemostasis) was more frequent in patients in whom no suctioning was used; as for the rates of postoperative primary bleeding after adenoidectomy, they were similar in both groups of patients, regardless of the technique used for haemostasis. *Conclusions*: The use of continuous suctioning during adenoidectomy haemostasis significantly shortens total surgical and haemostasis time, reduces intraoperative blood loss, and reduces the incidence of haemostasis failure (with the consequent need for bipolar electrocautery haemostasis).

Keywords: operative time; haemostasis time; adenoidectomy; continuous suctioning; primary postadenoidectomy hemorrhage

1. Introduction

Adenoidectomy is one of the most commonly performed surgical procedures in paediatric ENT [1,2]. In children, these procedures are sometimes the first major surgical challenge to their haemostatic system. Adenoidectomy is indicated for obstructive sleep apnea or recurrent infections of the adenoid mass and neighbouring organs [1]; adenotonsillectomy's incidence has dramatically increased over the last 20 years due to its utility in preventing obstructive sleep apnea and its negative side-effects (cognitive and behavioural disorders, learning difficulties, nocturnal enuresis, hypertension) [2].

Although generally accepted as a safe procedure by most surgeons, postoperative bleeding remains the most significant and scarring complication of adenoidectomy. Postadenotonsillectomy (PAT) bleeding, although rare (cited incidence of 0.5–4.2%) [1,2], requires immediate treatment and can be life-threatening to the patient, whereas intraoperative bleeding remains a challenge to the surgeon, requiring immediate action to control it.

Citation: Epure, V.; Hainarosie, R.; Gheorghe, D.C. Efficacy of Continuous Suctioning in Adenoidectomy Haemostasis—Clinical Study. *Medicina* 2023, 59, 1534. https://doi.org/10.3390/medicina59091534

Academic Editor: Steven M. Parnes

Received: 9 June 2023
Revised: 3 August 2023
Accepted: 23 August 2023
Published: 24 August 2023

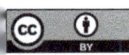

Copyright: © 2023 by the authors. Licensee MDPI, Basel, Switzerland. This article is an open access article distributed under the terms and conditions of the Creative Commons Attribution (CC BY) license (https://creativecommons.org/licenses/by/4.0/).

Decreasing postoperative pain, reducing the operative and haemostasis duration, and minimising intraoperative and postoperative haemorrhage risk have brought attention to new surgical techniques and instrumentation. Different techniques are nowadays used for paediatric adenoidectomy: cold surgery—the conventional curettage (so-called blind curettage) with Beckmann curette; microdebrider (shaver) or endoscopic—assisted adenoidectomy; hot methods—electrocautery adenoidectomy [3,4], adenoidectomy with radiofrequency (coblation) [3,4], each method presenting its own advantages and possible side-effects.

Most authors agree that operative time and blood loss are significantly reduced in the case of electrocautery used in adenoidectomy surgery [5–8]. Whereas some authors report no complications after electrocautery adenoidectomy [9,10], others report a higher risk of secondary (delayed) haemorrhage and a greater incidence of neck pain (referred pain at the back of the child's head) after bipolar electrocautery use (incidence up to 12%) [2,4,5,11], prolonged nasal obstruction, and velopharyngeal insufficiency symptoms.

Most authors agree that electrocautery use during adenoidectomy or adenotonsillectomy, regardless of duration of use, produces notable side-effects such as delayed epithelisation of the surgical bed [5–7,9,12]; all electrosurgical lesions demonstrate some adjacent areas of desiccation, coagulation, and carbonisation, regardless of the power, duration, or waveform used (radiofrequency included) [11–13].

Knowing the worrisome side-effects of electrocautery use in performing haemostasis for adenoidectomy, alternative methods to reduce blood loss and haemostasis time in adenoidectomy were investigated. Surgeons have started to use different biomaterials or topical agents at the end of surgical procedures in order to speed up haemostasis; however, there are always issues related to materials' availability or costs and the personal preferences of the surgeon. Haemostasis during adenoidectomy can be spontaneous, aided by gauze packings in the nasopharynx (simple or with vasoconstrictor agents as pseudoefedrine, xylometasoline, epiephrine dilution [10], tranexamic acid [14]), irrigation with hydrogen peroxide [15] or saline solutions at different temperatures [16,17], applying fibrin-based biomaterials or oxidised cellulose [18,19]. Applications of bipolar electrocautery or posterior nasal packing [19] are used as final solutions when all previous methods for haemostasis fail. Continuous suctioning has been used by some surgeons during adenoidectomy haemostasis; however, no documentation of its haemostatic effect has been made.

While various haemostatic techniques used during adenoidectomy have been studied [8,12–19], there is limited evidence of the efficacy of continuous suctioning during adenoidectomy haemostasis [20–26]. This study refers to intraoperative postadenoidectomy bleeding and ways to control it effectively. The aim of this study was to evaluate if continuous suctioning during adenoidectomy (creating a local "cold air effect"), a costless and easily accessible method, is efficient for shortening haemostasis and operative time and reducing intraoperative blood loss. The effect of suctioning used intraoperatively on the incidence of early postadenoidectomy haemorrhage was also studied in our enrolled children.

2. Methods

We conducted a prospective randomised controlled study in the ENT Department of a tertiary Children's Hospital between November 2022 and January 2023, involving children undergoing adenoidectomy. The aim of our study was to assess the cause—effect relationship between an intervention (use of continuous suctioning during adenoidectomy) and outcome (duration of haemostasis, total operative time, intraoperative bleeding, and incidence of early postoperative bleeding).

Our Hospital's Ethics Committee has approved this clinical study (53792/12 December 2022). After explaining the procedures and objectives of the study, parents' written consent was obtained in each case for preoperative blood tests, surgery, general anaesthesia, and inclusion in this study.

In our study, patient records were anonymised, data were collected in an Excel database, and it was analysed. The investigators for this study introduced in the OR protocols for adenoidectomies the exact measurements of the operative time, haemostasis time, and number of gauze packings used intraoperatively for each adenoidectomy procedure. The use of bipolar electrocautery to complete haemostasis was recorded for each patient in their surgical protocol.

Inclusion and exclusion criteria. 140 children were included in this study, divided into two groups. Children aged 0 to 18 years were enrolled if they met the following inclusion criteria: 1—child admitted to the Paediatric ENT Department of our hospital; 2—indication of adenoidectomy under general anaesthesia (due to obstructive sleep apnea or severe recurrent upper respiratory tract infections; recurrent acute otitis media or chronic serous otitis media); 3—laboratory tests (blood markers) performed preoperatively by our hospital's laboratory with no major coagulation abnormalities reported; 4—simple adenoidectomy procedures performed between November 2022 and January 2023 by the same 3 ENT experienced consultants; 5—adenoidectomies performed only on 2 days per week (Wednesdays and Fridays) during the trial period.

Adenoidectomies performed by any surgeon in the department on other weekdays were excluded. Adenoidectomies with myringotomy tube insertion or adenotonsillectomies were excluded from our study. Adenoidectomies performed by other surgeons, even if during the same 6-month period in the same department, were excluded.

The two analysed groups were defined by the presence or absence of a specific intervention (use of continuous suctioning). Group A enrolled children for whom continuous suctioning was used at the end of the adenoidectomy procedure. Group B consisted of children in whom no continuous suctioning was used during an adenoidectomy. Children were randomly recruited by the leading investigator from children undergoing adenoidectomy in our department over a 6-month period and assigned randomly to one of the two groups.

Patients were randomly assigned to groups A or B preoperatively. The leading investigator chose intervention days such that all enrolled surgeons used continuous suction on these specific days, while they used other haemostatic methods during the rest of the study (cotton packings, electrocautery). As a result, every surgeon out of the three participating in our study performed adenoidectomy with or without the application of continuous suctioning during this study period, but on different days. This was decided in order to eliminate bias and ensure the randomisation of the participants.

All adenoidectomies were performed under general anaesthesia with orotracheal intubation by three different surgeons, consultants with over 15 years of similar surgical experience, using the same technique and identical equipment, as well as the same anaesthesia procedure. General anaesthesia was performed with sevoflurane induction, and maintenance is carried out accordingly with intravenous propofol along with sevoflurane as needed. After initial endoscopic evaluation of the child's nasopharynx (drug-induced sleep endoscopy), classic cold instrument adenoidectomy was performed in all cases (Beckmann's curette adenoidectomy technique) under direct vision (hyperextension of the child's neck, unilateral Nelaton's probe used to retract the soft palate anteriorly and cranially for enhanced direct visualisation of the nasopharynx). Digital palpation of the adenoid mass and nasopharynx was routinely performed prior to and after the procedure in order to ensure complete excision of the adenoid mass. Endoscopic control is always used to assist adenoidectomy when local anatomy makes the inspection of the child's upper rhinopharynx (near the choanae) impossible. After complete resection of the adenoid mass, haemostasis follows these steps: a cotton packing is introduced in the nasopharynx twice (each left in place for a maximum of 1 min), then another packing is soaked in vasoconstrictor medication (epinephrine dilution 1/10), then direct irrigation with saline solution at room temperature (approximately 10 mL). In patients from group A, continuous suctioning via a metallic probe for 3–5 min was applied to the nasopharynx, set at 150 mbar/hPa. No action was taken in group B patients—cotton packings (without other haemostatic solutions) were used as needed until local bleeding stopped or the surgeon decided to use electrocautery for haemostasis.

No other haemostatic materials such as hydrogen peroxide, xylometasoline, topical tranexamic acid, or fibrin-based haemostatic powder were used either in groups A or B to enhance haemostasis. In cases of failure of haemostasis (over 10 min of haemostasis duration, failure of the saline irrigation solutions to clear or localise persistent bleeding from the nasopharynx), the consequent minimal use of bipolar electrocautery to complete haemostasis was allowed. In our department, we use bipolar electrocautery at the lowest setting for coagulation for as short a time as possible, intermittently (at 30 W for a maximum of 2 s).

After surgery, children were monitored in our intensive care unit next to the operating theatre for 20 min, until they were awake and stable, then returned to the clinical ward. Children are encouraged to start early oral intake of clear liquids. The adenoidectomy patient is then supervised for approximately 6 h before discharge. Patients living within 1 hs distance from the hospital are discharged on the same day if no early postoperative bleeding occurs and if they have successfully restarted oral feeding.

Group A (continuous suctioning) enrolled 70 patients in whom continuous suctioning via a metallic probe with a perforated tip was used during adenoidectomy haemostasis. Group B enrolled 70 patients—in whom no continuous suctioning was used during haemostasis.

Suctioning method. We typically use a large metallic tube with a wide tip (approximately 1 cm in diameter) and multiple orifices at its end; the instrument is used both for suctioning from the nasopharynx and as a tongue depressor (Figure 1—the first 2 probes from left were used in our study). The suctioning pressure is set at a low level (150 mbar/hPa). Preferably, the suctioning from the child's nasopharynx during adenoidectomy haemostasis involves keeping the probe's tip at a few millimeters distance from the surrounding nasopharyngeal walls. This way, the metallic probe avoids direct contact with the mucosa and produces a local mucosal turbinary air flow through the nasopharynx, resulting in moderately lower local temperatures and thus stimulating vasoconstriction in the area. The duration of continuous suctioning is 3–5 min for each patient in group A.

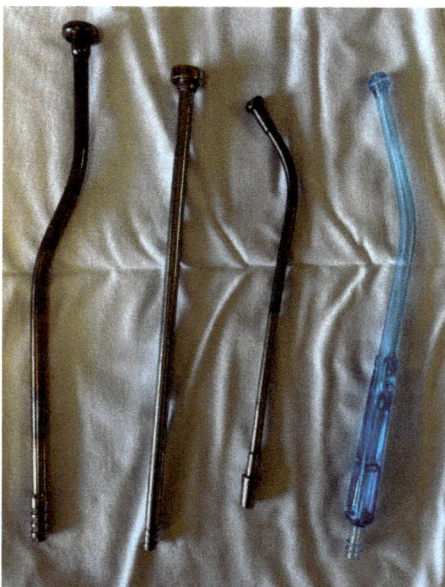

Figure 1. The metallic tubes used for continuous suctioning in our study. The pressure for suctioning is set at 150 mbar.

Outcome variables. Two of the investigators measured and recorded the studied variables in all the patients enrolled in this study: total operative time (time was measured beginning with the first surgical gesture, after retraction of the soft palate, until adenoidectomy completely ended and all instruments were retracted from the operated child's nasopharynx), haemostasis time (defined as the time elapsed after complete excision of the adenoid mass to completion of surgery, when surgical instruments are entirely withdrawn from the child's mouth and nose), and the number of cotton packings used intraoperatively (in order to assess semiquantitatively the blood loss; a packing is considered used if at least 80% soaked in blood). The need for electrocautery use was defined as failure of haemostasis (over 10 min of haemostatic time and/or intense localised and persistent bleeding from the adenoidectomy area) and consequent use of bipolar electrocautery to complete haemostasis. The need for electrocautery use was noted for each group (yes/no answer). Early postadenoidectomy haemorrhage (occurring in the first 24 h postoperatively) in both groups was inferred from OR surgical protocols (yes/no answer) and was retrospectively included in our database. These variables, together with the age and sex of each patient, were used to complete our Excel database.

Choosing the studied sample size followed calculations performed by our statistical analyst and economic reasons. Moreover, it was the number of patients operated on by the 3 designated surgeons on 2 days per week during the study period of 6 months. A statistical analysis was performed on our database to compare the results between the two groups. The R project for statistical computing (R version 4.1.3), Welch's Two Sample t-test, and Pearson's Chi-squared test with Yates' continuity correction were used to compare results between the two groups. A $p < 0.05$ was considered statistically significant.

3. Results

A Welch Two-Sample t-test was used to compare variables between the two groups—group A (70 patients in whom we used continuous suctioning in order to control postadenoidectomy bleeding) (continuous suctioning group) and group B (70 patients with spontaneous postadenoidectomy haemostasis) (no suctioning group). In all the patients, adenoidectomy was performed with cold steel instruments and eventually bipolar electrocautery for bleeding control.

Analysing patients' ages, distributions are similar between the two groups: the mean age in group A was 4.91 years (1–14 years) and in group B was 4.87 years (1–11 years). The difference was not statistically significant ($p = 0.912$), thus the two groups were similar and comparable. Group A consisted of 26 girls and 44 boys, while Group B consisted of 31 girls and 39 boys.

The mean operative time (duration of the adenoidectomy procedure) in group A (continuous suctioning group) was 11.48 min (688.57 s) (with variations between 5.57–22.49 min), while in group B it was 14.49 min (869.72 s) (with variations between 5.10 and 24.14 min). The difference was statistically significant ($p = 0.00001733$, t = -4.4988, df = 107.75).

The average haemostasis times were 8.67 min (520.54 s) in the A group (continuous suctioning group) (range between 3.44 and 13.00 min) and 10.97 min (658.06 s) respectively in group B (range between 2.17 and 23.29 min). The difference between the two groups was statistically significant ($p = 0.0007169$, t = -3.4399, df = 101.27).

A graphical representation of surgery duration with haemostasis, with continuous suctioning and without suctioning is found in Figure 2.

The assessment of quantitative intraoperative blood loss by recording the number of cotton packings used showed an average of 6.04 for group A patients and 8.68, respectively, for group B patients. The difference was statistically significant ($p = 0.00000007763$, t = -5.8318, df = 93.687). A graphic representation of the number of packings used intraoperatively versus total operative time, with and without continuous suctioning, can be found in Figure 3.

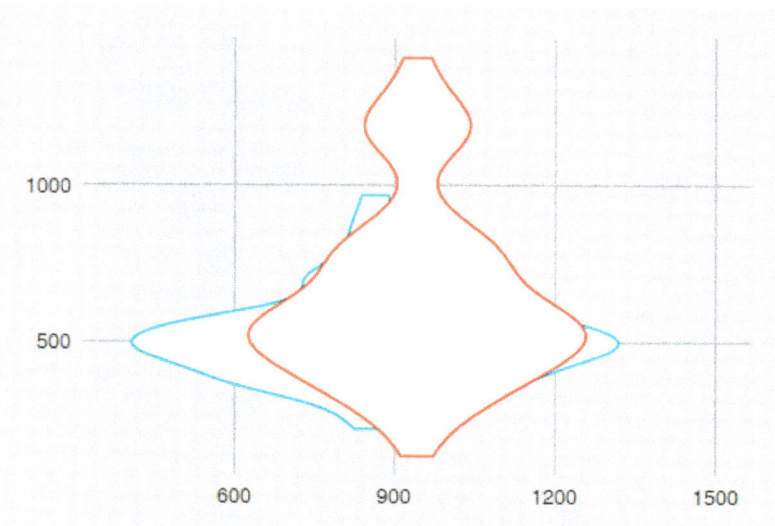

Figure 2. Duration of adenoidectomy procedure versus duration of haemostasis, with continuous suctioning (blue colour) and without suctioning (red colour).

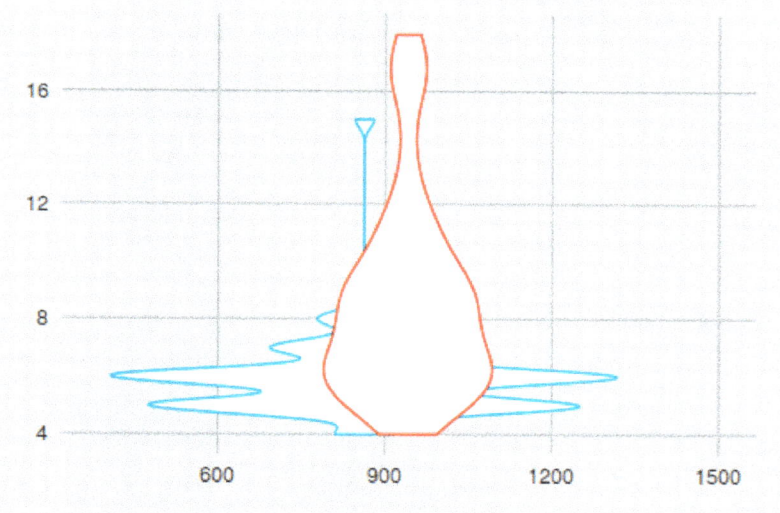

Figure 3. The number of gauze packings used intraoperatively versus total operative time, with (blue colour) and without suctioning (red colour).

Failure of haemostasis and the need for bipolar electrocautery application to the nasopharynx occurred in 4 patients in group A (4 out of 70 patients) and in 22 patients in group B (22 out of the total 70 patients). The difference was statistically significant ($p = 0.0002202$, X-squared = 13.65, df = 1) (Figure 4).

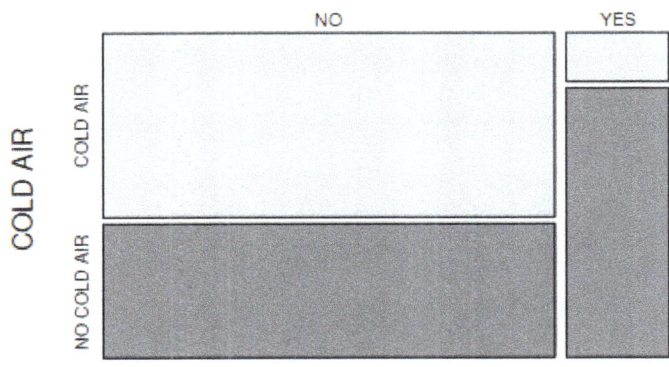

Figure 4. Failure of haemostasis and need for bipolar electrocautery use for haemostasis in groups A and B.

Early postadenoidectomy haemorrhage (occurring in the first 24 h after aderoidectomy) was noted in 3 cases in group A and in 2 cases in group B. This difference between groups was not statistically significant (X-squared = 0, df = 1, $p = 1$), regardless of the use of continuous suctioning (Figure 5).

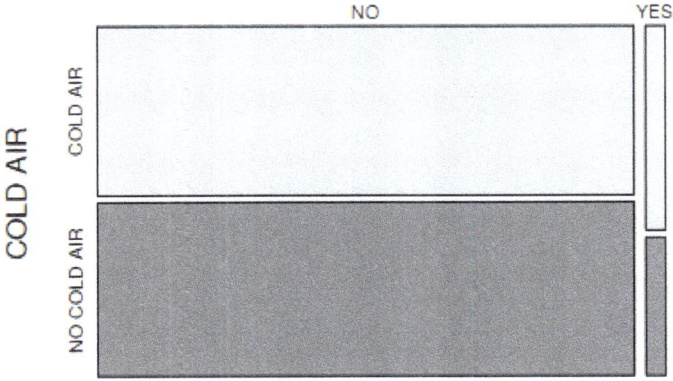

Figure 5. Incidence of early postadenoidectomy haemorrhage in groups A and B.

The structure of the two groups of patients and the results of our study are summarised in Table 1.

Table 1. Structure of the two groups of children, measured variables with comparison, and statistical significance of differences.

	Group A	Group B	Statistical Significance ($p < 0.05$)
Mean age of children	4.91 years (1–14)	4.87 years (1–11)	NO ($p = 0.912$)
Sex	26 F, 44 M	31 F, 39 M	
Mean operative time	11.48 min	14.49 min	YES ($p = 0.00001733$)
Mean haemostasis time	8.67 min	10.97 min	YES ($p = 0.00007169$)

Table 1. *Cont.*

	Group A	Group B	Statistical Significance ($p < 0.05$)
Number of packings used	6.04	8.68	YES ($p = 0.00000007763$)
Failure of haemostasis/use of electrocautery intraoperatively	4/70	22/70	YES ($p = 0.0002202$)
Primary postoperative haemorrhage/use of electrocautery postoperatively	3/70	2/70	NO ($p = 1$)

4. Discussion

There are many studies in the literature regarding the haemostatic effect of different topical agents for bleeding control during adenoidectomy. Most authors agree that topical agents such as hydrogen peroxide, tranexamic acid, saline solutions, and vasoconstrictor/epinephrine dilutions applied locally to the nasopharynx seem to be the most effective in controlling haemostasis after such surgery [8,14–19]. Moreover, a multitude of active fibrin-based topical biomaterials and calcium alginate dressings are used on a large scale to control bleeding during adenoidectomy and accelerate mucosal healing [18]. All these topical agents involve supplementary costs, and their use is largely dependent on the ENT surgeon's preferences and or experience and on the availability of materials from the hospital's supply [9,18].

One study regarding the effect of saline solution irrigation during adenoidectomy haemostasis reported that saline solutions are effective haemostatic agents, especially at hot temperatures (50 °C). The haemostatic effect of hot saline solutions (at 50 °C) was significantly higher compared to the use of cold saline solutions (at 4 °C) [16,17].

We could not find any studies regarding the use of continuous suctioning—a simpler and costless method to stop bleeding during adenoidectomy that is readily available during surgery. No side effects were noted regarding cold air use. Studies investigating lowering the local temperature (for vasoconstriction) at the nasopharyngeal level during adenoidectomy haemostasis report using irrigation of the nasopharynx with cold (4 °C) saline solutions. Most authors agree that cold solutions are less effective in controlling blood loss after adenoidectomy compared with hot solutions [16,17].

Many studies have been conducted to investigate the effects of hypothermia on haemostasis in vitro and in vivo, and these have yielded contradictory results. One of these studies found that mild hypothermia during surgery significantly increases blood loss by 16% (4–26%) and increases the relative risk of transfusion [20]. Other studies conclude that mild hypothermia (temperature >33 °C) is safe from the standpoint of bleeding and might induce increased ADP-stimulated platelet aggregation and increased platelet reactivity (whereas deep hypothermia, i.e., temperature <33 °C, might decrease platelet aggregation). Under normal conditions, blood flow is maximal at the centre of the vessel, and platelets are marginalised to the periphery, close to the scene of injury, thus promoting platelet-endothelial interaction. Mild hypothermia increases the viscosity of blood, thus the marginalisation effect of platelets is more prominent in a hypothermic situation; Higher blood viscosity during hypothermia decreases blood flow velocity, which facilitates the formation of a platelet plug because the forces that tend to draw the platelet plug away from the vessel wall are decreased [18,19]. These pro-coagulative factors are not easily measurable in vitro but seem to be present during hypothermia in vivo [22,23].

As studies show, when the local body temperature drops below 37 °C, platelets become more predisposed to activation by thrombotic stimuli, an event known as priming. The enhanced ability of platelets to prime at peripheral blood sites, where temperatures are lower and the chances of trauma are higher, is thought to have evolved as a protective and adaptive effect against bleeding in humans, whereas more central body sites have greater protection against thrombosis [23].

On exposure to cold, some authors report a marked increase in the affinity of the postjunctional alpha-adrenoreceptors for norepinephrine, resulting in a powerful vasoconstriction and consequent cessation of blood flow to the peripheric tissues (this phenomenon, called hunting reaction was first seen in dogs, then in humans) [24]; the local effects of lowering the temperature to a traumatised region of the body (and consequent enhancing effects on haemostasis) differ from systemic effects of longer exposure of humans to low temperatures, as most of the authors report low temperatures to increase morbidity and mortality in cardiovascular and cerebrovascular patients (by increasing blood pressure via sympathetic nervous system activation) [25].

In the endeavour of offering some explanation for the haemostatis effect of continuous suctioning, we measured the local nasopharyngeal temperature in some of our patients. The protocol of our study did not include assessing the local temperature of every patient enrolled in this study. The mean local temperature we measured intraoperatively at the adenoid area after use of cold air suctioning for 3 min (the device set at 150 mbar) in some of our patients is 34.4 °C, corresponding to mild hypothermia; our study reports enhanced haemostasis in these children, corresponding to data from the literature regarding the effects of mild hypothermia on haemostasis.

Using a metallic suctioning tube at the patient's nasopharyngeal level is not the only way to create locally mild hypothermia, as this effect ("cold air effect") can be reproduced regardless of the suctioning probe's material (plastic as well) and form.

After statistically analysing the data collected in our study and comparing the two groups, we found that the mean operative time during adenoidectomy, mean haemostasis time, and the mean intraoperative blood loss were significantly lower in children in whom continuous suctioning was used during haemostasis. Moreover, the need for electrocautery use because of haemostasis failure is higher in group B of patients in the absence of cold air suction use during adenoidectomy haemostasis. Absolutely no side-effects were noted in our patients in group A (continuous suctioning).

Choosing the studied sample size followed calculations performed by our statistical analyst. Moreover, it was the number of patients operated on by the three designated surgeons on 2 days per week during the study period of 6 months. The sample was small enough to be economically efficient and large enough to draw conclusions that warrant further extension of this study to larger samples of patients.

The mean operative time (duration of the adenoidectomy procedure) in group A (continuous suctioning group) was 11.48 min, while in group B it was 14.49 min; the difference is statistically significant ($p < 0.05$). According to our results, using cold air during adenoidectomy haemostasis reduces operative time by up to 3 min! On an individual level, shortening the total operative time by 3 min might seem unimportant in paediatric adenoidectomy; however, this means shortening the operation by 25%. These findings also prove that continuous suctioning can shorten the total operative time in adenoidectomy, which is the aim of the present study. Shortening the total operative time by 25% can gain importance in a department where the number of daily adenoidectomy procedures is high.

The average haemostasis times were 8.67 min in group A (cold air) and 10.97 min in group B. The comparison of these values is statistically significant ($p < 0.05$). According to our results, using cold air during adenoidectomy haemostasis reduces haemostasis time by up to 2 min!

The number of cotton packings used (reflecting in a semiquantitative manner the intraoperative blood loss) for group A patients was on average 6.04, while for group B patients it was on average 8.68. The comparison between these mean values is also statistically significant ($p < 0.05$). According to our results, using cold air during adenoidectomy haemostasis reduces intraoperative blood loss. Assessment of intraoperative blood loss using the number of packings used intraoperatively for each procedure is a semiquantitative, rapid, and easily reproducible method. Blood suctioned from the patient's nasopharynx is collected in a large graded device; however, individual, exact measuring of blood loss (in mL) for every procedure is difficult in patients from group B, in whom we do not use suction at all.

Failure of haemostasis and the need for bipolar electrocautery application to the nasopharynx were recorded in four patients in group A (4 out of 70 patients) and in 22 patients in group B (22 out of the total 70 patients). The difference is also statistically significant ($p < 0.05$). According to our results, using cold air suction during adenoidectomy haemostasis reduces the need for bipolar electrocautery, avoiding its significant side-effects.

In terms of early postadenoidectomy haemorrhage (during the first 24 h after surgery), there was no significant difference between group A and group B. Thus, we can conclude that cold air use does not interfere with early postoperative bleeding after adenoidectomy.

The dimensions of the adenoid mass were not taken into consideration in this study as an independent factor, as studies show operative time or postoperative haemorrhage risk do not correlate with the grade of hypertrophy of the adenoid mass [26].

Limitations of this study could be the number of enrolled patients (the effects of cold air suction during adenoidectomy haemostasis could benefit from studies on a larger number of patients; however, the size of our sample group is large enough to warrant statistical analysis and offer a correlation hypothesis). The fact that this study is based on a single—centre experience—with a consequently uniform surgical technique and general anaesthesia. The method for assessing intraoperative blood loss through counting the number of cotton packings used for each surgical procedure is a semiquantitative procedure that could eventually be perfected.

5. Conclusions

Local continuous suctioning at the level of the nasopharynx during adenoidectomy haemostasis (via suctioning tube) can be a costless and useful tool to promote immediate haemostasis, as it significantly shortens surgery and haemostasis time, lowers intraoperative blood loss, and reduces the need for electrocautery use in cases of persistent intraoperative bleeding.

Author Contributions: V.E.—conceptualisation, methodology, data curation, formal analysis, writing—original draft, reviewing; R.H.—validation, formal investigation, data curation, writing—review and editing; D.C.G.—methodology, formal analysis, software, resources, project supervision, writing—review and editing. All authors have read and agreed to the published version of the manuscript.

Funding: This research received no external funding.

Institutional Review Board Statement: This study was approved by the Ethics Committee of the Hospital (53792/12 December 2022).

Informed Consent Statement: Written informed consent was obtained from all the children's parents, both for surgery and for inclusion in this study.

Data Availability Statement: Data is available upon request to corresponding author.

Acknowledgments: The publication of this paper was supported by the Unversitiy of Medicine and Pharmacy Carol Davila, through the institutional program *Publish not Perish*.

Conflicts of Interest: The authors declare no conflict of interest.

Abbreviations

PAT postadenotonsillectomy bleeding
ENT Ear, Nose and Throat

References

1. Ikoma, R.; Sakane, S.; Niwa, K.; Kanetaka, S.; Kawano, T.; Oridate, N. Risk factor for posttonsillectomy hemorrhage. *Auris Nasus Larynx* **2014**, *41*, 376–379. [CrossRef] [PubMed]
2. Motta, S.; Testa, D.; Ferrillo, B.; Massimilla, E.A.; Varriale, R.; Barrella, T.; Motta, G.; Motta, G. Can a Surgical Technique Be a Risk for post-tonsillectomy Hemorrhage? Our Point of View. *Arch. Otorhinolaryngol. Head Neck Surg.* **2018**, *1*, 4.

3. Ferreira, M.S.; Mangussi-Gomes, J.; Ximendes, R.; Evangelista, A.R.; Miranda, E.L.; Garcia, L.B.; Stamm, A.C. Comparison of three different adenoidectomy techniques in children—Has the conventional technique been surpassed? *Int. J. Pediatr. Otorhinolaryngol.* **2018**, *104*, 145–149. [CrossRef] [PubMed]
4. Liu, T.; Ji, C.; Sun, Y.; Bai, W. Adverse effects of coblation or microdebrider in pediatric adenoidectomy: A retrospective analysis in 468 patients. *Laryngoscope Investig. Otolaryngol.* **2022**, *7*, 2154–2160. [CrossRef] [PubMed]
5. Clemens, J.; Mc Murray, J.S.; Willging, J.P. Electrocautery versus curette adenoidectomy: A comparison of postoperative results. *Int. J. Pediatr. Otorhinolaryngol.* **1998**, *43*, 115–122. [CrossRef]
6. Soumya, S.; Vissapragada, R.; Le, J.; Ooi, E.H. Halitosis and Pain Post Electrocautery Adenoidectomy. *Medicina* **2019**, *55*, 312. [CrossRef] [PubMed]
7. Stelter, K.; de Sousa, J.M.; Trotter, M.I. Adenotonsillectomy in children: A prospective, randomized study regarding use of bipolar electrocautery vs sharp dissection. *Otolaryngol. Head Neck Surg.* **2002**, *127*, 510–514.
8. Costa, D.J.; Mitchell, R. Adenoidectomy: Cold dissection vs. power-assisted techniques. *Otolaryngol. Head Neck Surg.* **1997**, *117*, 302–304.
9. Reed, J.; Sridhare, S.; Brietzke, S.E. Electrocautery adenoidectomy outcomes: A meta-analysis. *Otolaryngol. Head Neck Surg.* **2009**, *140*, 148–153. [CrossRef]
10. Teppo, H.; Virkkunen, H.; Revonta, M. Topical adrenaline in the control of intraoperative bleeding in adenoidectomy: A randomised, controlled trial. *Clin. Otolaryngol.* **2006**, *31*, 303–309. [CrossRef]
11. Epure, V.; Hainarosie, R.; Voiosu, C.; Gheorghe, D.C. Use and Abuse of Electrocautery in Adenoidectomy Hemostasis. *Medicina* **2023**, *59*, 739. [CrossRef]
12. Beriat, G.K.; Akmansu, S.H.; Ezerarslan, H.; Dogan, C.; Han, U.; Saglam, M.; Senel, O.O.; Kocaturk, S. The comparison of thermal tissue injuries caused by ultrasonic scalpel and electrocautery use in rabbit tongue tissue. *Bosn. J. Basic Med. Sci.* **2012**, *12*, 151–157. [CrossRef]
13. Henry, L.R.; Gal, T.J.; Hair, E.S. Does Increased Electrocautery during Adenoidectomy Lead to Neck Pain? *Otolaryngol. Head Neck Surg.* **2005**, *133*, 556–561. [CrossRef] [PubMed]
14. Albirmawy, O.A.; Saafan, M.E.; Shehata, E.M.; Basuni, A.S.; Eldaba, A.A. Topical application of tranexamic acid after adenoidectomy: A double-blind, prospective, randomized, controlled study. *Int. J. Otorhinolaryngol.* **2013**, *77*, 1139–1142. [CrossRef] [PubMed]
15. Altun, H.; Hanci, D.; Kumral, T.L.; Uyar, Y. The Hemostatic Efficacy of Hydrogen Peroxide Irrigation to Control Intraoperative Bleeding in Adenoidctomy. *Turk. Arch. Otorhinolaryngol.* **2018**, *56*, 193–198. [CrossRef]
16. Ozmen, S.; Ozmen, O.A. Hot saline irrrigation for control of intraoperative bleeding in adenoidctomy: A randomized controlled trial. *Otalaryngol. Head Neck Surg.* **2010**, *142*, 893–897. [CrossRef]
17. Hanci, D.; Sari, H.; Kumral, T.L.; Karaketir, S.; Ekincioglu, M.E.; Uyar, Y. Effects of saline irrigation at various temperatures on bleeding in adenoidectom. *B-ENT* **2019**, *15*, 367–370.
18. Liu, L.; Rodman, C.; Worobetz, N.E.; Johnson, J.; Elmaraghy, C.; Chiang, T. Topical biomaterials to prevent post-tonsillectomy hemorrhage. *J. Otolaryngol. Head Neck Surg.* **2019**, *48*, 45. [CrossRef]
19. El-Anwar, M.W.; Nofal, A.A.; Elmalt, A. Surgicel use in control of primary postadenoidectomy bleeding. *Ear Nose Throat J* **2017**, *96*, 372–375.
20. Kander, T.; Schött, U. Effect of hypothermia on haemostasis and bleeding risk: A narrative review. *J. Int. Med. Res.* **2019**, *47*, 3559–3568. [CrossRef]
21. Zhang, J.-N.; Wood, J.; Bergeron, A.L.; McBride, L.; Ball, C.; Yu, Q.; Pusiteri, A.E.; Holcomb, J.B.; Dong, J.-F. Effects of low temperature on shear-induced platelet aggregation and activation. *J. Trauma* **2004**, *57*, 216–223. [CrossRef] [PubMed]
22. Van Poucke, S.; Stevens, K.; Marcus, A.E.; Lancé, M. Hypothermia: Effects on platelet function and haemostasis. *Thromb. J.* **2004**, *12*, 31. [CrossRef] [PubMed]
23. Scharbert, G.; Kalb, M.; Marschalek, C.; Kozek-Langenecker, S.A. The Effects of Test Temperature and Storage Temperature on Platelet Aggregation: A Whole Blood In Vitro Study. *Obstet. Anesthesia Dig.* **2006**, *102*, 1280–1284. [CrossRef] [PubMed]
24. Sheperd, J.T.; Rusch, N.J.; Vanhoutte, P.M. Effect of cold air on the blood vessel wall. *Gen. Pharmacol.* **1983**, *14*, 61–64. [CrossRef]
25. Zhang, X.; Zhang, S.; Wang, C.; Wang, B.; Guo, P. Effects of Moderate Strength Cold Air Exposure on Blood Pressure and Biochemical Indicators among Cardiovascular and Cerebrovascular Patients. *Int. J. Environ. Res. Public Health* **2014**, *11*, 2472–2487. [CrossRef]
26. Wynn, R.; Rosenfeld, R.M. Outcomes in Suction Coagulator Adenoidectomy. *Arch. Otolaryngol. Head Neck Surg.* **2003**, *129*, 182–185. [CrossRef]

Disclaimer/Publisher's Note: The statements, opinions and data contained in all publications are solely those of the individual author(s) and contributor(s) and not of MDPI and/or the editor(s). MDPI and/or the editor(s) disclaim responsibility for any injury to people or property resulting from any ideas, methods, instructions or products referred to in the content.

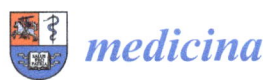

Review

Management of Aesthetic and Functional Deficits in Frontal Bone Trauma

Mihai Dumitru [1], Daniela Vrinceanu [1], Bogdan Banica [2], Romica Cergan [3,*], Iulian-Alexandru Taciuc [4], Felicia Manole [5] and Matei Popa-Cherecheanu [6]

[1] ENT Department, Carol Davila University of Medicine and Pharmacy, 050472 Bucharest, Romania
[2] OMF Surgery Department, Bucharest Emergency University Hospital, 050098 Bucharest, Romania
[3] Anatomy Department, Carol Davila University of Medicine and Pharmacy, 020021 Bucharest, Romania
[4] Department of Pathology, "Carol Davila" University of Medicine and Pharmacy, 050096 Bucharest, Romania
[5] Department of ENT, Faculty of Medicine, University of Oradea, 410073 Oradea, Romania
[6] Department of Cardiovascular Surgery, "Prof. Dr. Agrippa Ionescu" Emergency Clinical Hospital, 011356 Bucharest, Romania
* Correspondence: r.cergan@gmail.com

Abstract: Frontal bone trauma has an increasing incidence and prevalence due to the wide-scale use of personal mobility devices such as motorcycles, electric bicycles, and scooters. Usually, the patients are involved in high-velocity accidents and the resulting lesions could be life-threatening. Moreover, there are immediate and long-term aesthetic and functional deficits resulting from such pathology. The immediate complications range from local infections in the frontal sinus to infections propagating inside the central nervous system, or the presence of cerebrospinal fluid leaks and vision impairment. We review current trends and available guidelines regarding the management of cases with frontal bone trauma. Treatment options taken into consideration are a conservative attitude towards minor lesions or aggressive surgical management of complex fractures involving the anterior and posterior frontal sinus walls. We illustrate and propose different approaches in the management of cases with long-term complications after frontal bone trauma. The team attending to these patients should unite otorhinolaryngologists, neurosurgeons, ophthalmologists, and maxillofacial surgeons. Take-home message: Only such complex interdisciplinary teams of trained specialists can provide a higher standard of care for complex trauma cases and limit the possible exposure to further legal actions or even malpractice.

Keywords: bone; complications; frontal; management; otorhinolaryngology; trauma

1. Introduction

The recent use of Big Data algorithms for analyzing populations for the incidence and prevalence of head trauma cases revealed that the percentage of nasal bone fractures declined, the number of frontal bone fractures remained somewhat constant, whereas those of orbital fractures increased from 2011 to 2016 in a study published based on the Korean population [1]. Moreover in another 8 years retrospective cohort orbital trauma was confirmed in 23.6% of cases with concomitant soft tissue injuries and high risk of loss of vision or ocular motility [2]. This type of trauma presents a male predominance and a mean age of admission of 30 years [3].

Even from the 17th-century trauma to the frontal bone implied medical and legal aspects and still nowadays the distinction between medical/forensic autopsy and anatomical dissections for scientific research can be challenging [4].

The mechanism of trauma production ranges from accidents (automobiles, involuntary falls), human violence (with blunt or sharp objects), or self-inflicted [5].

The force of the impact is important in producing frontal sinus fractures with the involvement of both anterior and posterior sinus walls, like in the cases of animal kicks [6]

Gunshots, although rare, have a clear legal aspect, and unfortunately, when the trajectory affects the frontal sinus the outcome is almost fatal [7].

Unfortunately, there are even some cases of self-inflicted trauma to the head and neck region, and suicide attempts should not be excluded when analyzing a case with frontal bone trauma [8,9].

Frontal sinus fracture management depends on the functional deficit and life-threatening lesions and due to the potential aesthetic implications, the appropriate course of action is still controversial [10].

The arsenal of possible surgical approaches begins with primary closures, the use of osteosynthesis materials, or autologous tissues, sometimes the limit being only the imagination and innovative spirit of the surgical team [11,12].

The complications after such fractures range from local wound infection to nasal bleedings, short episodes of cerebrospinal fluid (CSF) leaks, orbital involvement, and even aesthetic deficits in the long term [13].

We have reviewed the current state-of-the-art practice in the management of aesthetic and functional deficits in frontal bone trauma. Following these guidelines will help clinicians understand the possible future medical and legal implications of these cases and assure proper informed consent on behalf of their patients. Moreover, these complex cases require input from various specialties and cooperation between different surgical departments.

The novelty of the present review resides in the endeavor of uniting the input from multiple specialties to align the guidelines followed by different departments. The objective is to provide a unified response and management of the head trauma cases and diminish the exposure to malpractice. This unified response starts from the very moment of admission, when unfortunately, cases tend to undergo multiple consults or are supervised by the first specialist present into the emergency department. In many cases involving the eyesight the first responder is the ophthalmologist, but further successful management of the patient and surgical planning is better performed by the ENT surgeon or the OMF surgeon [14].

2. Classification of Frontal Bone Fractures

Frontal bone (FB) fractures are found in about 12% of craniomaxillofacial trauma patients. This kind of trauma is a high kinetic energy trauma and subsequently has a high risk of cerebral damage [15].

Anterior wall fractures may be classified as anterior wall fractures with no displacement; anterior wall fractures with displacement but intact frontal sinus outflow tract (FSOT); or anterior wall fractures with displacement and FSOT injury [16].

Posterior wall fractures may be classified as posterior wall fracture without displacement and no cerebrospinal fluid (CSF) leak; posterior wall fractures without displacement and positive CSF leak; posterior wall fracture with displacement and no CSF leak; or posterior wall fracture with displacement and positive CSF leak [17].

3. Complications of Frontal Bone Fractures

Infection of the sinus, which causes sinusitis, may give rise to serious complications due to the proximity of the frontal sinus (FS) to the cranial cavity, orbit, and nasal cavity. Complications can develop into orbital cellulitis, epidural abscess, subdural abscess, and frontal lobe abscess. These complications may develop immediately or later after the traumatic episode [18].

Immediate complications in the fractures of the superior wall of the orbit with the involvement of the FS may occur within up to 6 months from the trauma—frontal sinusitis, meningitis, brain abscess, cavernous sinus thrombosis, cerebrospinal leak, diplopia, blindness, limitation of eye movement, neurosensory deficiency in the territory of the supraorbital nerves [19]. Late complications can occur more than 6 months after the trauma—formation of mucocele or mucopiocele, late frontal sinusitis, secondary brain abscess, and aesthetic defects.

4. Management of Frontal Bone Fractures (FBF)

The aims of FBF treatment are the restoration of facial appearance, the restoration of skull integrity and protection of the brain, and the prevention of late complications. The most important factor in the management of FBF is the involvement of the frontal sinus (FS). Despite the relative frequency of FS injuries, there is no consensus about their optimal management and numerous treatment algorithms were published in recent years [20].

A complicating factor is the involvement of the nasofrontal duct (FND). Its obstruction can lead to mucus retention and late infectious complications like frontal mucocele. So, the therapeutic options for frontal sinus fractures depend on the involvement of the anterior and posterior walls, and the functional integrity of the frontonasal duct [21].

Conservative treatment is indicated in cases where the fractures are strictly limited to the anterior wall of the frontal sinus and it presents a minimal displacement, without involving the frontonasal duct [22].

Reduction and osteosynthesis in displaced fractures are necessary but maintain FND permeability [23]. Displaced anterior wall fracture usually leads to a simple aesthetic deformity (Figure 1). Such a fracture needs surgery for correction. We performed surgery using the trans-eyebrow approach (Figure 2).

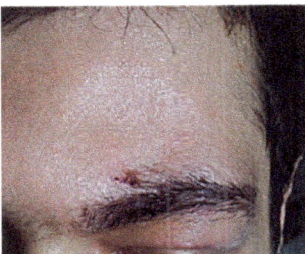

Figure 1. Left frontal sinus fracture with displacement.

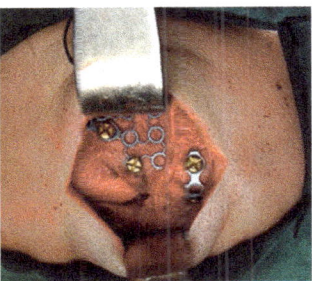

Figure 2. Osteosynthesis of a left frontal sinus fracture with displacement.

When we have a complex frontal orbital fracture, it becomes necessary a coronal approach for reduction and osteosynthesis [24]. This enables a wide exposure of the fracture site with the possibility of repositioning the bone fragments in an anatomic position and insertion of osteosynthesis devices (Figures 3 and 4). In the case of small bone fragments, individual positioning is difficult and the optimal approach is ablation and reconstruction with titanium mesh (Figures 5 and 6).

Exclusion of the frontal sinus by obliterating it in case the FND permeability is compromised but the posterior wall is intact. In this case, all the remaining mucous lining of the frontal sinus is completely cleared, and the frontonasal duct is obliterated with bone and periosteum. The sinus is obliterated with muscle, fat, or bone—without a consensus in the literature on the materials used for this purpose [25].

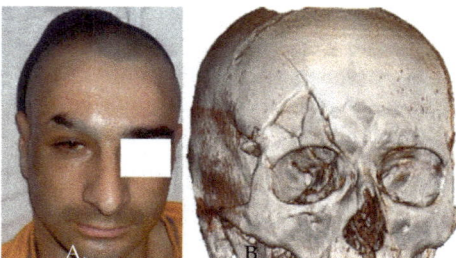

Figure 3. Human aggression using an axe resulting in right frontal sinus fracture with displacement—(**A**) clinical aspect; (**B**) 3D CT reconstruction.

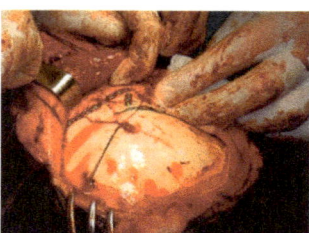

Figure 4. Coronal approach with surgical reduction and osteosynthesis of a right frontal sinus fracture with multiple fragments displacement.

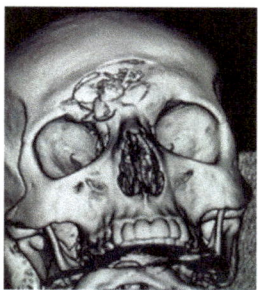

Figure 5. 3D CT reconstruction of a right frontal fracture with displacement.

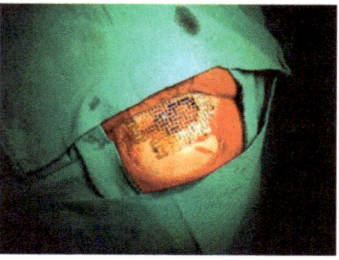

Figure 6. Surgical aspect of a right frontal sinus fracture with displacement benefiting from the use of a titanium mesh reconstruction.

The fourth method of treatment is the cranialization of the frontal sinus, namely the disintegration of the posterior wall of the frontal sinus, obliteration of the frontonasal duct, complete closure of the sinus mucosa, and obliteration of the sinus with bone, fat, or muscle [26]. Posterior wall fracture usually results from high-impact injury and bears a risk of placing the intracranial content in direct communication with the nasal cavity. In posterior wall fracture, it is compulsory a mixed team formed by neurosurgeon, maxillofacial surgeon, and ENT surgeon [27].

Cranialization of the frontal sinus is the most radical method of FS fracture management. the procedure with complete removal of the posterior table. In effect, it increases the volume of the anterior cranial fossa at the expense of cranialized FS, and the brain can expand into this additional extradural dead space. Because intracranial space is entered, and there is a possibility of encountering dura and brain injury, cranialization should always be performed in cooperation with a neurosurgeon [28].

Autogenous bone graft for FS obliteration was first described. Cancellous bone grafts, most often harvested from the ilium, have been widely used as a filler material. Cancellous bone promotes re-ossification from both the periphery of the defect and centrally. Another advantage of cancellous bone over adipose or muscle tissue for obliteration is that it is easier to distinguish radiographically in the postoperative period between resorption, infection, and mucocele formation. Much more comfortable and safer is to harvest bone chips from the adjacent calvarium. It can be done using a bone scraper. In case the harvested amount of bone is not sufficient for filling a large sinus. it can be augmented by an admixture of bone substitutes such as a demineralized bone matrix [29].

5. Management of Mucoceles after Trauma to the Frontal Sinus

The occurrence of a frontal mucocele after trauma is a complication that may appear late after the moment of the trauma, even after a decade. There were some cases described after 35 years of trauma moment. Given this aspect, the patient should undergo a periodic evaluation for local tumefaction, double vision, eyelid ptosis, and local pain at palpation [30].

Frontal sinus mucoceles are cysts with the wall neighboring the periosteum lined with respiratory epithelium and containing fluid transforming into sterile puss. They are affecting patients over fifty and the cause is disruption of the drainage pathway. Up to one-third of the cases appear after trauma [31].

Clinically the patients present with eyelid ptosis and deformity of the superior eyebrow appearing for a long period without local inflammation. Sometimes the patients were initially admitted to neurosurgery departments with the reconstruction of the defects using metal plates (Figure 7).

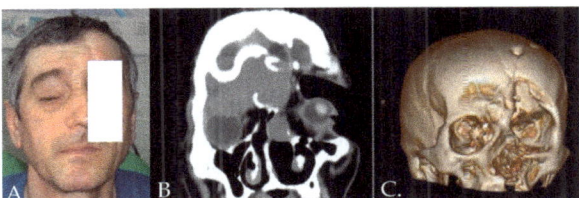

Figure 7. Right frontal sinus mucocele developed after trauma with right orbital involvement—(**A**) clinical aspect; (**B**) CT scan; (**C**) 3D reconstruction.

Treatment targets complete removal of the cyst, and closure of the sinus cavity and frontal-nasal duct with fascia, temporal muscle, and autologous bone. Usually, a coronal approach is preferred with osteotomy superior to the eyebrow arch to preserve local bony landmarks [32].

One important aspect is the involvement of the orbit roof. This bony landmark requires fixation by titanium plates (Figure 8). Commonly the patient evolution after surgery is uneventful without further impairment of the eye movements (Figure 9).

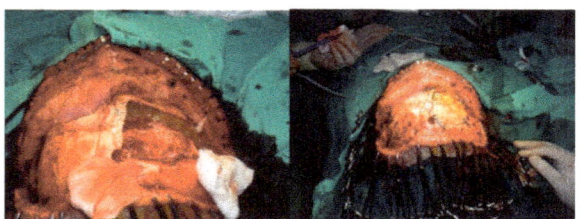

Figure 8. Giant right frontal sinus mucocele—surgical ablation, cranialization of the right frontal sinus, and reconstruction with bone flap.

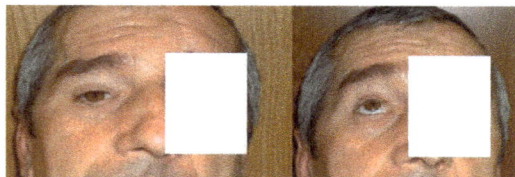

Figure 9. Recovery after surgical ablation of a post-traumatic mucocele, preservation of the esthetic aspect, and eye movements.

6. Medico-Legal Aspects

For underage patients the informed consent of legal guardians is compulsory, and the parents must be aware of the fact that the trauma itself and the reconstructive procedures performed in the hospital are likely to interfere with the normal development of the viscerocranium with unforeseeable long-term possible complications [33]. Possible litigations between the patients and the healthcare system may arise from the quality of the osteosynthesis materials used during the reconstructive procedures after trauma, although current titanium mesh implants seem to have a high safety profile [34]. Moreover, the team caring for the trauma patient should be as thorough as possible in documenting possible hidden lesions or secondary pathology to prevent future medicolegal prosecution [35]. Ultimately achieving both functional and good aesthetic results are desirable, but the patient should be aware of the fact that the pathology was an emergency with a life-threatening outcome and that the aesthetic aspects may be improved through further procedures after complete recovery [36].

7. Discussions

The most recent approach to managing head trauma cases is the use computational simulation to improve the outcome of surgical bone reconstruction. Moreover these complex cases associate multiple bone trauma at the level of the limbs [37].

Obviously there are various manufacturers of osteosynthesis equipment, but in all the images used to illustrate various bone fractures reconstructions we used Stryker, Berlin, Germany, titanium products for osteosynthesis in CMF surgery [38].

One modern approach is the use of engineered nanomaterials for closure of fractures. However, there is debate regarding the potential for adverse effects and inform product usage for individuals whose ocular health may be compromised by injury, disease, or surgical intervention [39].

One limitation of the present review is the scarce availability of data regarding the mortality due to frontal bone trauma. The mortality in such lesions should be divided in pre-hospital mortality and in-hospital mortality. The later type should be also analised taking into account conservative treatment or complex surgical procedures [40].

8. Conclusions

Treatment options in cases with frontal sinus fractures depend on the involvement of the anterior or posterior sinus walls and the functional integrity of the sinus communication drainage duct. One option is the complete closure of the sinus cavity if the normal drainage cannot be reinstated. Thus, we assure a clear barrier between the viscerocranium and neurocranium preventing potentially deadly meningitis. These cases require extended follow-up for long-term complications even decades after the trauma. In our experience maintaining the patency of the FND and of the NLD ensures a low risk for developing long term complications such as frontal sinus mucoceles or obstructive dacryocystitis. Following the example of skull base surgery training programs designed for ENT-surgeons and neurosurgeons teams performing endoscopic four hand surgery, there is a need for training programs designed for teams reuniting one specialist from each field of medical practice involved in head trauma cases: ENT surgeon, ophthalmologist, OMF surgeon, neurosurgeon at least.

Author Contributions: Conceptualization, M.D., D.V. and B.B.; methodology, M.D., D.V. and R.C.; software, R.C., I.-A.T. and F.M.; validation, D.V., R.C. and M.P.-C.; formal analysis, I.-A.T., F.M. and M.P.-C.; investigation, B.B., F.M. and M.P.-C.; resources, B.B., I.-A.T. and F.M.; data curation, R.C., F.M. and M.P.-C.; writing—original draft preparation, M.D., D.V. and B.B.; writing—review and editing, M.D., D.V. and B.B; visualization, I.-A.T.; supervision, R.C.; project administration, F.M.; funding acquisition, M.P.-C. All authors have read and agreed to the published version of the manuscript.

Funding: This research received no external funding.

Institutional Review Board Statement: Not applicable.

Informed Consent Statement: The study was conducted following the Declaration of Helsinki.

Data Availability Statement: All information presented in this review is documented by relevant references.

Acknowledgments: We acknowledge Cristina Andreescu from the Department of Foreign Languages at Carol Davila University of Medicine and Pharmacy, Bucharest, Romania for her kind support in revising the grammatical and language issues throughout the manuscript.

Conflicts of Interest: The authors declare no conflict of interest.

References

1. Park, C.-H.; Chung, K.J.; Kim, T.G.; Lee, J.H.; Kim, I.-K.; Kim, Y.-H. Big Data Statistical Analysis of Facial Fractures in Korea. *J. Korean Med. Sci.* **2020**, *35*, e57. [CrossRef] [PubMed]
2. Goelz, L.; Syperek, A.; Heske, S.; Mutze, S.; Hosten, N.; Kirsch, M. Retrospective Cohort Study of Frequency and Patterns of Orbital Injuries on Whole-Body CT with Maxillofacial Multi-Slice CT. *Tomography* **2021**, *7*, 373–386. [CrossRef] [PubMed]
3. Minja, I.K.; Wilson, M.L.; Shaikh, M.A.; Perea-Lowery, L. Head and Neck Trauma in a Rapidly Growing African Metropolis A Two-Year Audit of Hospital Admissions. *Int. J. Environ. Res. Public Health* **2019**, *16*, 4930. [CrossRef] [PubMed]
4. Scianò, F.; Zedda, N.; Mongillo, J.; Gualdi-Russo, E.; Bramanti, B. Autopsy or anatomical dissection: Evidence of a craniotomy in a 17th–eighteenth century burial site (Ravenna, Italy). *Forensic Sci. Med. Pathol.* **2021**, *17*, 157–160. [CrossRef]
5. Anghel, I.; Anghel, A.; Soreanu, C.; Dumitru, M. Craniofacial trauma produced by a violent mechanism. Coltea ENT Clinic experience. *Rom. J. Leg. Med.* **2012**, *20*, 215–218. [CrossRef]
6. Onișor-Gligor, F.; Țenț, P.A.; Bran, S.; Juncar, M. A Naso-Orbito-Ethmoid (NOE) Fracture Associated with Bilateral Anterior and Posterior Frontal Sinus Wall Fractures Caused by a Horse Kick—Case Report and Short Literature Review. *Medicina* **2019**, *55*, 731. [CrossRef]
7. Qi, H.; Li, K. Civilian gunshot wounds to the head: A case report, clinical management, and literature review. *Chin. Neurosurg. J.* **2021**, *7*, 12. [CrossRef]
8. Zhu, R.C.; Yoshida, M.C.; Kopp, M.; Lin, N. Treatment of a self-inflicted intracranial nail gun injury. *BMJ Case Rep.* **2021**, *14*, e237122. [CrossRef]
9. Vrinceanu, D.; Banica, B.; Papacocea, R.; Papacocea, T. Self-inflicted laryngeal penetrating wounds with suicidal intention: Two clinical cases. *Rom. J. Leg. Med.* **2018**, *26*, 16–20.
10. Jing, X.L.; Luce, E. Frontal Sinus Fractures: Management and Complications. *Craniomaxillofac. Trauma Reconstr.* **2019**, *12*, 241–248. [CrossRef]

11. Seok, H.; Im, S.-B.; Hwang, S.-C. Reconstruction of Anterior Skull Base Fracture Using Autologous Fractured Fragments: A Simple Stitching-Up Technique. *Korean J. Neurotrauma* **2021**, *17*, 25–33. [CrossRef] [PubMed]
12. Vrinceanu, D.; Banica, B.; Cirstoiu, C.F.; Papacocea, R.; Papacocea, T. 3D anatomically shaped titanium implant for the reconstruction of an orbital floor fracture with large posterior defect: A case report. *Rom. J. Mater.* **2018**, *48*, 407–411.
13. Pereira, R.A.; Barbosa, O.; Basílio, A.P.; Santana, A.S.; De Paula, D.; Marangon, H.M., Jr. Surgical decompression of the orbit due to frontal bone and roof of the orbit fractures—A case report. *Ann. Maxillofac. Surg.* **2020**, *10*, 495–500. [CrossRef]
14. Hsu, C.-R.; Lee, L.-C.; Chen, Y.-H.; Chien, K.-H. Early Intervention in Orbital Floor Fractures: Postoperative Ocular Motility and Diplopia Outcomes. *J. Pers. Med.* **2022**, *12*, 671. [CrossRef]
15. Bae, I.-S.; Kim, J.M.; Cheong, J.H.; Ryu, J.I.; Choi, K.-S.; Han, M.-H. Does the skull Hounsfield unit predict shunt dependent hydrocephalus after decompressive craniectomy for traumatic acute subdural hematoma? *PLoS ONE* **2020**, *15*, e0232631. [CrossRef] [PubMed]
16. Kim, Y.H.; Kim, B.-K. Approach to Frontal Sinus Outflow Tract Injury. *Arch. Craniofacial Surg.* **2017**, *18*, 1–4. [CrossRef] [PubMed]
17. Jeyaraj, P. Frontal bone fractures and frontal sinus injuries: Treatment paradigms. *Ann. Maxillofac. Surg.* **2019**, *9*, 261–282. [CrossRef]
18. Hakim, D.D.L.; Faried, A.; Nurhadiya, A.; Laymena, E.H.; Arifin, M.Z.; Imron, A.; Abdulrachman, I. Infected open depressed skull fracture complicated with tetanus grade I in an unimmunized child: A rare case report with literature review. *Int. J. Emerg. Med.* **2021**, *14*, 25. [CrossRef]
19. Irawati, Y.; Casalita, V. Management of ocular dystopia and lacrimal pathway obstruction in old multiple midfacial fractures: Case report. *Niger. J. Clin. Pract.* **2019**, *22*, 1307–1310. [CrossRef]
20. Abu Shqara, F.; Nseir, S.; Krasovsky, A.; Rachmiel, A. Surgical dilemmas in multiple facial fractures—Coronal flap versus minimally invasive: Case report and literature review. *Ann. Maxillofac. Surg.* **2021**, *11*, 191–194. [CrossRef]
21. Yakirevitch, A.; Bedrin, L.; Alon, E.E.; Yoffe, T.; Wolf, M.; Yahalom, R. Relation between preoperative computed tomographic criteria of injury to the nasofrontal outflow tract and operative findings in fractures of the frontal sinus. *Br. J. Oral Maxillofac. Surg.* **2013**, *51*, 799–802. [CrossRef] [PubMed]
22. Raghu, K.; Sathyanarayanan, R.; Deepika, S.; Sarath, K. Management of frontal sinus injuries. *Ann. Maxillofac. Surg.* **2018**, *8*, 276–280. [CrossRef] [PubMed]
23. Kim, J.; Choi, H. A Review of Subbrow Approach in the Management of Non-Complicated Anterior Table Frontal Sinus Fracture. *Arch. Craniofacial Surg.* **2016**, *17*, 186–189. [CrossRef] [PubMed]
24. Yun, S.; Na, Y. Panfacial bone fracture: Cephalic to caudal. *Arch. Craniofacial Surg.* **2018**, *19*, 1–2. [CrossRef] [PubMed]
25. Pajic, S.S.; Antic, S.; Vukicevic, A.M.; Djordjevic, N.; Jovicic, G.; Savic, Z.; Saveljic, I.; Janović, A.; Pesic, Z.; Djuric, M.; et al. Trauma of the Frontal Region Is Influenced by the Volume of Frontal Sinuses. A Finite Element Study. *Front. Physiol.* **2017**, *8*, 493. [CrossRef]
26. Braun, T.L.; Truong, T.A.; Schultz, K. Frontal Sinus Fractures. *Semin. Plast. Surg.* **2017**, *31*, 80–84. [CrossRef]
27. Da Silva, J.R.; Mourão, C.F.D.A.B.; Júnior, H.V.D.R.; Magacho, L.F.; Moraes, G.F.D.; Homsi, N. Treatment of frontal bone fracture sequelae through inversion of the bone fragment. *Rev. Colégio Bras. Cir.* **2016**, *43*, 472–475. [CrossRef]
28. Arnold, M.A.; Tatum, S.A. 3rd. Frontal Sinus Fractures: Evolving Clinical Considerations and Surgical Approaches. *Craniomaxillofac. Trauma Reconstr.* **2019**, *12*, 85–94. [CrossRef]
29. Binhammer, A.; Jakubowski, J.; Antonyshyn, O.; Binhammer, P. Comparative Cost-Effectiveness of Cranioplasty Implants. *Plast. Surg.* **2020**, *28*, 29–39. [CrossRef]
30. Plantier, D.B.; Neto, D.B.; Pinna, F.D.R.; Voegels, R.L. Mucocele: Clinical Characteristics and Outcomes in 46 Operated Patients. *Int. Arch. Otorhinolaryngol.* **2019**, *23*, 88–91. [CrossRef]
31. Eudaly, M.; Kraus, C.K. Frontal Mucocele following Previous Facial Trauma with Hardware Reconstruction. *Case Rep. Emerg. Med.* **2016**, *2016*, 4236421. [CrossRef] [PubMed]
32. Fujioka, M. Influence of Skull Base or Frontal Bone Fracture on the Result of Treatment for Le Fort Type Maxillofacial Fractures: Outcomes of Le Fort IV Fractures. *J. Emerg. Trauma Shock.* **2019**, *12*, 71–72. [CrossRef]
33. Wijaya, A.T.; Ayusta, I.M.D.; Niryana, I.W. Air gun wound: Bihemispheric penetrating brain injury in a paediatric patient. *BJR|Case Rep.* **2018**, *5*, 20180070. [CrossRef]
34. Chattopadhyay, C. Reconstruction of Acquired Frontal Bone Defects Using Titanium Mesh Implants: A Retrospective Study. *J. Maxillofac. Oral Surg.* **2019**, *18*, 34–39. [CrossRef]
35. Petetta, C.; Santovito, D.; Tattoli, L.; Melloni, N.D.; Bertoni, M.; Di Vella, G. Forensic and Clinical Issues in a Case of Motorcycle Blunt Trauma and Bilateral Carotid Artery Dissection. *Ann. Vasc. Surg.* **2020**, *64*, 409.e11–409.e16. [CrossRef]
36. Delaney, S.W. Treatment strategies for frontal sinus anterior table fractures and contour deformities. *J. Plast. Reconstr. Aesthetic Surg.* **2016**, *69*, 1037–1045. [CrossRef] [PubMed]
37. Ammarullah, M.I.; Santoso, G.; Sugiharto, S.; Supriyono, T.; Wibowo, D.B.; Kurdi, O.; Tauviqirrahman, M.; Jamari, J. Minimizing Risk of Failure from Ceramic-on-Ceramic Total Hip Prosthesis by Selecting Ceramic Materials Based on Tresca Stress. *Sustainability* **2022**, *14*, 13413. [CrossRef]
38. Available online: https://www.stryker.com/content/dam/stryker/craniomaxillofacial/products/universalmp/resources/CMF%20Maxillofacial%20Portfolio%20-%20Brochure%20(EN).pdf (accessed on 19 November 2022).

39. Cosert, K.M.; Kim, S.; Jalilian, I.; Chang, M.; Gates, B.L.; Pinkerton, K.E.; Van Winkle, L.S.; Raghunathan, V.K.; Leonard, B.C.; Thomasy, S.M. Metallic Engineered Nanomaterials and Ocular Toxicity: A Current Perspective. *Pharmaceutics* **2022**, *14*, 931. [CrossRef]
40. Stirparo, G.; Ristagno, G.; Bellini, L.; Bonora, F.; Pagliosa, A.; Migliari, M.; Andreassi, A.; Signorelli, C.; Sechi, G.M.; Fagoni, N. Changes to the Major Trauma Pre-Hospital Emergency Medical System Network before and during the 2019 COVID-19 Pandemic. *J. Clin. Med.* **2022**, *11*, 6748. [CrossRef]

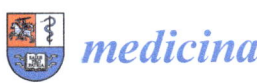

Article

Multidisciplinary Therapeutic Management in Complex Cervical Trauma

Florentina Severin [1,†], Andrei-Mihail Rosu [1,†], Mirela Tiglis [2], Laura-Elisabeta Checherita [1], Gina Stegaru [1], Mihail Dan Cobzeanu [1], Razvan Hainarosie [3,*], Bogdan Mihail Cobzeanu [1,*] and Octavian Dragos Palade [1]

1. Surgery Department, University of Medicine and Pharmacy "Grigore T. Popa", 700115 Iasi, Romania; florentina-s-severin@umfiasi.ro (F.S.)
2. Department of Anesthesia and Intensive Care, Emergency Clinical Hospital of Bucharest, 014461 Bucharest, Romania
3. Surgery Department, University of Medicine and Pharmacy "Carol Davila", 37 Dionisie Lupu Str., 020021 Bucharest, Romania
* Correspondence: razvan.hainarosie@umfcd.ro (R.H.); bogdan-mihail.cobzeanu@umfiasi.ro (B.M.C.)
† These authors contributed equally to this work.

Abstract: *Background and Objectives*: In the current literature, mandatory surgical exploration is a controversial topic, with some advocating for it and others against it, proposing a selective conservative management. This multidisciplinary therapeutic approach is based on clinical examination and serial paraclinical explorations associated with supportive drug treatment. *Materials and Methods*: The study group consisted of 103 patients with complex cervical trauma pathology produced by various mechanisms such as car or domestic accidents, aggression, ballistic trauma, self-inflicted attempts, hanging or strangulation hospitalized in the Ear, Nose and Throat (E.N.T.) Clinic, at "St. Spiridon" Iași Hospital, between 2012 and 2016. *Results*: The universal clinical indication for urgent surgical exploration of the patient with complex cervical trauma is the presence of the following symptoms: unstable vital signs, significant pulsatile bleeding, hematoma with a substantial increase in size, shock, airway obstruction, open airway wound, hematemesis, or hemoptysis. In this context, we considered it worthwhile to research the management of complex cervical trauma in a reference university medical center, alongside the analysis of the patient's characteristics under different aspects (demographic, pathological aspects, therapeutic). *Conclusions*: Complex cervical trauma has a variety of clinical aspects, with a variable evolution, which involves multidisciplinary therapeutic management. The increasing trauma rate is one of the main public health problems, requiring epidemiological studies, and the implementation of control strategies.

Keywords: otorhinolaryngology; surgery; multidisciplinary treatment; complex cervical trauma

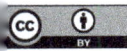

1. Introduction

The management of cervical trauma has been a topic of great interest and controversy over the years. The need for surgical exploration of all cervical wounds' dates back to the time of the Second World War (WWII). However, the evolution of the emergency medical system and paraclinical investigations has contributed to the improvement of global statistics regarding the mortality and morbidity of this pathology.

Currently, studies reported by various authors show similar mortality and morbidity regarding the approach of clinical surveillance and non-exploratory diagnosis in selected cases versus surgical management for all patients. The universal clinical indication for urgent surgical exploration of the patient with complex cervical trauma is the presence of the following symptoms: unstable vital signs, significant pulsatile bleeding, hematoma with a substantial increase in size, shock, airway obstruction, open airway wound, hematemesis, or hemoptysis [1]. Proponents of mandatory surgical management argue that any injury that penetrates the platysma should be explored in the operating room. In particular, zone II is mainly due to the rich content of critical neurovascular structures.

On the other hand, in the last five years, the current otolaryngology opinion issues the hypothesis, with already quite a few followers, in favor of selective surgical management. Paraclinical examinations are required, which include angiography, esophagography, panendoscopy, and computed tomography. Explorations are indicated only in hemodynamically and respiratory stable patients. This management strategy is preferably performed only in hospital facilities with appropriate logistics [2].

We present a retrospective and prospective study of complex cervical trauma pathology secondary to various accidents or aggressions, which required surgical interventions. Our main objectives were to analyze the management of complex cervical trauma in a reference university medical center, and the analysis of the patient's characteristics under different aspects (demographic, pathological aspects, therapeutic).

2. Materials and Methods

The study group was made up of 103 patients admitted to the Ear, Nose and Throat (E.N.T.) Clinic, "St. Spiridon", Iasi, between 2012–2016, with complex cervical trauma pathology produced by various mechanisms, such as car accidents, domestic accidents, assaults, ballistic trauma, self-inflicted attempts, hanging or strangulation. However, this study was partially limited by the fact that information on particular patients was incomplete, due to the retrospective nature of the research and the lack of uniformity regarding the description of the operative technique, along with the results of the paraclinical investigations performed, as there was no existing standardized protocol; a situation that could bring some damage to the data identified on this study. The study was started in 2014 and it consisted of two parts. The patients included in the retrospective study were those admitted to the ENT clinic of "Saint Spiridon" Hospital, Iasi, in the period 2012–2014. Likewise, the patients included the prospective study were those patients admitted to the ENT Clinic in during 2014–2016. We defined the complex cervical trauma as the lesions that are penetrating platysma and involve at least the superior aero-digestive tract, vascular, neurologic, thyroidian or salivary gland structures.

The data were centralized in an SPSS 18.0 database and processed with the statistical functions to which they lend themselves at the significance threshold of 95%. Using specific statistical methods, it was possible to calculate the mean value and the standard deviation (SD); quantitative variables were compared using the Student's t-test, and the Chi-square test assessed quantitative parameters. The ANOVA test was used to evaluate descriptive statistical indicators: minimum, maximum, mean, median, standard deviation, standard error of the mean, and variance. The Skewness, Kurtosis ($-2 < p < 2$) method tests the normality of the series of values. In calculating the significant difference between the two means, the Student's t-test considers the measurement of variability and the weight of the observations. F-test (ANOVA) was used to compare values with normal distributions in three or more groups. The Pearson correlation coefficient was used to establish the existence of correlations, and their intensity between various numerical variables studied. The type of correlation was expressed by the sign of the Pearson correlation coefficient, and the power of the link between the variables was represented by its value. Statistical significance was set at the $p < 0.05$ threshold for a 95% confidence interval. Univariate and multivariate analysis by logistic regression was used to determine the variables correlated with the presence or absence of the studied events, identifying statistically significant independent parameters.

General inclusion criteria had in view the information selected from the observation sheets and fell into the following categories: demographics data, epidemiological characteristics, lesion appearance and mechanism, location cervical corresponding to the defined areas of the neck, the type and extent of the damaged tissues, paraclinical investigations carried out, associated pathologies or relapses, therapeutic approach, complications along with the data obtained from the periodic consultations performed upon discharge from the hospital.

General exclusion criteria were under 18 years of age, the patient's refusal to participate, the presence of previous cervical trauma, but without pathological lesions or only superficial lesions without being accompanied by the above-mentioned symptoms.

3. Results

The patients selected for this study presented with closed and open penetrating cervical traumatic injuries caused by self-inflicted, interpersonal aggression and accidental mechanism. The symptoms and clinical signs identified varied according to the location of the injury and the affected visceral or extra-visceral structure, and the concomitant existence of other traumas with other sites. Dysphonia, dyspnea, various degrees of acute respiratory failure, cervical subcutaneous emphysema, and a mid-cervical blowing wound are characteristic elements of the involvement of the laryngotracheal axis. Pharyngoesophageal damage is characterized by dysphagia and subcutaneous emphysema. A descending injury from zone I is associated with acute respiratory distress, pneumothorax or hemothorax, signs of cardiac tamponade suggesting damage to the apex of the lung and the vessels at the base of the neck, nerve involvement of the cervical plexus or cranial nerves, which may decrease the sensitivity and motility of the superior limbs. In parallel with the clinical examination, respiratory and cardiac vital signs were monitored, blood samples were taken, and the indication was established regarding paraclinical investigations or the need for emergency surgical exploration depending on the stability of Surgical explorations.

In the study group, made up of 103 patients hospitalized in the ENT clinic, the age varied between 17 and 78 years, the average age was 43 years (standard deviation = 15.57), registering a slightly higher average value in the male sex (43.41 vs. 42.09 years; $p = 0.793$). patients come more frequently from rural areas (56.6%), they are predominantly male (89.6%), under the age of 45 (55.7%); the lesional determining mechanism is noted more frequently through aggression (39.6%), followed by the self-inflicted mechanism (39.6%) and the accidental mechanism (22.6%).

In this study, the cases that required surgical intervention were characterized by complex aero-digestive, thyroid, vascular, and polytrauma injuries. Thus, the following were identified: section of the thyrohyoid membrane with involvement of the hypopharynx (11 cases), fracture of the laryngeal cartilages with dilaceration of the epiglottis, vocal cords and pyriform sinuses (14 cases), dilacerations with retrocricoid hematomas (5 cases), sectioning of the cricothyroid membrane and interest partial or total cricoid cartilage (7 cases), sectioning of the crico-tracheal membrane and tracheal rings (7 cases), sectioning of the superficial jugular veins (31 cases), involvement of the internal jugular vein (6 cases), involvement of the thyroid gland (6 cases), involvement of the submandibular gland (5 cases), polytraumas due to traffic accidents or falls from a height with complex thoracic, abdominal, craniofacial and limb injuries (11 cases) (Figure 1).

From the total number of vascular lesions of the anterior, external, and internal jugular veins, the following lesions were identified: contusions, adventitial lesions, and complete or partial sections, to which is added a case of penetrating wound involving the thoracic duct. These injuries required parietal reconstruction and vascular ligature to perform hemostasis, depending on the case, through specific techniques (Figure 2).

Regarding the arterial lesions of the carotid system, adventitious contusion-type lesions of the common and external carotid arteries and pseudoaneurysm-type lesions at the level of the common carotid artery were identified in our study (Figure 3).

As for the penetrating hypopharyngeal lesions, in the entire study group, penetrating lesions of the pharyngeal wall were identified only at the level of the piriform sinuses with the development of parapharyngeal hematomas that had a posterior prevertebral extension and determined compressive phenomena with the onset of acute upper respiratory insufficiency and dysphagia (Figure 4).

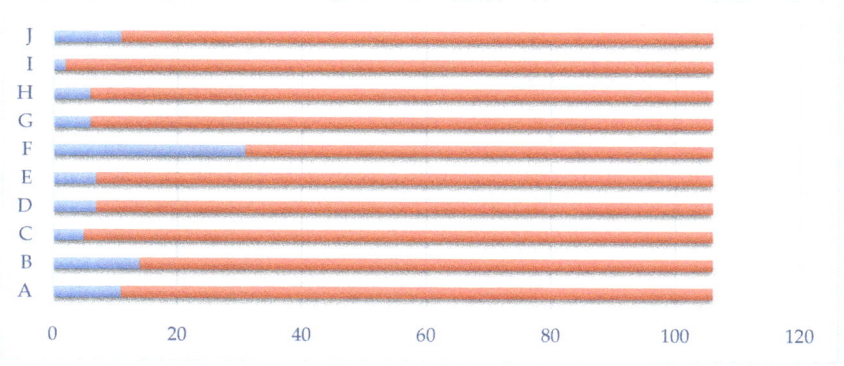

Figure 1. Distribution of complex aero-digestive cervical trauma cases and associated injuries. A—section of the thyrohyoid membrane with the interest of the hypopharynx. B—fracture of the laryngeal cartilages with laceration of the epiglottis, vocal cords, and pyriform sinuses. C—dilacerations with retrocricoid hematomas. D—sectioning of the cricothyroid membrane and partial or total involvement of the cricoid cartilage. E—sectioning of the crico-tracheal membrane and the tracheal rings. F—dissection of the superficial jugular veins. G—internal jugular vein involvement. H—thyroid gland interest and I—the interest of the submandibular gland. J—Polytraumatism.

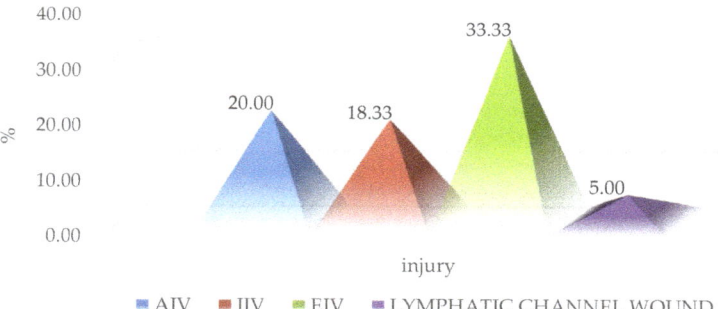

Figure 2. Distribution of venous lesions that required surgical treatment. (AJV = anterior jugular vein, IVJ = internal jugular vein, EJV = external jugular vein).

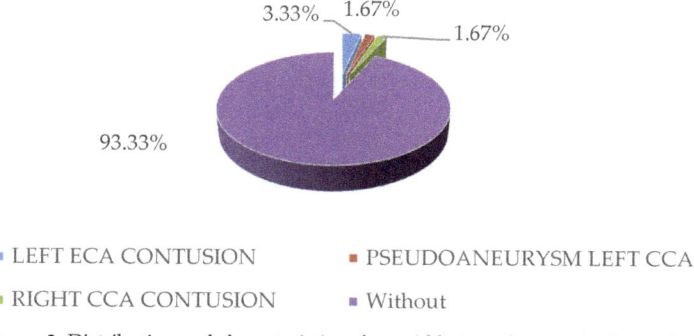

Figure 3. Distribution and characteristics of carotid lesions that required specific surgical treatment. (ECA = external carotid artery, CCA = common carotid artery).

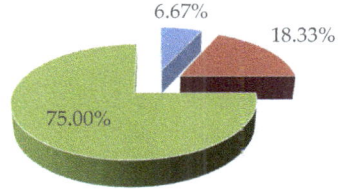

- PARAPHARYNGEAL HEMATOMAS
- PYRIFORM SINUS INJURIES
- NO INJURIES

Figure 4. Distribution and characteristics of hypopharyngeal and parapharyngeal lesions that required surgical therapeutic management.

The appearance of traumatic laryngeal lesions identified both clinically, paraclinical, and intraoperatively is very diverse, including lesions of the mucosa, vocal cords, laryngeal cartilages, thyrohyoid and cricothyroid membrane, as illustrated in Figure 5 and on which specific therapeutic intervention was performed, both surgically and medically.

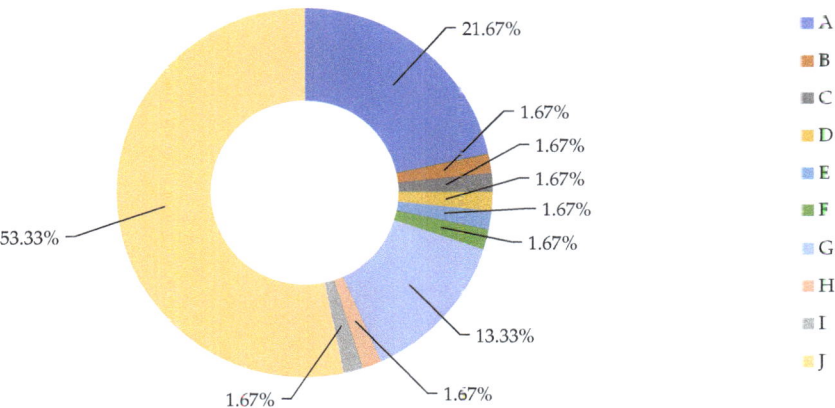

Figure 5. Distribution and characteristics of traumatic laryngeal injuries that required a surgical therapeutic approach. A—vocal cord injuries. B—arytenoid cartilage injuries. C—cricoid cartilage fracture. D—cricotracheal membrane section. E—section thyroyidian membrane. F—paralaryngian hematoma. G—total or partial thyroid cartilage fractures. H—section thyrohyoid membrane, epiglottic exposure, and laryngeal continuity solution. I—continuity solution at the laryngeal level with the appearance of cervical emphysema. J—no laryngeal injuries.

Surgical exploration under general anesthesia was performed in 42 of the 103 patients in the study group (39.6%), more frequently in males (44.1% vs. 27.3%; $p = 0.656$), age group under 45 years (40.7% vs. 38.3%; $p = 0.803$) and with a rural background (37% vs. 41.7%; $p = 0.623$) (Figure 6).

Regarding the mechanism of production of traumatic injuries, the statistical analysis shows that the use of surgical exploration through general anesthesia was more common in patients with penetrating injuries produced by aggression and accidentally (27.3% vs. 45.2% and 50%; $p = 0.05$) (Figure 7).

Surgical exploration of penetrating wounds under local anesthesia was performed in 28 of the patients in the study group (26.4%), more frequently in females (36.4% vs. 28.3%; $p = 0.443$), age group over 45 years (23.7% vs. 29.8%; $p = 0.483$) and the urban environment (34.8% vs. 20%; $p = 0.688$) (Figure 8).

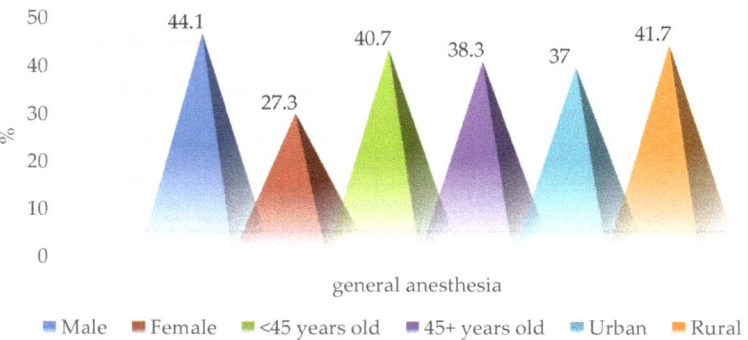

Figure 6. Epidemiological characteristics of patients with surgical exploration performed under general anesthesia.

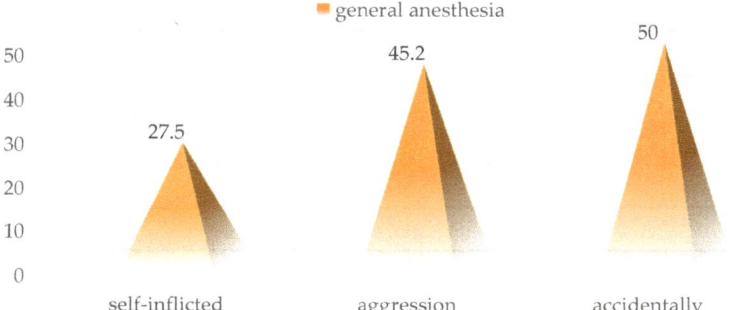

Figure 7. Distribution of cases surgically explored under general anesthesia according to the injury mechanism.

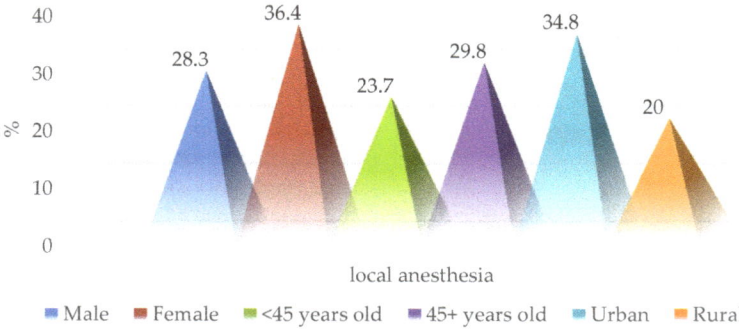

Figure 8. Epidemiological characteristics of patients with surgical exploration performed under local anesthesia.

Tracheostomy was performed in 17 patients included in the study (16%) without significant differences between sexes, age groups, or place of residence (Figure 9). In addition, the need to secure the airway by performing a tracheostomy was not statistically significantly correlated with a specific injury mechanism determining cervical trauma (7.5% vs. 23.8% and 16.7%; $p = 0.117$) (Figure 10).

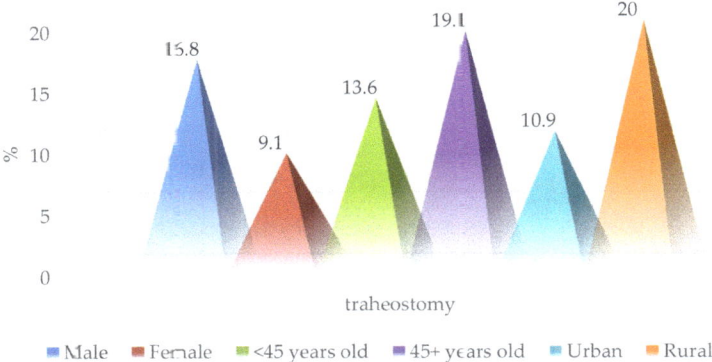

Figure 9. Epidemiological characteristics of patients who underwent tracheostomy.

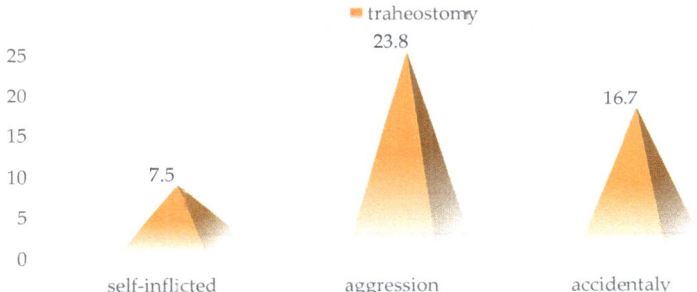

Figure 10. Distribution of cases in the batch in which tracheostomy was performed according to the lesion mechanism.

Complex penetrating traumatic injuries of the aero-digestive tract require local digestive rest and the application of a nasogastric tube. However, the recommendation to apply the nasogastric tube was not statistically significantly correlated with the lesion mechanism, which produced the penetrating traumatic injury (15% vs. 14.3% and 12.5%; $p = 0.961$) (Figure 11).

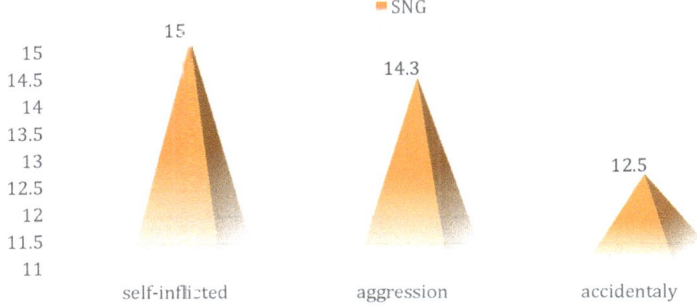

Figure 11. Distribution of cases in the batch to which SNG was applied according to the lesion mechanism.

Conservative therapeutic management, consisting of observation, serial clinical examination, paraclinical explorations, and supportive drug treatment, was carried out in 38 of the selected patients (35.8%) without significant differences between sexes, age groups, or the place of residence (Figure 12).

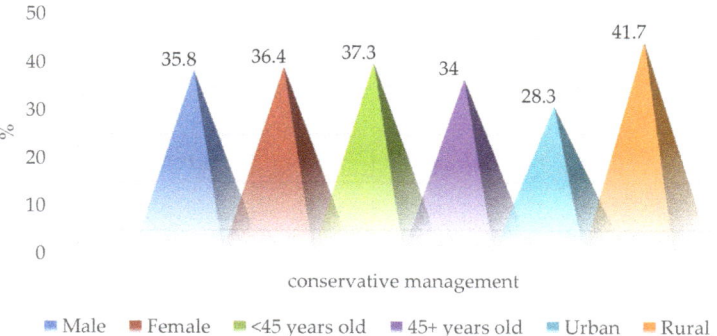

Figure 12. Epidemiological characteristics of patients with conservative management.

The conservative therapeutic approach correlated statistically significantly with the self-inflicted mechanism (60% vs. 26.2% and 12.5%; $p = 0.001$) (Figure 13).

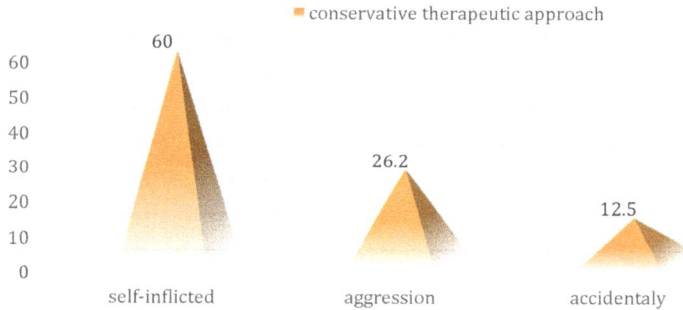

Figure 13. Distribution of cases in the batch with indications for conservative management according to the lesion mechanism.

The need for the administration of supportive drug treatment was identified in 102 patients from the group (96.2%), without significant differences between sexes, age groups, or the place of residence (Figure 14).

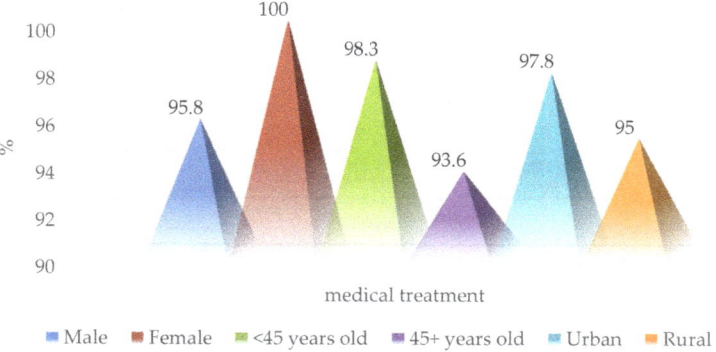

Figure 14. Epidemiological characteristics of patients who received medical treatment.

Postoperative complications were noted in 6 patients (5.7%), all male, five aged over 45 years, and five from rural areas. The postoperative complications identified were the following: partial dehiscence of the postoperative wound, parotid salivary fistula, postoperative wound infection with Enterobacter, stroke, pneumococcal pneumonia, post-traumatic left genital edema, dysphonia, and torticollis.

4. Discussion

The essential therapeutic attitude in complex cervical trauma is ensuring the airways' safety through orotracheal intubation or emergency tracheostomy and hemostasis control, followed by clinical and paraclinical investigations, then exploration and reconstructive surgical treatment. In cases where the hemodynamically unstable patient could not be investigated paraclinical and presented traumatic injuries with a penetrating character, urgent surgical exploration is required. This exploration can be performed under general anesthesia with orotracheal intubation, tracheostomy, or local anesthesia.

The importance of first aid, as well as emergency therapeutic measures in other health facilities, must include primary hemostasis and the proper support of cardio-respiratory parameters. Transport must be ensured in safe conditions and as soon as possible, considering the complications that can occur in the first hours after the trauma. In emergencies, the airway was secured (freeing the oral cavity of secretions and blood, possibly intubating the patient or tracheotomy), immobilizing the cervical spine, accessing the venous lines, and obtaining a correct anamnesis regarding the circumstances of the accident, the associated diseases, the state of consciousness. Intubation through the cervical area is indicated when there are injuries to the oral cavity, pharynx, or larynx. Orotracheal intubation can accentuate pharyngolaryngeal lesions, causing the extension of some lesions from the level of the piriform sinus to the mediastinum. In lesions with significant cervical tissue destruction, intubation was performed through the continuity solution at the level of the sectioned thyrohyoid membrane.

According to the European Manual of Medicine, Otorhinolaryngology, Head and Neck Surgery, the standard of investigation and exploration procedures in the case of cervical traumatology is applied depending on the presence or not of the hemodynamic and neurological stability criteria. The unstable patient will be provided with an airway simultaneously with the treatment of shock and cervical surgical exploration; postoperative achievement of hemodynamic stability and neurological will allow additional endoscopic and imaging investigations to be performed. The symptomatically stable patient is subjected to endoscopic, imaging and interventional angiographic investigations to determine the lesion balance and establish subsequent to the therapeutic conduct.

Depending on the symptomatology and clinical examination of the patients with cervical trauma selected for this study, the following methods of paraclinical exploration were used: cervical and thoracic X-ray, Doppler cervical and soft part ultrasound, craniocerebral, cervical and thoracic computed tomographic scan, computed tomographic angiography, naso-pharyngo-laryngeal and upper digestive endoscopic exploration. Cervical and chest X-rays identify cervical soft tissue emphysema, fractures, tracheal lacerations, foreign body retention, hemothorax, pneumothorax, mediastinal emphysema. Computed tomography, ultrasound of the cervical soft parts and Doppler, angiography, or pharyngoesophageal transit with contrast material are performed when complex lesions are suspected. Panendoscopic exploration (laryngeal, pharyngo-esophageal and tracheo-bronchoscopy) are used in the case of complex lesions of the aerodigestive axis. The use of the rigid endoscope is superior to the flexible one in upper esophageal lesions.

For patients with aero-digestive lesions depending on the severity of the symptoms and the injury complexity, the therapeutic attitude involved a medical treatment associated with the surgical one. Patients with mild laryngeal and tracheal injuries, without respiratory changes or signs of laryngeal fractures, were hospitalized and kept under observation for at least 24–48 h (since there is a potential risk of further respiratory dysfunction, through the expansion of edema, in the interval of time, which follows the trauma). The treatment was conservative, with medicinal support, and consisted of administering antibiotic therapy, steroid anti-inflammatories, aerosols, oxygen therapy, and air humidification. During hospitalization, it is indicated to carry out serial evaluations clinically and through nasopharyngo-laryngeal fiberoscopy.

In the case of patients with variable respiratory disorders associated with laryngeal mucosa lesions, edema, and hematomas, the intervention was performed by performing a tracheotomy under local anesthesia and an endoscopic lesion assessment after the induction of general anesthesia. 3–5 days postoperatively, the tracheotomy was suppressed, during which the patient received supportive drug treatment. The presentation at admission with signs and different degrees of acute respiratory insufficiency associated with extensive laryngeal lesions of the mucosa, edema, and endolaryngeal hematomas, alteration of the mobility of the vocal cords or different degrees of comminution of cartilaginous fractures required the surgical therapeutic approach. This was performed in the following sequence: tracheotomy, endolarynx exploration through direct laryngoscopy, cervical wound exploration, and laryngeal approach through thyrotomy or the thyroid cartilage fracture path. Lesions of the laryngeal mucosa were repaired by sutures with absorbable 4-0 or 5-0 threads without exposing cartilaginous areas. Depending on each case's lesion, the foot of the epiglottis, the ventricular band, or the vocal cords were reinserted, the aryepiglottic fold was restored, and the laryngeal fractures were reduced by suturing with non-absorbable threads. Anchorage of the superior and inferior retrocricoid ends was required. In cases with significant loss of substance, the larynx was restored with different muscles plasties. Anchorage of the hyoid with separate wires to the external laryngeal perichondrium was performed to achieve adequate laryngeal tightness and statics. Surgical therapeutic management was associated with antibiotic treatment, steroid anti-inflammatories, aerosols, and oxygen therapy. Suppression of the tracheal cannula was performed after 10–12 days.

The most severe cases with poor prognosis were characterized by extensive destructive lesions, loss of soft and cartilaginous substance, vocal cord disinsertion, or crico-tracheal disjunction associated with severe acute respiratory failure. These required emergency surgical exploration, laryngeal reconstruction, and recalibration. Recalibration was performed by fitting and maintaining a Montgomery tube for two weeks. Again, appropriate laryngeal calibration is recommended, with scar management in major debridement and mucosal restoration to avoid stenoses.

In cases with hypopharyngeal lesions of varying degrees of complexity, a careful clinical examination was performed, digestive rest was indicated with the application of a nasogastric tube, and depending on the severity of the lesion, surgical reconstruction as quickly as possible (ideally within the first 6–8 h from trauma) associated with performing a tracheotomy. The suturing of the pharyngeal wall was performed in two planes, serous and mucous. Hypopharyngoesophageal injuries are severe and require immediate recognition and treatment. A muscle flap can be used as a sleeve and isolates the upper digestive tract to avoid the formation of pharyngo-cutaneous or eso-tracheal fistulas. Pharyngeal plastic surgery was performed with prevertebral aponeurosis and subhyoid muscles. They are ideal for preventing post-operative suppurative or stenotic complications. Significant is the prompt correction of metabolic and hydro-electrolytic imbalances in the pre-, intra-, and post-operative periods, such as the administration of correct broad-spectrum antibiotic therapy, anti-inflammatories, and proton pump and H2 receptor inhibitors to prevent regional complications and sequelae. Maintaining the nasogastric feeding tube is indicated in cases where pharyngeal sutures were performed and in the remission of fistulas for 3–4 weeks.

Depending on the complexity of the traumatic aero-digestive injury, digestive rest through a nasogastric tube and respiratory rest through tracheotomy for 7–14 days are necessary conditions for resuming normal swallowing, breathing, and phonation. In addition, aspiration drainage is applied and maintained to avoid the formation of postoperative hematomas and seromas to smooth the tissue planes.

Cervical wounds involving various tissues and the cervical visceral aerodigestive axis require an established protocol for a multidisciplinary team approach. This team consists of the otolaryngologist, anesthesia and intensive care physician, emergency physician, and other specialties depending on the injuries associated with different body segments.

Vascular lesions in the zone I required collaboration with the thoracic surgery department, with the performance of mediastinotomy and thoracotomy to perform hemostasis. The identification following the radiological examination of hemothorax, pneumothorax, or pneumomediastinum required proper drainage of air and blood collections. In one case with plurivisceral involvement and basicervical venous vascular section, the thoracic duct was also involved, along with anterior mediastinal lesions in the left half. This case also involved collaboration with the thoracic surgeon. In zone III, the lesions required the performance of a median mandibulotomy to expose the parapharyngeal space to evacuate hematomas with an obstructive dyspneic character or to have access to the vasculo-nervous structures at the base of the skull. In the case of cases involving the submandibular gland, excision of the torn tissues, suturing of the glandular body, or total or partial excisions of it were necessary.

Cervical venous injuries (jugular vein and thyro-lingo-facial venous trunk) were resolved by ligation and adventitial sutures except when both internal jugular veins were involved when an attempt was made to restore the continuity of one of them. In the case of the carotid artery injury, it was important to fix it by adventitial sutures, end-to-end anastomosis, or by applying a graft with the help of vascular surgery colleagues (two cases).

In the case of complex cervical trauma produced by a closed or penetrating mechanism, which involved the thyroid, the following aspects were identified: expansive anterior cervical hematoma, compressive on the respiratory axis with phenomena of acute respiratory failure, which required its emergency drainage; cervical wounds with thyroid and laryngeal involvement with bleeding, which flood the respiratory tract, causing the exacerbation of respiratory failure phenomena and which required the performance of protective tracheotomy and the securing of the airway associated with the removal of crushed glandular tissues or different degrees of subtotal thyroidectomy. In addition, in 7 of the cases included in the study group, the glandular suture of the suture type with slow resorbable thread was performed.

The postoperative occurrence of fever, tachycardia, chest pain, widening of the radiographic mediastinum, subcutaneous emphysema, bleeding wound, the onset of neurological deficits, or the development of a hematoma requires imaging and surgical re-exploration.

All cervical aero-digestive traumas, regardless of complexity, were carefully recorded in terms of local examination, the evolution of symptoms and vital or biological constants, imaging and endoscopic examination, and exploratory and surgical reconstruction protocols.

The clinical management of complex cervical trauma has changed over time towards a conservative approach. Even so, the need for surgical exploration in patients with traumatic penetrating injuries of the aerodigestive tract or great vessels should be based on clinical elements and reliable indicators for indicating an open exploration.

The number of medical and medical-surgical specialties involved and the diagnostic assessment of patients with traumatic neck injuries requires developing and implementing a multidisciplinary institutional protocol with national applicability. In addition, it could support the ways of indicating paraclinical diagnostic procedures, such as flexible rasopharyngo-laryngeal fiberoscopy, plain radiography, and esophagography, as well as computed tomography, but also the clear indications of surgical versus conservative treatment.

Since Ambroise Pare ligated both carotid arteries and the jugular vein of a soldier with polytrauma of the neck in 1552, the therapeutic approach to complex penetrating cervical trauma has been one of the controversial topics in trauma surgery. There has not yet been a consensus on this. Surgical exploration of all neck injuries beyond the platysma muscle significantly reduced mortality during World War II [3], but 89% of interventions did not identify deep visceral injuries [4]. In 1969, Monson et al. divided the cervical region into the three zones used in the management of trauma diagnostic protocol [5]. Legerwood et al. in 1980 and Narrod et al. in 1984 showed that the absence of severe clinical signs of hemodynamic instability in penetrating limb trauma quite clearly excludes arterial injuries, which require surgical treatment [6,7]. They extrapolated this reasoning to the diagnosis and treatment algorithm of cervical trauma with vascular involvement, revealing that some arterial lesions may be missed in the diagnosis and may result in potentially life-threatening vascular accidents.

In the 1990s, two studies focused on clinical examination to identify severe signs of vascular involvement in zone II cervical trauma and the need for an indication for reparative surgical exploration [8,9]. In addition, the clinical examination is more than 99% accurate in diagnosing these lesions with a false-negative rate comparable to angiography [9]. Furthermore, clinical examination is faster, less expensive, and involves few medical staff. Even so, it is less likely to be able to detect minor lesions such as intimal vascular irregularities, pseudoaneurysms, and arteriovenous fistulas compared to angiographic exploration. Most of these lesions are of no clinical significance [10]. Therefore, routine angiography's additional costs and morbidity are difficult to justify.

Some studies even promote mandatory surgical exploration of all penetrating cervical wounds based on low morbidity and reduced hospital days. This approach has been described as cost-effective and characterized by higher accuracy than contrast-enhanced imaging studies [10].

For patients with high suspicion of penetrating laryngotracheal injury, detailed clinical examination is mandatory. Trauma of the upper aerodigestive tract is suspected in face of dysphonia or stridor, subcutaneous emphysema appearance, or blowing wound presence, and the main objective is to ensure and maintain the upper airway patency. In a retrospective study including 748 patients with this type of injury, only 11% of cases required immediate airway control, raising questions about the importance of conservative measures [11]. Surgical wound management is indicated if there is a significant change in the laryngotracheal anatomy. In such cases, orotracheal intubation may worsen the existing injuries; therefore, tracheostomy under local anesthesia is recommended, even at the site of the accident.

Metheny et al. believe that nasogastric tube placement and feeding is more effective than parenteral nutrition in most patients with critical aero-digestive traumatic injury because it preserves the integrity of the bowel and causes fewer infectious complications. However, nasogastric tube feeding has been associated with risks like other therapies. The most serious potential complication is the tracheobronchial aspiration of gastric contents, with the risk of developing a series of clinically silent microaspirations [12].

As we emphasized before, starting with WWII, the main recommendation was to surgically explore the neck for any traumatic lesion that involves the platysma [13]. Over the years, various research showed that this may be associated with a significant number morbidity. An article from the late 1970s showed that 56% of surgical neck explorations were non-therapeutic [14]. The modernization of imaging technologies made the selective approach of neck exploration more common. In this matter, an important study showed that 207 of 312 patients (66%) presenting with penetrating neck injuries were able to be managed conservatively, due to a thorough physical examination, along with angiography/esophageal exploration. Only one patient appeared to have an esophageal lesion missed on the initial examination and required repeat exploration [10]

Nowadays, the advantages of a selective nonoperative management for penetrating cervical trauma have been established, but there remain some circumstances when immediate operative exploration is mandatory, such as significant airway or major vascular injuries [10]. In 2011, Burgess et al. [15] reviewed the specialized literature regarding managing traumatic cervical injuries with a penetrating character and the institution of mandatory or selective surgical treatment.

In the case of our study, all cervical traumas beyond the platysma were surgically explored under general or local anesthesia with the identification and surgical reconstruction of the lesion. The indication of paraclinical imaging studies was influenced by the hemodynamic status and the need to secure the airway by orotracheal intubation or tracheostomy. In addition, complex aero-digestive lesions required digestive rest and the placement of a nasogastric tube, with the administration of food through this route or the association with the parenteral administration of the necessary nutrients. In cases of reduced complexity, conservative management and supportive drug treatment of traumatic and associated pathology were associated, as appropriate.

Early recognition and management of the complications of penetrating cervical wounds are essential in reducing the mortality and morbidity of these injuries. Prevention of these complications depends on the initial therapeutic actions of securing the airway by intubation or tracheostomy, prompt control of bleeding, protection of the head and neck, accurate and rapid lesion diagnosis, and surgical treatment according to the indication [16]. Additionally, in this study, 89.7% of selected patients were identified with uncomplicated healing, while in our study, the rate was 94.3%, close to other studies [16,17].

5. Conclusions

The first evaluation of complex cervical trauma is part of the standard Advanced Trauma Life Support (ATLS) protocol, an essential element on which the vital prognosis depends: securing the airways by orotracheal intubation or tracheostomy. The prehospital period should not be prolonged by performing the ATLS protocol and involves simultaneously balancing vital signs. These elements can dramatically change the patient's prognosis, transforming him from dying to savable. An unstable hemodynamic status and an airway, which requires emergency stabilization, determined the performance of the lesion balance by performing emergency surgical exploration and involves multidisciplinary therapeutic management, followed by reconstructive surgical treatment at the same operative time or a second time. Optimizing a multidisciplinary emergency medical system will lead to improving global statistics regarding this pathology's mortality and morbidity.

Author Contributions: Conceptualization, F.S. and O.D.P.; methodology, B.M.C. and M.D.C.; software, A.-M.R.; validation, F.S. and A.-M.R.; formal analysis, R.H.; investigation, F.S. and A.-M.R. resources, B.M.C., M.D.C. and L.-E.C. data curation, A.-M.R., L.-E.C., M.T. and G.S. writing—original draft preparation, F.S.; writing—review and editing, A.-M.R. and M.T.; visualization, R.H. and M.T. supervision, O.D.P.; These authors contributed equally to this work—F.S. and A.-M.R. All authors have read and agreed to the published version of the manuscript.

Funding: This research received no external funding.

Institutional Review Board Statement: The study was conducted in accordance with the Declaration of Helsinki and approved by the Ethics Committee of University of Medicine and Pharmacy "Grigore T. Popa" (no.22991/17 October 2016) and "St. Spiridon" Iași Hospital(no.52806/15 November 2016).

Informed Consent Statement: Informed consent was obtained from all subjects involved in the study.

Data Availability Statement: Database is available, upon reasonable request, to the corresponding authors.

Acknowledgments: We had the support of the English Department from the University of Medicine and Pharmacy "Grigore T. Popa" Iasi for the English proofreading.

Conflicts of Interest The authors declare no conflict of interest.

References

1. Bent, J.P., 3rd; Silver, J.R.; Porubsky, E.S. Acute laryngeal trauma: A review of 77 patients. *Otolaryngol. Head Neck Surg.* **1993**, *109 Pt 1*, 441–449. [CrossRef] [PubMed]
2. Greaves, N. Gunshot bullet embolus with pellet migration from the left brachiocephalic vein to the right ventricle: A case report. *Scand. J. Trauma Resusc. Emerg. Med.* **2010**, *18*, 36–40. [CrossRef] [PubMed]
3. Monson, D.O.; Saletta, J.D.; Freeark, R.J. Carotid vertebral trauma. *J. Trauma* **1969**, *9*, 987–999. [CrossRef] [PubMed]
4. Azuaje, R.E.; Jacobson, L.E.; Glover, J.; Gomez, G.A.; Rodman, G.H., Jr.; Broadie, T.A.; Simons, C.J.; Bjerke, H.S. Reliability of physical examination as a predictor of vascular injury after penetrating neck trauma. *Am. Surg.* **2003**, *69*, 804–807. [CrossRef] [PubMed]
5. Merion, R.M.; Harness, J.K.; Ramsburgh, S.R.; Thompson, N.W. Selective management of penetrating neck trauma. Costs implication. *Arch. Surg.* **1981**, *116*, 691–696. [CrossRef] [PubMed]

6. Narrod, J.A.; Moore, E.E. Selective management of penetrating neck injuries. A prospective study. *Arch. Surg.* **1984**, *119*, 574–578. [CrossRef] [PubMed]
7. Sekharan, J.; Dennis, J.W.; Veldenz, H.C.; Miranda, F.; Frykberg, E.R. Continued experience with physical examination alone for evaluation and management of penetrating zone 2 neck injuries: Results of 145 cases. *J. Vasc. Surg.* **2000**, *32*, 483–498. [CrossRef] [PubMed]
8. Das, J. Trauma to the Neck and Aerodigestive Tract. In *Trauma in Otolaryngology*; Das, J., Ed.; Springer Nature: Singapore, 2018; pp. 117–143.
9. Pakarinen, T.K.; Leppäniemi, A.; Sihvo, E.; Hiltunen, K.M.; Salo, J. Management of cervical stab wounds in low volume trauma centres: Systematic physical examination and low threshold for adjunctive studies, or surgical exploration. *Injury* **2006**, *37*, 440–447. [CrossRef] [PubMed]
10. Ahmed, N.; Massier, C.; Tassie, J.; Whalen, J.; Chung, R. Diagnosis of penetrating injuries of the pharynx and esophagus in the severely injured patient. *J. Trauma* **2009**, *67*, 152–154. [CrossRef] [PubMed]
11. Tallon, J.M.; Ahmed, J.M.; Sealy, B. Airway management in penetrating neck trauma at a Canadian tertiary trauma center. *Can. J. Emerg. Med.* **2007**, *9*, 101–104. [CrossRef] [PubMed]
12. Fox, C.J.; Gillespie, D.L.; Weber, M.A.; Cox, M.W.; Hawksworth, J.S.; Cryer, C.M.; Rich, N.M.; O'Donnell, S.D. Delayed evaluation of combat-related penetrating neck trauma. *J. Vasc. Surg.* **2006**, *44*, 86–93. [CrossRef] [PubMed]
13. Nason, R.W.; Assuras, G.N.; Gray, P.R.; Lipschitz, J.; Burns, C.M. Penetrating neck injuries: Analysis of experience from a Canadian trauma center. *Can. J. Surg.* **2001**, *44*, 122–126. [PubMed]
14. Biffl, W.I.; Moore, E.E.; Rehese, D.H. Selective management of penetrating neck trauma based on cervical level of injury. *Am. J. Surg.* **1997**, *174*, 678–682. [CrossRef] [PubMed]
15. Burgess, C.A.; Dale, O.T.; Almeyda, R.; Corbridge, R.J. An evidence-based review of the assessment and management of penetrating neck trauma. *Clin. Otolaryngol.* **2012**, *37*, 44–52. [CrossRef] [PubMed]
16. Aich, M.; Alam, A.K.; Talukder, D.C.; Sarder, M.R.; Fakir, A.Y.; Hossain, M. Cut throat injury: Review of 67 cases. *Bangladesh J. Otorhinolaryngol.* **2011**, *17*, 5–13. [CrossRef]
17. Teng, S.X.; Molina, P.E. Acute alcohol intoxication prolongs neuroinflammation without exacerbating neurobehavioral dysfunction following mild traumatic brain injury. *J. Neurotrauma* **2014**, *31*, 378–386. [CrossRef] [PubMed]

Disclaimer/Publisher's Note: The statements, opinions and data contained in all publications are solely those of the individual author(s) and contributor(s) and not of MDPI and/or the editor(s). MDPI and/or the editor(s) disclaim responsibility for any injury to people or property resulting from any ideas, methods, instructions or products referred to in the content.

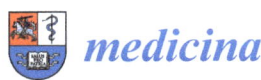

Article

Patterns and Characteristics of Midface Fractures in North-Eastern Romania

Andrei-Mihail Roșu [1,†], Florentina Severin [1,†], Oana Cristina Roșu [2], Bogdan Mihail Cobzeanu [1], Stefan Gherasimescu [1], Florin Petrică Sava [1], Dragoș Octavian Palade [1,*], Cristian Ilie Drochioi [1,*], Victor Vlad Costan [1] and Mihail Dan Cobzeanu [1]

1 Surgical Department, Faculty of Medicine University of Medicine and Pharmacy "Grigore T. Popa", 700115 Iași, Romania
2 Emergency Clinical County Hospital, 730006 Vaslui, Romania
* Correspondence: octavian.palade@umfiasi.ro (D.O.P.); ilie-cristian.drochioi@umfiasi.ro (C.I.D.)
† These authors contributed equally to this work.

Abstract: Midface fractures are common injuries that are the result of interpersonal violence, traffic accidents, falls, work-related accidents, sports-related accidents, or animal aggression. In the northeastern part of Romania, these injuries are a significant health concern that, if left untreated, may lead to functional and esthetic sequelae. *Background and Objectives*: This study aims to update the statistical data available to help promote a different lifestyle, with awareness campaigns to prevent aggression, accidents, and domestic violence. *Materials and Methods*: This research was conducted over five years and included 651 patients of both sexes, with ages between 3 and 95 years, that addressed our center for midface fracture treatment. *Results*: The authors of this study found that men are more predisposed to fractures of the middle third of the face, with anterior laterofacial fractures being the most common type of fracture. Interpersonal violence was the most incriminated etiology for all midface fractures. *Conclusions*: The present study regarding midfacial fractures shows similar results compared to the medical literature. These findings could help promote a different lifestyle, with awareness campaigns to prevent aggression, accidents, and domestic violence.

Keywords: midface fractures; interpersonal violence; trauma; maxillofacial fracture

Citation: Roșu, A.-M.; Severin, F.; Roșu, O.C.; Cobzeanu, B.M.; Gherasimescu, S.; Sava, F.P.; Palade, D.O.; Drochici, C.I.; Costan, V.V.; Cobzeanu, M.D. Patterns and Characteristics of Midface Fractures in North-Eastern Romania. *Medicina* 2023, 59, 510. https://doi.org/10.3390/medicina59030510

Academic Editors: Adriana Neagos, Daniela Vrinceanu, Codrut Sarafoleanu and Mahmut Tayyar Kalciogu

Received: 1 February 2023
Revised: 25 February 2023
Accepted: 3 March 2023
Published: 6 March 2023

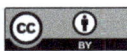

Copyright: © 2023 by the authors. Licensee MDPI, Basel, Switzerland. This article is an open access article distributed under the terms and conditions of the Creative Commons Attribution (CC BY) license (https://creativecommons.org/licenses/by/4.0/).

1. Introduction

Traumatic pathology is the main cause of mortality in adults under 40 years of age, and a significant part of trauma cases are in the maxillofacial area [1,2].

Of all the injuries that can result after trauma to the cephalic extremity, midface fractures represent an important medical and social problem due to the frequency, complexity, and socio-economic impact they involve. They can have multiple consequences, both aesthetic and functional. In addition to facial deformity, they can cause a malocclusion, difficulty mobilizing the mandible with masticatory problems, diplopia, epiphora, nasal obstruction, respiratory disorders, but also sensory disorders or paresthesia [2,3].

Midface fractures are a common type of injury that can occur due to various causes, such as falls, interpersonal violence, car accidents, and sports injuries. These fractures can affect the nose, cheekbones, and maxillary bone and can cause significant physical and emotional distress for the affected individuals, including facial deformities, functional impairment, and long-term scarring.

In the northeastern part of Romania, midface fractures are a significant health concern, with a high incidence rate among the population. This is likely due to a combination of factors, including the prevalence of high-risk activities and certain factors in the region, such as a high rate of alcohol consumption.

Understanding the epidemiology of midface fractures in the northeastern part of Romania is essential for developing effective prevention and treatment strategies to address this health issue.

In the last years, there has been an increasing interest in understanding the prevalence and patterns of midface fractures in different populations. Therefore, it was considered necessary to carry out a retrospective descriptive statistical study that aims to update the epidemiological characteristics of midface trauma between the years 2015 and 2020, also including the general lock-down period during the COVID-19 pandemic in the northeastern area of Romania.

Midface fractures represent a significant medical and social problem due to their frequency, complexity, and socio-economic impact. It was stated that severe midface fractures protect the brain and torso from major traumatic injuries by dissipating the energy of the impact. A study conducted in the United States over the period 1989–2013, including 20,971 patients with trauma, concluded that severe midface fractures were associated with lower rates of hemorrhagic brain injuries and lower rates of thoracic and abdominal post-traumatic complications [4].

In most cases, a multidisciplinary approach is required, as well as modern diagnostic methods and innovative surgical techniques. In the era of technological medicine and permanent advances, the three-dimensional reconstruction of affected structures based on advanced medical imaging is being discussed, with the aim of more thorough and efficient preparation of operative steps [5].

In the present study, the authors aimed to investigate the prevalence of midface fractures in the northeastern part of Romania. This region has a diverse population with a mix of urban and rural areas, and previous studies have shown that the incidence of midface fractures can vary significantly between different regions. Therefore, this study aims to contribute to a better understanding of the epidemiology of these injuries and to aid the development of preventive measures and treatment strategies.

2. Materials and Methods

Within the Emergency Clinical Hospital "Sf. Spiridon" Iași, a retrospective study, aims to establish the epidemiological data from 2015 to 2020 related to midface fractures. Thus, the data on the background, environment, sex, and age of the patients who were treated in the hospital for fractures of the middle third of the face was collected, as well as the type of fracture, the etiology, the need for surgical treatment and the necessary hospitalization period.

Laterofacial fractures interest the zygoma and the zygomatic arch. Centrofacial fractures affect the nasal skeleton and the upper frontomaxillary processes. Oclusofacial fractures are also known as LeFort fractures. LeFort type I fracture affects the anterior maxilla, lateral nasal wall, and pterygoid plates. The LeFort type II fracture line passes through the nasal bones, causing fractures along the nasal bridge, frontal maxilla, lacrimal bones, orbital floor and inferior rim near the inferior orbital foramen, through the anterior wall of the maxillary sinus, and through the pterygoid plates. Lefort type III fractures determine the separation of the midface from the base of the skull, and the fracture line affects the nasal bridge, the medial orbital wall, the orbital floor, passes along the lateral orbital wall, through the zygomatic arch, ethmoid bone, and pterygoid processes.

A number of 651 subjects aged between 3 and 95 were included, patients of both sexes who suffered a midfacial trauma.

This study was carried out with the approval of the "Sf. Spiridon" Iași Emergency Clinical Hospital ethics committee, as well as of the "Grigore T. Popa" University of Medicine and Pharmacy Iași, in compliance with the European General Data Protection Regulation (GDPR) convention and the legislation in force on the protection of personal data.

The data was analyzed statistically using IBM SPSS Statistics 26 (IBM Corp. Released 2019, IBM SPSS Statistics for Windows, Version 26.0. Armonk, NY, USA: IBM Corp.) and Microsoft Excel 2023 (Microsoft Corporation. (2023), Microsoft Excel for Mac, Version 16.70,

Redmond, Washington, United States. Retrieved from https://office.microsoft.com/excel, accessed on 21 January 2023) using descriptive statistic (average values, maximum values, 25th and 75th percentiles respectively), the ANOVA test, chi-square test and the study of the correlation between different phenomena was carried out using the correlation coefficient r (Pearson).

3. Results

Out of the total number of patients included in the study, 87 were females, representing 13.36%, and 564, respectively 86.63%, were males; with a distribution of 6.48 to 1 in favor of the male sex with the mean age for female participants being 46.83 (min—5 years, max—95 years) and 40,49 for the male group (min—3 years, max—89 years)

Additionally, the age groups 21–30 years (140 patients), 31–40 years (133 patients), and 41–50 years (117 patients) prevailed in the case of midface traumas. Additionally, 45.01% (mean age 40.97; CI 38.82–43.11; Min 5; Max 95) of subjects were from an urban environment, with 38.25% being male and 6.76% female, while 54.99% (age mean 41.33; CI 39.52–43.13; Min 3; Max 89) were from the rural area, of which 48.39% males and 6.51% females (Figure 1). From the studied lot, a total of 462 (70.81%) patients admitted to our service required surgical treatment, while 189 (29.19%) were treated conservatively (Table 1).

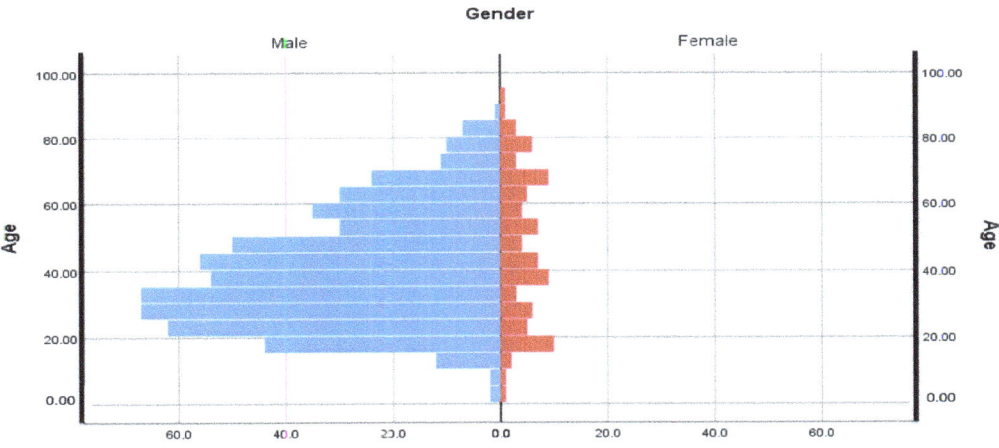

Figure 1. Distribution of the studied lot according to gender and age.

Table 1. Descriptive indicators depending on the type of treatment.

	Gender	N	%	Mean Age	Std. Dev.	Min.	Max.	p
medical treatment	female	32	11.90	47.75	24.20	5	89	0.513
	male	157	88.10	40.19	17.00	3	85	
	TOTAL	189	100.00	41.47	18.53	3	89	
surgical treatment	female	55	16.93	46.30	21.55	13	95	0.102
	male	407	83.07	40.33	17.05	8	89	
	TOTAL	462	100.00	41.04	17.72	8	95	

Regarding the etiology of midface trauma, the first place was occupied by interpersonal violence, representing 46.85% of cases, followed by traffic accidents. In the last places, we found work and sports-related accidents (Figure 2). When the lot was divided according to gender, the predominance of interpersonal violence was maintained in the case of male participants. In contrast, for most female participants, midface trauma was caused by traffic accidents (Figure 3).

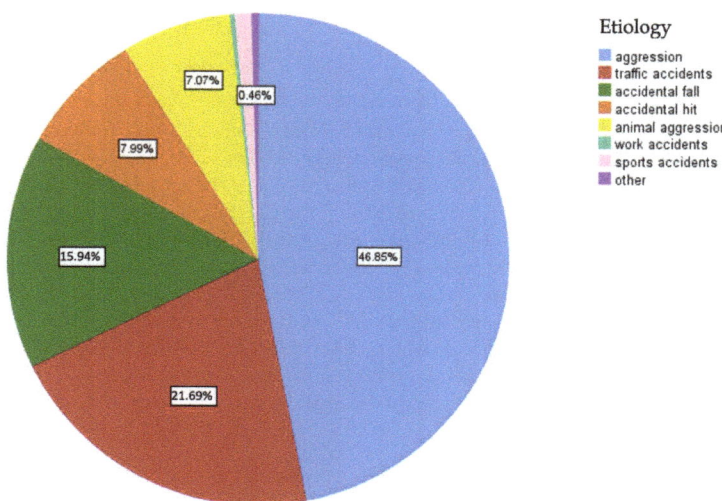

Figure 2. Chart reflecting the etiology of midface trauma in the studied lot.

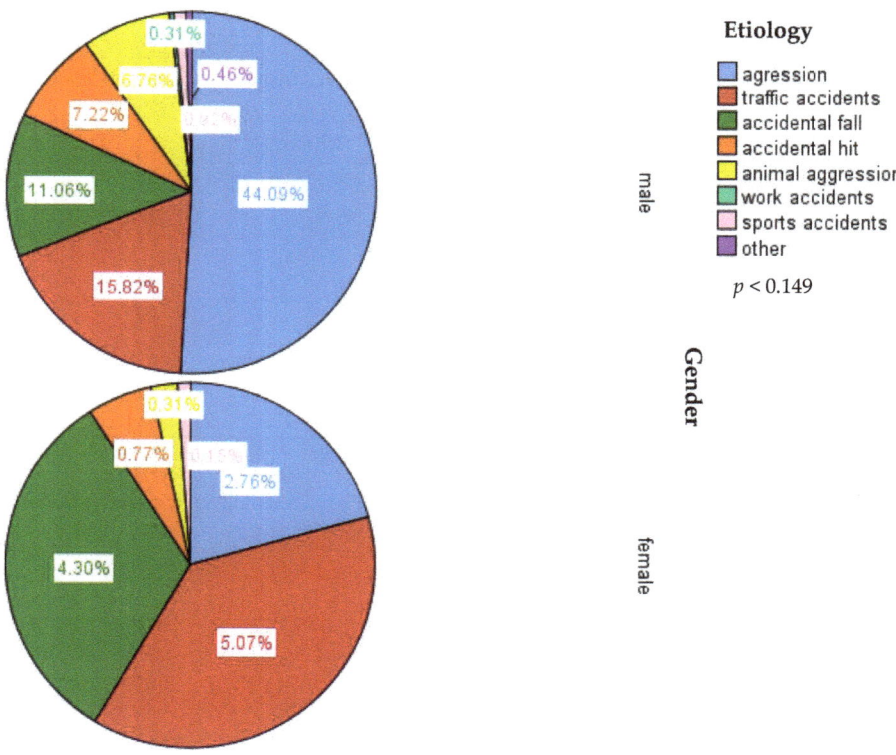

Figure 3. Etiology for midface trauma between gender.

When comparing the number of hospital attendance by gender for the COVID-19 pandemic lock-down period with the same period from the previous year, the authors found no significant differences between female and male patients that were admitted to the hospital ($p = 0.886$) with a total number of patients of 16 admitted between march and may 2019 and 14 for the same period in 2020.

As for the different types of midface fractures, our study found that the most frequent, representing 44% of the total cases, were anterior laterofacial fractures, followed by antero-posterior laterofacial fractures and nose fractures, each representing 13%. On the other hand, the least encountered types of midface fractures were NOE (naso-orbio-ethmoidal) complex and LeFort type I fractures (Figure 4A,B). In addition, this study found that hospital admission for midface fractures had a continuous drop over the studied period, although the number of female patients was similar for each year in the documented period (Figure 5).

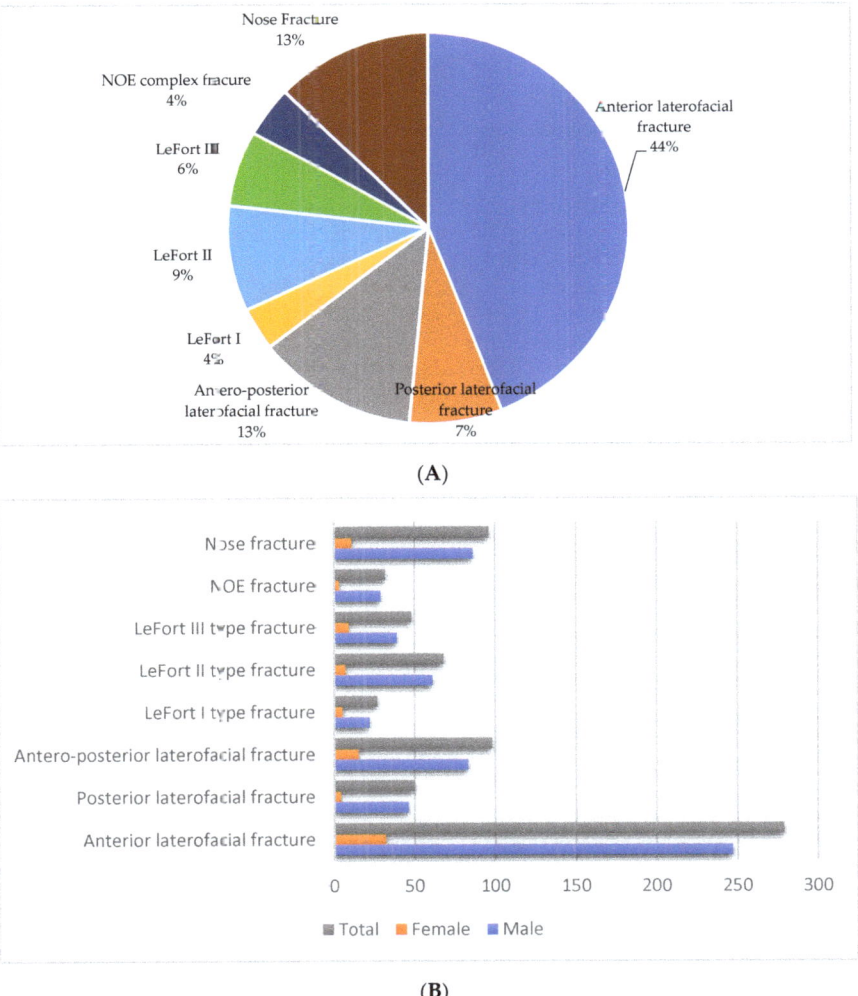

Figure 4. (A) Types of midface fractures represented as a percentage, (B) Types of midface fractures according to gender.

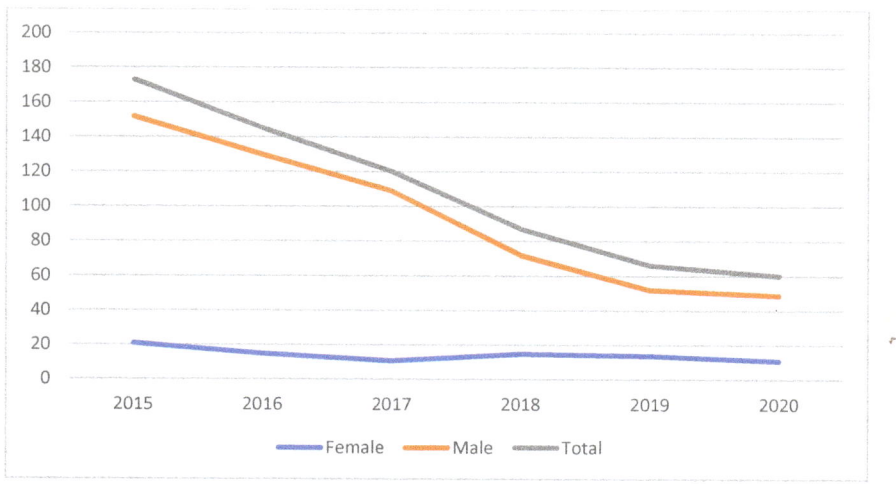

Figure 5. The number of cases of midfacial trauma over the years of the studied period.

4. Discussion

Our study found that most of the midface trauma cases were anterior laterofacial fractures representing 44%, followed by anteroposterior laterofacial fractures and nose fractures, each representing 13%. LeFort type II and LeFort type III fractures expressed 9% and respectively 6% of the total studied lot, with LeFort type I and NOE complex fractures each representing 4% of the cases. Men were especially at risk, surpassing the female patients, with a ratio of 6.48 to 1, with adults between 21 and 50 years old comprising more than 80% of the total patients included in this study.

The values of male to female ratio differ greatly in the specialized literature, depending on the area where the studies were conducted. Thus, a lower value of only 1.8:1 was recorded in Italy in 2017 in a study that followed trauma in the maxillo-facial region over a period of 15 years and included 1720 patients in the research [6]. Another study carried out in Europe, this time in Austria in 2003, reported a ratio of 2.1:1 (male: female) [2]; in Amsterdam, in 2013, the stated ratio was 2.6:1 [1], and in China, the male: female ratio was 3.5:1 [7]. A ratio similar to that obtained in our study (6.4:1) was reported by a survey conducted in the Arab countries around the Persian Gulf in 2021, which included more than 19,000 patients [8]. Higher values with a ratio of 8:1 were reported by India [5], but also in Africa, where this ratio reaches 12:1 in certain areas [9]. These large differences between the number of men and women with facial fractures could be explained by socio-economic, cultural, and educational factors.

A study realized in 2015 comparing data from multiple centers enrolled in the European Maxillofacial Trauma project about the demographics, cause, and characteristics of maxillofacial trauma showed a male-to-female ratio of 3.6:1 overall. Still, the ratio varied from center to center, with the highest ratio (9,4:1) present in Kyiv, Ukraine, and the lowest in Amsterdam, The Netherlands (2.2:1). Additionally, the mean age varied from 29.9 years in Dundee, Scotland, UK to 43.9 in Ljubljana, Slovenia. Interpersonal violence (39%) was the most incriminated etiology, followed by falls (31%), traffic accidents (11%), sport-related injuries (11%), and work-related injuries (3%) [10].

Regarding the etiology of midface traumas, for the entire studied group, the first place was occupied by interpersonal violence with 46.85% of cases, followed by traffic accidents at 21.69%, accidental falls at 15.94%, accidental hits at 7.99%, and aggression caused by animals with a percentage of 7.07%. In the last places, we found accidents at work and those resulting from sports activities. After dividing the group according to gender, we noticed that, for male participants, the situation reflected the global trend, with aggression being by far the most frequent etiology, followed by traffic accidents, falls, and accidental hits, while for female patients, the most cases of midface trauma were caused by traffic accidents, followed by accidental falls and, in 3rd place, by assault. Regarding the etiology of these fractures in the general population and, subsequently, by gender, numerous studies have been conducted worldwide at different time periods. We can thus try to outline an etiological hierarchy of midfacial fractures, although the results of the studies are extremely varied from one geographic region to another.

In European countries, interpersonal violence is also the most incriminated etiology, but with a lower percentage than that objectified by our study (39% vs. 46.85%), followed by falls (31%), traffic accidents (11%), sports-related injuries (11%) and work accidents (3%) [10]. Other countries reported different results, as follows: in the Netherlands (2013), the most frequent etiology was represented by traffic accidents, regardless of the patient's gender, followed by interpersonal violence for men, respectively, by falls in the case of women. For those who consumed alcohol, aggression was most frequently incriminated [1]. On the other hand, in Italy in 2017, in a study carried out over a period of 15 years on 1720 patients, the hierarchy of etiologies looked like this: in first place were road accidents (57.1%), followed by interpersonal violence (21.7%), falls (14.2%), work accidents (3.5%), respectively sports accidents (3.3%) [6]. Another study from Italy conducted in 2013 also mentions road accidents as the main etiology of facial fractures [11]. We find that there are differences depending on the specifics of the area; thus, in Austria in 2003, a study carried out on a group of 9543 patients described a completely different order of etiologies: initially, daily activities were incriminated (38%)—including falls, followed by sports accidents (31%), then interpersonal violence and traffic accidents, each with 12%, 5% work accidents, and 2% other causes. 19% of the patients included in the study were foreigners, with the Austrian Alps being a highly frequented area for winter sports [2]. In Croatia, authors reported falls as the main etiology, followed by aggression for men and traffic accidents for women. [12]. The same study also describes a difference regarding age, with interpersonal violence more frequent among young people, with falls being the prerogative of adults over 50.

A study that analyzed the clinical patterns and characteristics of midfacial fractures over a period of 10 years, this time in the western Romanian population, found that the most common types of fracture were laterofacial (50%) and nasal bone fractures (22.93%), with LeFort type fractures being the least encountered, representing 0.83% for LeFort type I, 1.03% for LeFort Type II and 0.83 for LeFort type III from a total of 397 patients [13]. Another study from the same part of the country found that midface fractures affect most commonly the male sex and patients from the urban area (54.35%) aged between 20 and 29 years old, with the most incriminated etiology being assault, followed by fall trauma and road traffic accidents [14]. The fact that the second most incriminated etiology from the north-eastern part of the country is road traffic accidents, and for the western part is accidental falls could be explained by a more developed transport infrastructure in the western part of the country.

Regarding the background, the current study mentions that 45.01% of the subjects are from urban areas, while 54.99% are from rural areas. Another interesting observation would be the similar percentage of women from both backgrounds (6.76% in the urban environment versus 6.51% in the rural environment), thus not supporting the statement that domestic violence is more frequent in the rural environment. On the other hand, there is a greater number of men coming from the rural environment, 48.39% of the whole lot, compared to 38.25% from the urban environment. This can be explained by the level of education, the more frequent consumption of alcoholic beverages, but also their involvement in raising animals or other activities within the household.

Our study's results showed a continuous drop of the hospital attendance rate for midface fractures over the studied period. This can be attributed to a better implementation of public safety rules, better management of alcohol consumption and stricter traffic regulations, the implementation of a better diagnostic protocol utilizing cone beam computer tomography instead of conventional radiographic studies, and the cases of maxillofacial trauma being directed to other healthcare centers in the region. This phenomenon may also be explained by the lawmaker's concern for citizens' safety, whcih led to tougher sentences for acts of aggression (including interpersonal violence and road traffic accidents) directed to members of the family or for those committed by inebriated authors [15].

The authors compared the data regarding hospital attendance for midfacial trauma during the COVID-19 general lockdown with the same period of the previous year, but the results showed no significant difference. In contrast, another recently published study concerning the effect of the COVID-19 pandemic on midface fractures found a decrease in hospital admissions for facial trauma, approximately seven times lower, comparing the number of patients from March to April 2019 with the same period in 2020 [16].

Interpersonal violence was the most incriminated cause of midface trauma, followed by traffic accidents and accidental falls. It must be noted that men were more affected by violence, while the leading cause for women was traffic accidents. Other studies in the literature show a different predominance in the etiology of facial fractures: an Indian study conducted in 2019 on 944 patients with facial trauma, with 19% midface fractures, found that the leading cause was by far road traffic accidents [17]. The same predominance of road traffic accidents is mentioned in another study from Saudi Arabia (2019) [18] and India (2022) [19].

The current study also underlines the predominance of young male adults, with a peak incidence between the 2nd and 3rd decade of life. Most studies report the same conclusions, with young people in their 20s and 30s having an active lifestyle and engaging in many outdoor activities [8]. The average age for female patients was 46.83 years (minimum age—5 years, maximum age—95 years) and 40.49 years for male patients (minimum age—3 years, and maximum age—89 years). In general, most studies on the epidemiology of fractures in the oro-maxillo-facial region describe an older average age for female patients, something also highlighted in a study from Italy from 2017, where the average age for women with facial fractures is 59.5 years [6]. For Europe, a varying average age of the whole lot can be observed, regardless of sex, from 29.9 years in Dundee, Scotland, UK, to 43.9 in Ljubljana, Slovenia [10]. Reviewing data from the literature, we find that the predominance of young adults in the group of patients with facial trauma has not changed over time, being described in Sweden in 1980 [20] and in Scotland (1985) [21].

Although children are more prone to craniofacial trauma, the absence of sinus pneumatization, the bone elasticity, the thickness of the periosteum, and the retruded position of the face in relation to the neurocranium offer a greater degree of protection [22]. In our study, only 58 patients were children (maximum age of 18 years), representing 8.91% of the entire lot. A total number of 38 children received surgical treatment, representing 65,51%. A smaller percentage was mentioned in a study conducted in Indianapolis, Indiana, in 2019, on 218 pediatric patients, showing that only a quarter (25.2%) of the hospitalized children needed surgical intervention, the rest receiving conservative treatment [23].

Craniofacial trauma is common in all age groups. The cause is closely related to age, sex, and alcohol consumption, and it determines the type and severity of the injury. Hussain states that accidental falls are the primary cause of injuries in elderly patients, while interpersonal violence and traffic accidents are responsible for injuries in patients between 15 and 50 years of age. Physical violence most often involves young adults, and fights usually occur between strangers who have consumed excessive amounts of alcohol. Women are assaulted by people known to them, in most cases, their life partners; pedestrians are prone to skull fractures, vehicle occupants involved in traffic accidents suffer midfacial fractures, and cyclists have mandibular fractures [24].

Our study found that the most common types of fractures affecting the midface were those involving the zygomatic complex, namely laterofacial fractures (75.58%) followed by oclusofacial fractures (LeFort type fractures) (21.81%) and centrofacial fractures (19.66%). Other authors reported that fractures of the zygomatic complex accounted for 62.5% of the total number of midface fractures, followed by LeFort II type fractures (23%), multiple fractures of the midface (10%), LeFort I type fractures (6%), LeFort III fractures (4.5%), and naso-orbito-ethmoid complex fractures (4%) [25].

Fractures of the NOE complex are the result of forces applied to the middle third of the face. Due to the violence of the impact required to cause these fractures, other facial, cranial, or body lesions may be present. Traffic accidents, more often those involving an occupant not wearing a seat belt at the time of impact, are the most common causes of trauma affecting the NOE complex, representing 4% of all adult skull fractures [26,27], the most frequently affected being young male adults. This corresponds with the results of our study.

Midface fractures' treatment follows similar principles to the treatment of other systemic fractures but presents a series of particularities due to the complexity of the facial anatomy [28], with authors stating that the restoration of the facial vertical buttresses restores the load-bearing structure of the midface, while the rehabilitation of the horizontal buttresses recovers the aesthetic aspect.

The authors of this study found that 461 (70.81%) required and received surgical treatment consisting of open reduction and internal fixation with titanium miniplates and/or mesh for selected cases of laterofacial or nose fractures, while 189 (29.19%) patients admitted in our center were treated conservatively. Our results are similar to other studies. Manodph et al. found that 73.56% of the entire lot (3611 patients) required surgery [29], while Wouter et al. reported similar percentages in a tertiary trauma center from the Netherlands where, over a period of 5 years, 293 (74%) patients received surgical treatment for midface fractures [30]. A higher percentage of 85.4% was mentioned in a study from Nepal in 2021 [31] and in Berlin, Germany, where 89.5% of patients with midface fractures were treated surgically in 2019 [32]

5. Conclusions

The present study regarding midfacial fractures shows similar results compared to the medical literature, with certain particularities: a male predominance with more than 80% of the current lot, a high incidence of interpersonal violence and traffic accidents, as well as high frequency of anterior laterofacial fractures, compared to other types. In addition, we observed a continuous descending trend in the total number of hospitalizations.

Most of the patients received surgical treatment.

Given the increasing esthetic and functional demands, a continuous update of available resources is necessary for a better outcome for midface fracture cases.

Reviewing the literature shows an extremely high variability of etiological agents, influenced by numerous factors such as socio-economic status, cultural background, life habits, or level of education. These findings could help promote a different lifestyle with awareness campaigns to prevent aggression, accidents, and domestic violence. Further studies are needed for dynamic observation of changes in the epidemiology of midface fractures, to establish the effectiveness of preventive strategies, and also to note the impact of lifestyle on facial traumatic pathology.

Author Contributions: Conceptualization, A.-M.R. and D.O.P.; methodology, M.D.C. and V.V.C.; software, S.G. and B.M.C.; validation, F.S. and A.-M.R.; formal analysis, F.S.; investigation F.P.S and A.-M.R. resources, M.D.C. and V.V.C.; data curation, F.S.; writing—original draft preparation, A.-M.R.; writing—review and editing, A.-M.R and O.C.R.; visualization, C.I.D.; supervision, D.O.P. All authors have read and agreed to the published version of the manuscript.

Funding: This research received no external funding.

Institutional Review Board Statement: University of Medicine and Pharmacy "Grigore T. Popa" Iași nr. 26268/19.12.2019 and "Sf Spiridon" Hospital, Iași nr. 20/12.06.2020.

Informed Consent Statement: The informed consent was waved due to the fact the data was anonymized prior to manipulation.

Data Availability Statement: Data available on request.

Conflicts of Interest: The authors declare no conflict of interest.

References

1. Salentijn, E.G.; Bergh, B.V.D.; Forouzanfar, T. A ten-year analysis of midfacial fractures. *J. Cranio-Maxillofac. Surg.* **2013**, *41*, 630–636. [CrossRef] [PubMed]
2. Gassner, R.; Tuli, T.; Hächl, O.; Rudisch, A.; Ulmer, H. Cranio-maxillofacial trauma: A 10 year review of 9543 cases with 21067 injuries. *J. Cranio-Maxillofac. Surg.* **2003**, *31*, 51–61. [CrossRef] [PubMed]
3. Yamamoto, K.; Matsusue, Y.; Horita, S.; Murakami, K.; Sugiura, T.; Kirita, T. Clinical Analysis of Midfacial Fractures. *Mater. Socio Med.* **2014**, *26*, 21–25. [CrossRef]
4. Woriax, H.E.; Hamill, M.E.; Gilbert, C.M.; Reed, C.M.; Faulks, E.R.; Love, K.M.; Lollar, D.I.; Nussbaum, M.S.; Collier, B.R. Is the Face an Air Bag for the Brain and Torso? -The Potential Protective Effects of Severe Midface Fractures. *Am. Surg.* **2018**, *84*, 1299–1302. [CrossRef]
5. Satish, P.; Prasad, K.; Lalitha, R.M.; Ranganath, K.; Sagar, P. Analysis of the Changing Patterns of Midface Fractures Using 3D Computed Tomography: An Observational Study. *Craniomaxillofacial Trauma Reconstr.* **2017**, *11*, 265–272. [CrossRef]
6. Bonavolonta, P.; Orabona, G.D.; Abbate, V.; Vaira, L.A.; Faro, C.L.; Petrocelli, M.; Attanasi, F.; De Riu, G.; Iaconetta, G.; Califano, L. The epidemiological analysis of maxillofacial fractures in Italy: The experience of a single tertiary center with 1720 patients. *J. Cranio-Maxillofac. Surg.* **2017**, *45*, 1319–1326. [CrossRef] [PubMed]
7. Zhou, H.-H.; Liu, Q.; Yang, R.-T.; Li, Z.; Li, Z.-B. Maxillofacial Fractures in Women and Men: A 10-Year Retrospective Study. *J. Oral Maxillofac. Surg.* **2015**, *73*, 2181–2188. [CrossRef] [PubMed]
8. AlQahtani, F.; Bishawi, K.; Jaber, M.; Thomas, S. Maxillofacial trauma in the gulf countries: A systematic review. *Eur. J. Trauma Emerg. Surg.* **2020**, *47*, 397–406. [CrossRef] [PubMed]
9. Jaber, M.A.; AlQahtani, F.; Bishawi, K.; Kuriadom, S.T. Patterns of Maxillofacial Injuries in the Middle East and North Africa: A Systematic Review. *Int. Dent. J.* **2021**, *71*, 292–299. [CrossRef]
10. Boffano, P.; Roccia, F.; Zavattero, E.; Dediol, E.; Uglešić, V.; Kovačič, Ž.; Vesnaver, A.; Konstantinovic, V.; Petrović, M.; Stephens, J.; et al. European Maxillofacial Trauma (EURMAT) project: A multicentre and prospective study. *J. Cranio-Maxillofac. Surg.* **2015**, *43*, 62–70. [CrossRef] [PubMed]
11. Roccia, F.; Boffano, P.; Bianchi, F.A.; Ramieri, G. An 11-year review of dental injuries associated with maxillofacial fractures in Turin, Italy. *Oral Maxillofac. Surg.* **2012**, *17*, 269–274. [CrossRef] [PubMed]
12. Siber, S.; Matijević, M.; Sikora, M.; Leović, D.; Mumlek, I.; Macan, D. Assessment of Oro-Maxillofacial Trauma According to Gender, Age, Cause and Type of the Injury. *Acta Stomatol. Croat.* **2015**, *49*, 340–347. [CrossRef]
13. Tent, P.; Juncar, R.; Juncar, M. Clinical patterns and characteristics of midfacial fractures in western romanian population: A 10-year retrospective study. *Med. Oral Patol. Oral Y Cirugía Bucal* **2019**, *24*, e792–e798. [CrossRef] [PubMed]
14. Tent, P.A.; Juncar, R.I.; Lung, T.; Juncar, M. Midfacial fractures: A retrospective etiological study over a 10-year period in Western Romanian population. *Niger. J. Clin. Pract.* **2018**, *21*, 1570–1575.
15. Codul Penal al României, 21.06.1968, art. 181, 182, 184; Republicat și Modificat. Available online: https://legislatie.just.ro/Public/DetaliiDocument/38090 (accessed on 21 January 2023).
16. Kasem, A.; Redenski, I.; Oren, D.; Zoabi, A.; Srouji, S.; Kablan, F. Decline in Maxillofacial Injuries during the Pandemic: The Hidden Face of COVID-19. *J. Clin. Med.* **2022**, *12*, 128. [CrossRef]
17. Abhinav, R.P.; Selvarasu, K.; Maheswari, G.U.; Taltia, A.A. The patterns and etiology of maxillofacial trauma in South India. *Ann. Maxillofac. Surg.* **2019**, *9*, 114–117. [CrossRef] [PubMed]
18. Al-Bokhamseen, M.; Salma, R.; Al-Bodbaij, M. Patterns of maxillofacial fractures in Hofuf, Saudi Arabia: A 10-year retrospective case series. *Saudi Dent. J.* **2018**, *31*, 129–136. [CrossRef]
19. Menon, S.; Shivakotee, S.; Sham, M.; Kumar, V.; Archana, S. Midface fracture pattern in a tertiary care hospital—A prospective study. *Natl. J. Maxillofac. Surg.* **2022**, *13*, 238. [CrossRef]
20. Afzelius, L.-E.; Rosén, C. Facial fractures: A review of 368 cases. *Int. J. Oral Surg.* **1980**, *9*, 25–32. [CrossRef]
21. Ellis, E.; Moos, K.F.; El-Attar, A. Ten years of mandibular fractures: An analysis of 2137 cases. *Oral Surg. Oral Med. Oral Pathol.* **1985**, *59*, 120–129. [CrossRef]
22. Cole, P.; Kaufman, Y.; Hollier, L.H. Managing the Pediatric Facial Fracture. *Craniomaxillofac. Trauma Reconstr.* **2009**, *2*, 77–83. [CrossRef]
23. Kao, R.; Campiti, V.J.; Rabbani, C.C.; Ting, J.Y.; Sim, M.W.; Shipchandler, T.Z. Pediatric Midface Fractures: Outcomes and Complications of 218 Patients. *Laryngoscope Investig. Otolaryngol.* **2019**, *4*, 597–601. [CrossRef] [PubMed]
24. Hussain, K.B.; Wijetunge, D.B.M.; Grubnic, S.M.; Jackson, I.T.M. A Comprehensive Analysis of Craniofacial Trauma. *J. Trauma Inj. Infect. Crit. Care* **1994**, *36*, 34–47. [CrossRef]
25. Bulgaru Iliescu, D.; Enache, A.; Scripcaru, C.; Curcă, G. *Tratat de Traumatologie Medico-Legala*; Editura Revistei Timpul: Iasi, Romania, 2021; Volume 1, p. 369. ISBN 978-973-612-837-0.
26. Kelley, P.; Crawford, M.; Higuera, S.; Hollier, L.H. Two Hundred Ninety-Four Consecutive Facial Fractures in an Urban Trauma Center: Lessons Learned. *Plast. Reconstr. Surg.* **2005**, *116*, 42e–49e. [CrossRef] [PubMed]

27. Cabalag, M.S.; Wasiak, J.; Andrew, N.E.; Tang, J.; Kirby, J.C.; Morgan, D.J. Epidemiology and management of maxillofacial fractures in an Australian trauma centre. *J. Plast. Reconstr. Aesthetic Surg.* **2014**, *67*, 183–189. [CrossRef] [PubMed]
28. Wusiman, P.; Maimaitituerxun, B.; Guli; Saimaiti, A.; Moming, A. Epidemiology and Pattern of Oral and Maxillofacial Trauma. *J. Craniofacial Surg.* **2020**, *31*, e517–e520. [CrossRef]
29. Manodh, P.; Shankar, D.P.; Pradeep, D.; Santhosh, R.; Murugan, A. Incidence and patterns of maxillofacial trauma—A retrospective analysis of 3611 patients—An update. *Oral Maxillofac. Surg.* **2016**, *20*, 377–383. [CrossRef] [PubMed]
30. Van Hout, W.M.; Van Cann, E.M.; Abbink, J.H.; Koole, R. An epidemiological study of maxillofacial fractures requiring surgical treatment at a tertiary trauma centre between 2005 and 2010. *Br. J. Oral Maxillofac. Surg.* **2013**, *51*, 416–420. [CrossRef]
31. Chaurasia, N.K.; Upadhyaya, C.; Dulal, S. Etiology, Pattern, Treatment and Outcome of Maxillofacial Fractures at Dhulikhel Hospital. *Kathmandu Univ. Med. J.* **2021**, *19*, 356–360. [CrossRef]
32. Goedecke, M.; Thiem, D.G.E.; Schneider, D.; Frerich, B.; Kämmerer, P.W. Through the ages-Aetiological changes in maxillofacial trauma. *Dent. Traumatol.* **2019**, *35*, 115–120. [CrossRef]

Disclaimer/Publisher's Note: The statements, opinions and data contained in all publications are solely those of the individual author(s) and contributor(s) and not of MDPI and/or the editor(s). MDPI and/or the editor(s) disclaim responsibility for any injury to people or property resulting from any ideas, methods, instructions or products referred to in the content.

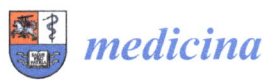

Case Report

Granulomatosis with Polyangiitis (GPA)—A Multidisciplinary Approach of a Case Report

Cornelia M. Trandafir [1,2], Nicolae Constantin Balica [1,2,*], Delia I. Horhat [1,2], Ion C. Mot [1,2], Cristian A. Sarau [3] and Marioara Poenaru [2]

1. Department of ENT, Victor Babeş University of Medicine and Pharmacy, 300041 Timisoara, Romania
2. ENT Department, SCMUT Hospital Timisoara, Bd. Revolutiei No. 6, 300054 Timisoara, Romania
3. Department of Medical Semiology I, Victor Babeş University of Medicine and Pharmacy, 300041 Timisoara, Romania
* Correspondence: balica@umft.ro; Fax: +02-56498205

Abstract: Granulomatosis with polyangiitis is an atypical, multisystem disease with unknown etiology that generally affects both genders equally, with a predominance in the Caucasian racial group for individuals in their fourth decade. The disease affects the small vessels of the respiratory system, lungs, and kidneys. ENT manifestations are common, but ocular involvement is also frequent and can occur as an initial harbinger of the disease. The signs and symptoms of the disease are non-pathognomonic and sometimes localized, but it carries a poor prognosis if left untreated. Early diagnosis of granulomatosis with polyangiitis can be difficult and is established by a clinical examination along with laboratory tests for anti-neutrophil cytoplasmic antibodies (ANCA) and anatomopathological exam results that showcase necrosis, granulomatous inflammation, and vasculitis. Although the ocular involvement is not life threatening, it can cause blindness and may also be a sign of the active form of this systemic fatal disease. Treatment strategies involving immunosuppression and adjuvant therapies improve the prognosis. In this article we present a rare case of a patient diagnosed with granulomatosis with polyangiitis in our ENT department in 2003, with a follow-up for 19 years in our clinic.

Keywords: otorhinolaryngology; granulomatosis with polyangiitis; interdisciplinary; vasculitis; ocular manifestations; diagnosis; treatment

Citation: Trandafir, C.M.; Balica, N.C.; Horhat, D.I.; Mot, I.C.; Sarau, C.A.; Poenaru, M. Granulomatosis with Polyangiitis (GPA)—A Multidisciplinary Approach of a Case Report. *Medicina* 2022, *58*, 1837. https://doi.org/10.3390/medicina58121837

Academic Editors: Adriana Neagos, Daniela Vrinceanu, Codrut Sarafoleanu and Mahmut Tayyar Kalcioglu

Received: 14 November 2022
Accepted: 12 December 2022
Published: 13 December 2022

Publisher's Note: MDPI stays neutral with regard to jurisdictional claims in published maps and institutional affiliations.

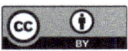

Copyright: © 2022 by the authors. Licensee MDPI, Basel, Switzerland. This article is an open access article distributed under the terms and conditions of the Creative Commons Attribution (CC BY) license (https://creativecommons.org/licenses/by/4.0/).

1. Introduction

Granulomatosis with polyangiitis (GPA) is a rare, immunologically mediated vasculitis associated with anti-neutrophil cytoplasmic antibodies (ANCA) [1]. It was first described in 1897 by McBride, with a further description in 1931 by Klinger, as a variant of polyarteritis nodosa, followed by Wegener in 1936 who characterized it for the first time as an individual, distinct syndrome, clinically and pathologically distinct from polyarteritis nodosa.

Its annual incidence is reported to be between 5 and 10 cases/1,000,000 population [2] and rarely seen in children and young adults. Remission occurs in 85–90% of treated patients [3]. The relapse rate within 5 years is 50% [4]. The risk of mortality is secondary to subglottic stenosis, rapidly progressing glomerulonephritis, or respiratory system involvement.

Although its etiology remains largely unknown, a few theories linked to genetic predisposition, environmental triggers, and the implication of infectious agents have been suggested [1,5].

The pathology is characterized by the development of a general, necrotizing, systemic vasculitis and a granulomatous inflammation pattern within the vessel wall and subendothelial space [6]. It usually affects the respiratory tract and kidneys; for that reason the acronym ELK (E—ear, nose and throat involvement; L—lung involvement; K—kidney involvement) is classically used.

Goldman and Churg proposed in 1954 a useful criteria to diagnose the condition: (1) the presence of granuloma in the upper airways; (2) necrotizing vasculitis; (3) glomerulonephritis [7].

GPA is traditionally considered a disease with a predilection for renal and pulmonary involvement.

Clinically, the patient complains of a wide spectrum of manifestations. They may present limited forms, involving one or two ELK areas, or a severe, generalized form due to the affliction of multiple organ systems (fever, acute pain, severe malaise, weakness) if left untreated. Renal involvement can be suspected if the patient has hematuria, proteinuria, or a cellular cast on the urine cytology, and can be manifested as acute kidney injury, chronic kidney injury, or renal failure [8,9].

An otolaryngologist plays an important role in its diagnosis and treatment [10]. The most common ENT manifestations include epistaxis, sinus inflammation, nasal obstruction, facial nerve palsy [11], and hearing loss [12]. Clinically, the literature reports septal perforation as the most common feature of damage and a prevalence of subglottic stenosis between 6 and 23% [13,14]. Other signs, such as mucosal ulcerations of the nose with bone and cartilage destruction, might be present with evolution of the disease.

Granulomatosis with polyangiitis can also have pulmonary [15], renal, cutaneous, cardiovascular, and neurological manifestations. GPA can affect any part of the eye, and orbital involvement may be the first and only sign of the disease. The ophthalmological symptomatology is also nonspecific, but the anterior segment of the eye and the orbit are usually involved, consisting of episcleritis, scleritis, conjunctivitis, blindness, and nasolacrimal obstruction. According to Pakrou et al., ophthalmic involvement can result in significant morbidity and even blindness [16]. A remarkable association between nasolacrimal obstruction and subglottic stenosis was reported in the literature by Robinson et al. [17].

Laboratory tests show elevated levels of anti-neutrophil cytoplasmic antibodies (ANCA) with a cytoplasmic staining pattern directed against proteinase 3 (PR3). Being related to disease activity, ANCAs have been identified as risk factors of GPA relapse and are currently used in the long-term follow-up process [18].

As the symptomatology is nonspecific, the exclusion of other granulomatous diseases (bacterial, viral, fungal) and other diseases with unspecified etiology diagnosis is usually needed.

Histologically, evidence of necrotizing granulomas usually indicates the diagnosis; however, treatment can be initiated even if a histological diagnosis cannot be made, if the clinical criteria of diagnosis are present and the c-ANCA titer is positive.

The treatment of GPA is through medication and is based on a combination of immunosuppressants divided into various phases, followed by a maintenance treatment once remission has been achieved.

2. Case Report

Female patient, 43 years old, previously diagnosed with granulomatosis with polyangiitis in our department in 2003 with a nasal and laryngeal determination, was admitted to the clinic for clinical-biological reassessment.

From her medical history, we know that she suffers from: granulomatosis with polyangiitis with ANCA–PR3 positive in remission, chronic secondary glomerulonephritis in remission, asthma, secondary hypertension, hypokalemia, mild secondary anemia, mixed dyslipidemia with triglyceride predominance, secondary hyperparathyroidism, septal perforation, nasal granuloma, subglottic stenosis, and hearing loss after repeated otitis for which she had tympanotomy and auditory prosthesis.

In light of her renal involvement (chronic secondary glomerulonephritis), she was treated by the nephrology department with a combination of corticoterapic treatment (prednisone) and cyclophosphamide. She was in remission under this pathognomonic treatment.

The nasal endoscopy revealed a single cavity by disappearance of the septal cartilage, an atrophic, friable, crust-covered mucosa, almost complete disappearance of the inferior and middle nasal turbinate, and rhino pharynx covered by gray crusts (Figure 1).

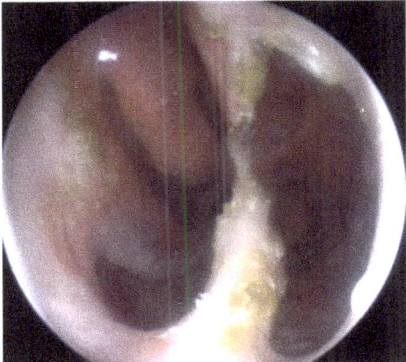

Figure 1. Nasal endoscopy.

The laryngeal endoscopy revealed subglottic stenosis and free vocal cords, which were mobile with breathing and phonation. The stenosis had not progressed since the last follow-up (Figure 2).

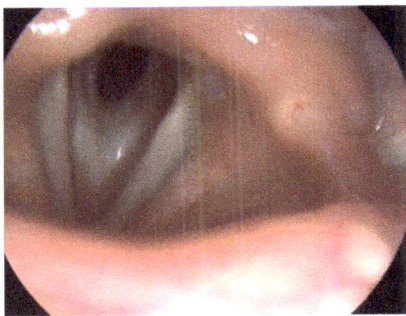

Figure 2. Subglottic stenosis.

The audiogram showed mixed hearing loss after repeated otitis for which she had tympanotomy (Figure 3).

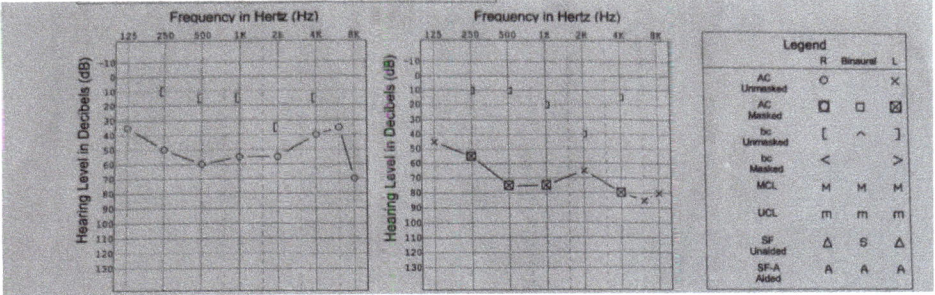

Figure 3. Hearing exam using an Itera II audiometer.

Ocular examination
BCVA (best corrected visual acuity) RE (right eye) = 20/25 (+1.00 dsf × −0.50 dcyl 10°)
BCVA LE (left eye) = 20/25 (+1.50 dsf × −0.50 dcyl 5°)
Normal ocular adnexa, normal eye motility.

The slit lamp examination revealed a normal aspect of the anterior pole. In order to correctly evaluate the posterior pole structures, a complex examination was performed that included: retino photography, ocular ultrasound, and optical coherence tomography (OCT) (Figures 4–7). The pathological findings highlighted by the ancillary tests were: discreet miliary drusen, a slight reduction of the thickness of the retinal nerve fiber layer in the LE, and a C/D ratio of 0.69/0.7. These pathological features are not specific to granulomatosis with polyangiitis.

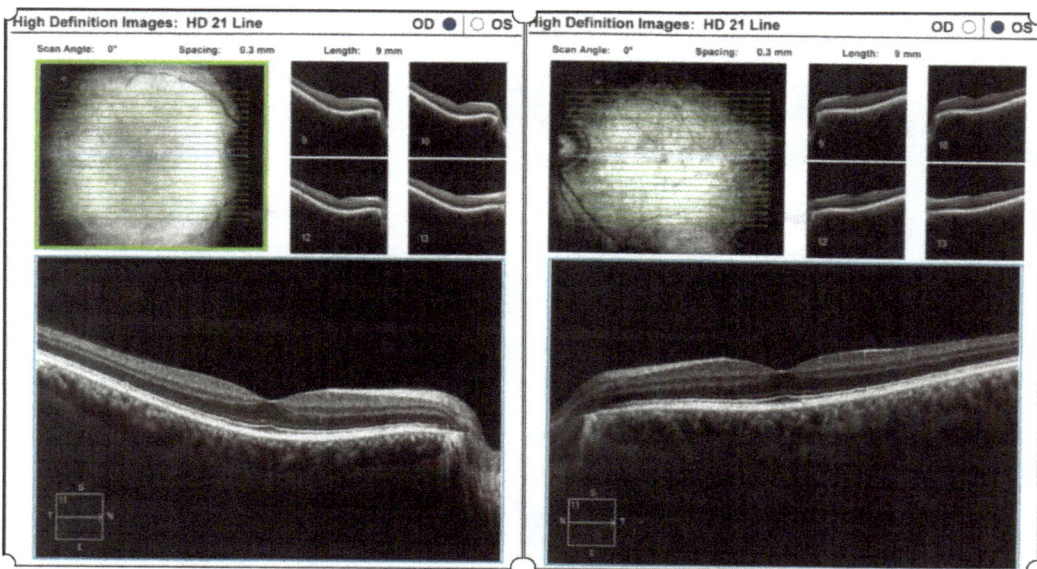

Figure 4. Optical coherence tomography.

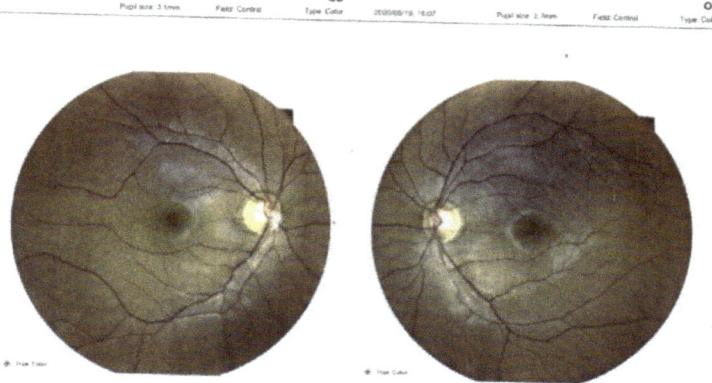

Figure 5. Retino photography.

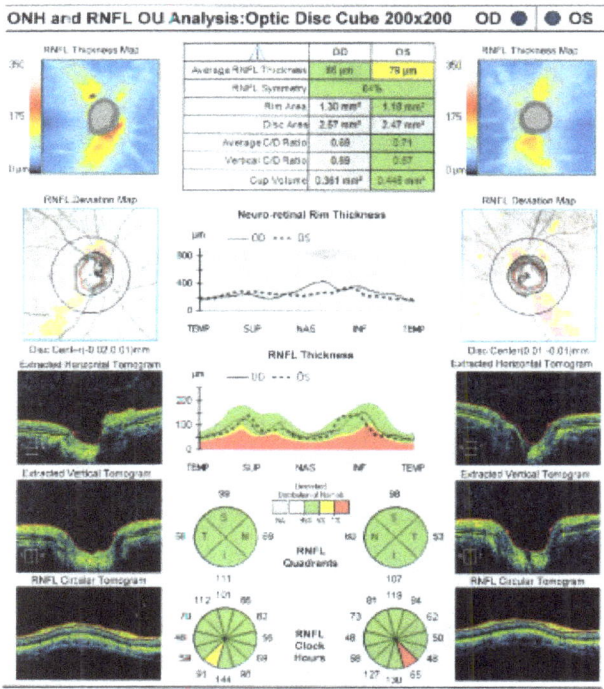

Figure 6. ONH and RNFL analyses.

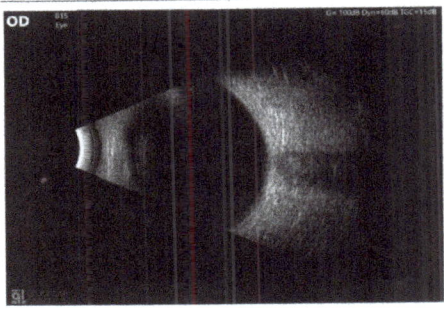

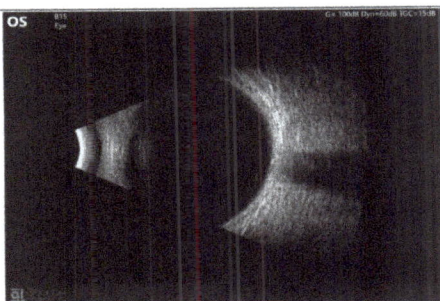

Figure 7. Ocular ultrasound.

3. Discussion

With an unknown etiology, granulomatosis with polyangiitis is a rare systemic disease characterized by granulomatous vasculitis of the small to medium sized vessels in almost any organ system [19], but it is usually seen in the upper respiratory tract and kidneys. The most common renal involvement is rapidly progressing, necrotizing glomerulonephritis [20]. GPA is associated with anti-neutrophil cytoplasmic antibodies (ANCA) [21].

It affects both genders equally in their fourth and fifth decades of life [22]. A prompt diagnosis and early treatment can reduce the morbidity and mortality of the disease.

Up to 85% of patients will present respiratory tract involvement as the first sign of the illness. Although the disease is usually seen in the upper respiratory tract, various manifestations occupying a wide distribution can be found. In some studies, 8–16% of patients presented ocular manifestations as the first symptoms, but orbital manifestations were eventually present in 50–87% of patients with GPA [16].

In the literature, the presence of c-ANCA with a cytoplasmic staining pattern directed against proteinase 3 (PR3) is present in 80% of cases [6], resulting in the development of systemic vasculitis and granulomatous inflammation. The biopsy results support the diagnosis with evidence of necrotizing granulomas and vasculitis [23].

Ocular involvement isa common manifestation in patients with vasculitis. It can include tarsal-conjunctival disease, episcleritis, scleritis, keratitis, uveitis, retinal disease, nasolacrimal disease, orbital disease, and adnexal disease. The classification made by Straatsma describes the ophthalmologic involvement as continuous or non-contiguous, based on the presence or absence of direct extension from the adjacent structures [24].

Orbital disease and eyelid involvement may manifest as inflammation and growth of tissue from the sinuses and is commonly seen after several years of disease progression. Injury to the ocular structures can be caused by compression activity by the tumor mass, orbital cellulitis expansion, or vascular injury. The inflammation may cause optic nerve compression and ischemic optic neuropathy with visual loss [25]. Hoffman et al. reported in the NIH series that almost one half of patients with optic nerve ischemia lost vision and that 52% of patients with GPA developed an ophthalmologic disease; thus, any sign of ocular inflammation may indicate relapse of the disease in other organs [22].

Proptosis can be seen in 15–20% of patients with granulomatosis with polyangiitis due to orbital inflammation. It is considered an important sign since the association of proptosis with renal or lung involvement is highly suggestive for diagnosis of the disease [26]. A few cases of diplopia had been described in the literature due to the inflammation of the orbital muscles, vasculitis of the vasa vasorum, and compression of the optic nerve [27]. Supplementary, orbital fistula, or orbital abscesses due to infection can also be encountered [28,29].

Granulomatosis with polyangiitis can affect the lacrimal drainage system and can cause nasolacrimal obstruction and dacryoadenitis, which lead to epiphora [30]. Dacryoadenitis can be the first sign of granulomatosis with polyangiitis, as reported by Howe et al. [31], which is often bilateral [32,33], and can be suggested in a patient with pain and edema of the eyelid and anterior orbit. The dacryoadenitis may cause ocular sicca syndrome [13,22,34]. A study of 226 patients reported that 13 patients had chronic dacryocystitis due to necrotizing and destructive rhino-sinusitis [35].

Conjunctivitis was reported in 16% of patients in a Robinson study [11]. It can cause chronic inflammation and ulcerative conjunctivitis, which can produce cicatricial changes in the ocular surface [36–38]. The patients may present symptoms such as red eye, foreign body sensation, and blurred vision [13].

Mild episcleritis can occur [39], but scleritis is the most common ophthalmologic diagnosis in 10% of patients with granulomatosis with polyangiitis. It can cause red eye and severe pain [40]. Bullen et al., reported scleritis and episcleritis in 7 and 3.5% of patients included in their study, respectively, while retinitis was diagnosed in 2.9% patients [13]. The involvement of the retina may vary from cotton-wool spots to intraretinal hemorrhages;

occlusion of retinal and choroidal circulation has been reported in patients with vasculitis [41,42]. Impaired prognosis for visual capacity was seen in retinal manifestations [43,44].

Corneal involvement may also be seen in GPA, manifested as peripheral ulcerative keratitis or interstitial keratitis [45]. An immunohistochemical exam can be performed since granulomatosis with polyangiitis has a particular presentation of peripheral ulcerative keratitis (PUK) with positive antibodies to a 66-kDa corneal epithelial antigen (BCEA-A). Scleritis is a common associated presentation alongside PUK due to conjoint blood supply [46].

Uveitis is rarely seen as an initial manifestation of GPA [47]. A cohort study found an incidence of 17.9% of uveitis in patients with ANCA-positive vasculitis. Meanwhile, 50% of patients with anterior uveitis had coexisting scleritis, suggesting that uveitis was a secondary manifestation [45]. Granulomatous panuveitis has been described as the first manifestation of GPA [48].

The causes of visual loss in patients with GPA are caused by compression of the optic nerve, vasculitis of the retinal and optic nerves, and also by complications from scleritis and keratitis. Multiple factors can impact visual prognosis, such as the development of the disease and initiation of early treatment [49].

Studies have shown that ocular pathology can either be the first sign of GPA, or it can appear later in the development of the disease, as presented earlier. With a multidisciplinary approach to this disease, an ophthalmologic examination is required because of the possible presentation of subglottic stenosis with tarsal-conjunctival disease in the progression of GPA.

In our case, after follow-up for 19 years, the patient presented with Sicca syncrome at the last ophthalmological examination during the COVID-19 period, for which she is receiving proper treatment.

As for treatment of GPA, combined glucocorticoids and cyclophosphamide have generally been demonstrated to achieve remission in the majority of patients, and several trials achieved remission with the combination of methotrexate and glucocorticoids [22,50]. A randomized trial supported the advantages of cyclosporine after remission induction. The literature shows some success in remission induction with the use of immunosuppressive agents such as rituximab, infliximab, and 15-deoxyspergualin. Despite different treatment strategies [51], relapses are often encountered [18,52]. Some risk factors for relapse and treatment resistance were identified and may be used to achieve a better prognosis [53].

4. Conclusions

Granulomatosis with polyangiitis is a rare and fatal disease without treatment. Early diagnosis and treatment are key to controlling its progression. Necrotizing granulomatous inflammation and vasculitis on a biopsy, along with the presence of ANCAs, provide support for the diagnosis of the disease. Various manifestations occupying a wide distribution may be found throughout disease progression. Regular ophthalmic examination is important since a multitude of manifestations can be present, as we have seen in this case report. For the best outcome in patient treatment, a multidisciplinary approach is required.

Author Contributions: Conceptualization M.P.; methodology I.C.M.; software C.M.T.; validation N.C.B.; formal analysis C.A.S.; investigation C.M.T., writing—original draft preparation C.M.T.; writing—review and editing N.C.B. and C.M.T.; visualization D.I.H.; All authors have read and agreed to the published version of the manuscript.

Funding: This research received no external funding.

Institutional Review Board Statement: The study was conducted in accordance with the Declaration of Helsinki and approved by the Ethics Committee of Universitatea de Medicina si Farmacie Victor Babes, Timisoara (CECS No 30/2015/rev November 2022).

Informed Consent Statement: Informed consent was obtained from the patient involved in the study.

Acknowledgments: All authors have equal contribution to the paper.

Conflicts of Interest: The authors declare no conflict of interest.

References

1. Harman, L.E.; Margo, C.E. Wegener's Granulomatosis. *Surv. Ophthalmol.* **1998**, *42*, 458–480. [CrossRef] [PubMed]
2. Scott, D.G.; Watts, R.A. Systemic vasculitis: Epidemiology, classification and environmental factors. *Ann. Rheum. Dis.* **2000**, *59*, 161–163. [CrossRef] [PubMed]
3. Miloslavsky, E.M.; Specks, U.; Merkel, P.A.; Seo, P.; Spiera, R.; Langford, C.A.; Hoffman, G.S.; Kallenberg, C.G.M.; St. Clair, E.W.; Tchao, N.K.; et al. Clinical Outcomes of Remission Induction Therapy for Severe Antineutrophil Cytoplasmic Antibody-Associated Vasculitis. *Arthritis Rheum.* **2013**, *65*, 2441–2449. [CrossRef] [PubMed]
4. Pagnoux, C.; Hogan, S.L.; Chin, H.; Jennette, J.C.; Falk, R.J.; Guillevin, L.; Nachman, P.H. Predictors of treatment resistance and relapse in anti-neutrophil cytoplasmic antibody-associated small-vessel vasculitis: Comparison of two independent cohorts. *Arthritis Rheum.* **2008**, *58*, 2908–2918. [CrossRef] [PubMed]
5. Stegeman, C.A.; Tervaert, J.W.C.; Sluiter, W.J.; Manson, W.L.; DeJong, P.E.; Kallenberg, C.G.M. Association of Chronic Nasal Carriage of Staphylococcus aureus and Higher Relapse Rates in Wegener Granulomatosis. *Ann. Intern. Med.* **1994**, *120*, 12–17. [CrossRef]
6. Yazici, H.; Husby, G.; Watts, R.A. Vasculitis. *Bailliere's Clin. Rheumatol.* **1997**, *11*, 191–450. [CrossRef]
7. Godman, G.C.; Churg, J. Wegener's granulomatosis: Pathology and review of the literature. *Arch. Pathol.* **1954**, *6*, 533–553.
8. Lutalo, P.M.K.; D'Cruz, D.P. Diagnosis and classification of granulomatosis with polyangiitis (aka Wegener's granulomatosis). *J. Autoimmun.* **2014**, *48–49*, 94–98. [CrossRef]
9. Seo, P.; Stone, J.H. The antineutrophil cytoplasmic antibody-associated vasculitides. *Am. J. Med.* **2004**, *117*, 39–50. [CrossRef]
10. Srouji, I.A.; Andrews, P.; Edwards, C.; Lund, V.J. Patterns of presentation and diagnosis of patients with Wegener's granulomatosis: ENT aspects. *J. Laryngol. Otol.* **2007**, *121*, 653–658. [CrossRef]
11. Iannella, G.; Greco, A.; Granata, G.; Manno, A.; Pasquariello, B.; Angeletti, D.; Didona, D.; Magliulo, G. Granulomatosis with polyangiitis and facial palsy: Literature review and insight in the autoimmune pathogenesis. *Autoimmun. Rev.* **2016**, *15*, 621–631. [CrossRef]
12. Cartin-Ceba, R.; Peikert, T.; Specks, U. Pathogenesis of ANCA-Associated Vasculitis. *Curr. Rheumatol. Rep.* **2012**, *14*, 481–493. [CrossRef]
13. Langford, C.A.; Sneller, M.C.; Hallahan, C.W.; Hoffman, G.S.; Kammerer, W.A.; Talar-Williams, C.; Fauci, A.S.; Lebovics, R.S. Clinical features and therapeutic management of subglottic stenosis in patients with Wegener's granulomatosis. *Arthritis Rheum.* **1996**, *39*, 1754–1760. [CrossRef]
14. Kornblut, A.D.; Wolff, S.M.; deFries, H.O. Wegener's granulomatosis. *Laryngoscope* **1980**, *90*, 1453–1465. [CrossRef]
15. Thickett, D.R.; Richter, A.G.; Nathani, N.; Perkins, G.; Harper, L. Pulmonary manifestations of anti-neutrophil cytoplasmic antibody (ANCA)-positive vasculitis. *Rheumatology* **2006**, *45*, 261–268. [CrossRef]
16. Pakrou, N.; Selva, D.; Leibovitch, I. Wegener's granulomatosis: Ophthalmic manifestations and management. *Semin. Arthritis Rheum.* **2006**, *35*, 284–292. [CrossRef]
17. Robinson, M.R.; Lee, S.S.; Sneller, M.C.; Lerner, R.; Langford, C.A.; Talar-Williams, C.; Cox, T.A.; Chan, C.C.; Smith, J.A. Tarsal-conjunctival disease associated with Wegener's granulomatosis. *Ophthalmology* **2003**, *110*, 1770–1780. [CrossRef]
18. Hogan, S.L.; Falk, R.J.; Chin, H.; Cai, J.; Jennette, C.E.; Jennette, J.C.; Nachman, P.H. Predictors of Relapse and Treatment Resistance in Antineutrophil Cytoplasmic Antibody-Associated Small-Vessel Vasculitis. *Ann. Itern. Med.* **2005**, *143*, 621–631. [CrossRef]
19. Peng, Y.J.; Fang, P.C.; Huang, W.T. Central retinal artery occlusion in Wegener's granulomatosis: A case report and review of the literature. *Can. J. Ophthalmol.* **2004**, *39*, 785–789. [CrossRef]
20. Grygiel-Gorniak, B.; Limphaibool, N.; Perkowska, K.; Puszczewicz, M. Clinical manifestations of granulomatosis with polyangiitis: Key considerations and major features. *Postgrad. Med.* **2018**, *130*, 581–596. [CrossRef]
21. Lee, P.Y.; Adil, E.A.; Irace, A.L.; Neff, L.; Son, M.B.F.; Lee, E.Y.; Perez-Atayde, A.; Rahbar, R. The presentation and management of granulomatosis with polyangiitis (Wegener's Granulomatosis) in the pediatric airway: GPA in the Pediatric Airway. *Laryngoscope* **2017**, *127*, 233–240. [CrossRef] [PubMed]
22. Tarabishy, A.B.; Schulte, M.; Papaliodis, G.N.; Hoffman, G.S. Wegener's granulomatosis: Clinical manifestations, differential diagnosis, and management of ocular and systemic disease. *Surv. Ophthalmol.* **2010**, *55*, 429–444. [CrossRef] [PubMed]
23. Jennette, J.C.; Falk, R.J. Small-Vessel Vasculitis. *N. Engl. J. Med.* **1997**, *337*, 1512–1523. [CrossRef] [PubMed]
24. Straatsma, B.R. Ocular manifestations of Wegener's granulomatosis. *Am. J. Ophthalmol.* **1957**, *144*, 789–799. [CrossRef] [PubMed]
25. Blaise, P.; Robe-Collignon, N.; Andris, C.; Rakic, J.-M. Wegener's granulomatosis and posterior ischemic optic neuropathy: Atypical associated conditions. *Eur. J. Intern. Med.* **2007**, *18*, 326–327. [CrossRef]
26. Hoffman, G.S.; Kerr, G.S.; Leavitt, R.Y.; Hallahan, C.W.; Lebovics, R.S.; Travis, W.D.; Rottem, M.; Fauci, A.S. Wegener granulomatosis: Ananalysis of 158 patients. *Ann. Intern. Med.* **1992**, *116*, 488–498. [CrossRef]
27. Loke, Y.K.; Tan, M.H. An unusual case of Wegener's granulomatosis. *Med. J. Malays.* **1998**, *53*, 107–109.
28. DeSilva, D.J.; Cole, C.; Luthert, P.; Olver, J.M. Masked orbital abscess in Wegener's granulomatosis. *Eye* **2007**, *21*, 246–248. [CrossRef]
29. Woo, T.L.; Francis, I.C.; Wilcsek, G.A.; Coroneo, M.T.; McNab, A.; Sullivan, T. Australasian orbital and adnexal Wegener's granulomatosis. *Ophthalmology* **2001**, *108*, 1535–1543. [CrossRef]
30. Ghanem, R.C.; Chang, N.; Aoki, L.; Santo, R.; Matayoshi, S. Vasculitis of the Lacrimal Sac Wallin Wegener Granulomatosis. *Ophthalmic Plast. Reconstr. Surg.* **2004**, *20*, 254–257. [CrossRef]

31. Howe, L.; D'Cruz, D.; Chopdar, A.; Hughes, G. Anterior ischaemic optic neuropathy in Wegener's granulomatosis. *Eur. J. Ophthalmol.* **1995**, *5*, 277–279. [CrossRef]
32. Boukes, R.J.; deVries-Knoppert, W.A. Lacrimal gland enlargement as one of the ocular manifestations of Wegener's granulomatosis. *Doc Ophthalmol.* **1985**, *59*, 21–26. [CrossRef]
33. Kiseleva, T.N.; Grusha, I.O.; Polunina, A.A.; Semenkova, E.N.; Abdurakhmanov, G.A.; Nikol'skaia, G.M. Involvement of lacrimal organs in Wegener's granulomatosis. *Vestn. Oftalmol.* **2009**, *125*, 33–36.
34. Hibino, M.; Kondo, T. Dacryoadenitis with Ptosis and diplopia as the Initial Presentation of Granulomatosis with Polyangiitis. *Intern. Med.* **2017**, *56*, 2649–2653. [CrossRef]
35. Ismailova, D.S.; Abramova, J.V.; Novikov, P.I.; Grusha, Y.O. Clinical features of different orbital manifestations of granulomatosis with polyangiitis. *Graefe's Archives. Clin. Exp. Ophthalmol.* **2018**, *256*, 1751–1756. [CrossRef]
36. Fortney, A.C.; Chodosh, J. Conjunctival Ulceration in Recurrent Wegener Granulomatosis. *Cornea* **2002**, *21*, 623–624. [CrossRef]
37. Meier, F.M.; Messmer, E.P.; Bernauer, W. Wegener's granulomatosis as a cause of cicatrizing conjunctivitis. *Br. J. Ophthalmol.* **2001**, *85*, 628. [CrossRef]
38. Jordan, D.R.; Zafar, A.; Brownstein, S.; Faraji, H. Cicatricial Conjunctival Inflammation with Trichiasis as the Presenting Feature of Wegener Granulomatosis. *Ophthalmic Plast. Reconstr. Surg.* **2006**, *22*, 69–71. [CrossRef]
39. Taylor, S.R.J.; Salama, A.D.; Pusey, C.D.; Lightman, S. Ocular manifestations of Wegener's granulomatosis. *Expert Rev. Ophthalmol.* **2007**, *2*, 91–103. [CrossRef]
40. Jabs, D.A.; Mudun, A.; Dunn, J.; Marsh, M.J. Episcleritis and scleritis: Clinical features and treatment results. *Am. J. Ophthalmol.* **2000**, *130*, 469–476. [CrossRef]
41. Lamprecht, P.; Lerin-Lozano, C.; Reinhold-Keller, E.; Nölle, B.; Gross, W.L. Retinal artery occlusion in Wegener's granulomatosis. *Rheumatology* **2000**, *39*, 928–929. [CrossRef] [PubMed]
42. Wong, S.C.; Boyce, R.L.; Dowd, T.C.; Fordham, J.N. Bilateral central retinal artery occlusion in Wegener's granulomatosis and α_1 antitrypsin deficiency. *Br. J. Ophthalmol.* **2002**, *86*, 476. [CrossRef] [PubMed]
43. Wang, M.; Khurana, R.N.; Sadda, S.R. Central retinal vein occlusion in Wegener's granulomatosis without retinal vasculitis. *Br. J. Ophthalmol.* **2006**, *90*, 1435–1436. [CrossRef] [PubMed]
44. Matlach, J.; Freiberg, F.J.; Gadeholt, C.; Göbel, W. Vasculitis like hemorrhagic retinal angiopathy in Wegener's granulomatosis. *BMC Res. Notes* **2013**, *6*, 364. [CrossRef] [PubMed]
45. Watkins, A.S.; Kempen, J.H.; Choi, D.; Liesegang, T.L.; Pujari, S.S.; Newcomb, C.; Nussenblatt, R.B.; Rosenbaum, J.T.; Thorne, J.E.; Foster, C.S.; et al. Ocular disease in patients with ANCA-positive vasculitis. *J. Ocul. Biol. Dis. Inform.* **2009**, *3*, 12–19. [CrossRef]
46. Perez, V.L.; Chavala, S.H.; Ahmed, M.; Chu, D.; Zafirakis, P.; Baltatzis, S.; Ocampo, V.; Foster, C. Ocular manifestations and concepts of systemic vasculitides. *Surv. Ophthalmol.* **2004**, *49*, 399–418. [CrossRef]
47. Samuelson, T.W.; Margo, C.E. Protracted uveitis as the initial manifestation of Wegener's granulomatosis. *Arch. Ophthalmol.* **1990**, *108*, 478–479. [CrossRef]
48. DuHuong, L.T.; Tran, T.H.; Piette, J.C. Granulomatous uveitis revealing Wegener's granulomatosis. *J. Rheumatol.* **2006**, *33*, 1209–1210.
49. Sfiniadaki, E.; Tsiara, I.; Theodossiadis, P.; Chatzirallli, I. Ocular Manifestations of Granulomatosis with Polyangiitis: A Review of the Literature. *Ophthalmol. Ther.* **2019**, *8*, 227–234. [CrossRef]
50. Reinhold-Keller, E.; Fink, C.O.E.; Herlyn, K.; Gross, W.L.; DeGroot, K. High rate of renal relapse in 71 patients with Wegener's granulomatosis under maintenance of remission with low-dose methotrexate. *Arthritis Rheum.* **2002**, *47*, 326–332. [CrossRef]
51. Comarmond, C.; Cacoub, P. What is the best treatment option for granulomatosis with polyangiitis? *Int. J. Clin. Rheumatol.* **2015**, *10*, 227–235. [CrossRef]
52. Langford, C.A.; Talar-Williams, C.; Barron, K.S.; Sneller, M.C. Use of acyclophosphamide-induction methotrexate-maintenance regimen for the treatment of Wegener's granulomatosis: Extended follow-up and rate of relapse. *Am. J. Med.* **2003**, *114*, 463–469. [CrossRef]
53. Karia, V.R.; Espinoza, L.R. Risk factors for treatment failures in antineutrophil cytoplasmic antibody-associated small-vessel vasculitis. *Curr. Rheumatol. Rep.* **2009**, *11*, 416–421. [CrossRef]

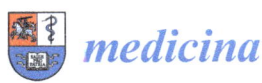

Article

Towards Regenerative Audiology: Immune Modulation of Adipose-Derived Mesenchymal Cells Preconditioned with Citric Acid-Coated Antioxidant-Functionalized Magnetic Nanoparticles

Adeline Josephine Cumpata [1,†], Dragos Peptanariu [2,†], Ana-Lacramioara Lungoci [2], Luminita Labusca [3,4,*], Mariana Pinteala [2] and Luminita Radulescu [1,5]

1. Doctoral School, "Grigore T. Popa" University of Medicine and Pharmacy, Universitatii Street 16, 700115 Iasi, Romania; adeline-josephine_d_cumpata@d.umfiasi.ro (A.J.C.); luminita.radulescu@umfiasi.ro (L.R.)
2. Centre of Advanced Research in Bionanoconjugates and Biopolymers "Petru Poni", Institute of Macromolecular Chemistry Aleea Grigore Ghica, Voda 41A, 700487 Iasi, Romania; peptanariu.dragos@icmpp.ro (D.P.)
3. Orthopedics and Traumatology Clinic, Emergency Hospital Saint Spiridon, 1 St Independentei Boulevard, 700111 Iasi, Romania
4. National Institute of Research and Development in Technical Physics Iasi Romania, 700111 Iasi, Romania
5. ENT Clinic Department, "Grigore T. Popa" University of Medicine and Pharmacy, Universitatii Street 16, 700115 Iasi, Romania
* Correspondence: llabusca@phys-iasi.ro
† These authors contributed equally to this work.

Abstract: *Introduction and Background*: Based on stem cells, bioactive molecules and supportive structures, regenerative medicine (RM) is promising for its potential impact on field of hearing loss by offering innovative solutions for hair cell rescue. Nanotechnology has recently been regarded as a powerful tool for accelerating the efficiency of RM therapeutic solutions. Adipose-derived mesenchymal cells (ADSCs) have already been tested in clinical trials for their regenerative and immunomodulatory potential in various medical fields; however, the advancement to bedside treatment has proven to be tedious. Innovative solutions are expected to circumvent regulatory and manufacturing issues related to living cell-based therapies. The objectives of the study were to test if human primary ADSCs preconditioned with magnetic nanoparticles coated with citric acid and functionalized with antioxidant protocatechuic acid (MNP-CA-PCA) retain their phenotypic features and if conditioned media elicit immune responses in vitro. MNP-CA-PCA was synthesized and characterized regarding size, colloidal stability as well as antioxidant release profile. Human primary ADSCs preconditioned with MNP-CA-PCA were tested for viability, surface marker expression and mesenchymal lineage differentiation potential. Conditioned media (CM) from ADSCs treated with MNP-CA-PCA were tested for Il-6 and IL-8 cytokine release using ELISA and inhibition of lectin-stimulated peripheral blood monocyte proliferation. *Results*: MNP-CA-PCA-preconditioned ADSCs display good viability and retain their specific mesenchymal stem cell phenotype. CM from ADSCs conditioned with MNP-CA-PCA do not display increased inflammatory cytokine release and do not induce proliferation of allergen-stimulated allogeneic peripheral blood monocytes in vitro. *Conclusions*: While further in vitro and in vivo tests are needed to validate these findings, the present results indicated that CM from ADSCs preconditioned with MNP-CA-PCA could be developed as possible cell-free therapies for rescuing auditory hair cells.

Keywords: hearing loss; adipose-derived mesenchymal cells; conditioned media; magnetic nanoparticles; protocatechuic acid; regenerative medicine

Citation: Cumpata, A.J.; Peptanariu, D.; Lungoci, A.-L.; Labusca, L.; Pinteala, M.; Radulescu, L. Towards Regenerative Audiology: Immune Modulation of Adipose-Derived Mesenchymal Cells Preconditioned with Citric Acid-Coated Antioxidant-Functionalized Magnetic Nanoparticles. *Medicina* 2023, 59, 587. https://doi.org/10.3390/medicina59030587

Academic Editors: Adriana Neagos, Daniela Vrinceanu, Codrut Sarafoleanu and Mahmut Tayyar Kalciogu

Received: 17 February 2023
Revised: 12 March 2023
Accepted: 14 March 2023
Published: 16 March 2023

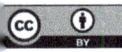

Copyright: © 2023 by the authors. Licensee MDPI, Basel, Switzerland. This article is an open access article distributed under the terms and conditions of the Creative Commons Attribution (CC BY) license (https://creativecommons.org/licenses/by/4.0/).

1. Introduction

Regenerative medicine (RM) involves the use of cells, bioactive molecules and supportive structures for replacing or substituting dysfunctional, lost organs or bodily functions [1]. With more than 20 years of basic and translational research and with the rapidly increasing number of clinical trials testing various regenerative strategies, RM is coming to age, already delivering therapies for so-far intractable diseases [2]. Recent developments in stem cell technology and nanomedicine have offered new perspectives introducing the possibility of rescue and regeneration of musculoskeletal tissues [3], sensory organs [4] and auditory epithelia [5] and to prevent or treat deafness of various causes in the adult and pediatric populations [6]. Differentiation methods to obtain hair cell-like cells seem to be effective; however, they proved to be technically challenging, costly and less amenable to large-scale manufacturing [7]. Mesenchymal stem cells (MSCs) are adult tissues which derive from a large variety of tissues of mesenchymal origin (such as bone marrow, adipose tissue, bone and synovium). MSCs assist regeneration mainly by means of the trophic and immunomodulatory effect generated by their paracrine activity. Adipose-derived mesenchymal cells (ADSCs) are MSCs derived from adipose tissue considered to be a convenient source for RM strategies due to their large-scale availability and phenotypic properties [8]. ADSCs were shown to express immunomodulatory and trophic effects in vitro as well as in vivo in an animal model investigating autoimmune and traumatic hearing loss [9]. Many issues in MSC/ADSC-based cell therapies remain unsolved, especially regarding cell survival after transplantation, accumulation within the target tissue as well as fate surveillance. The currently available clinically approved imaging methods are not able to detect a therapeutic cell population after implantation. Cell fate after implantation cannot be resolved non-invasively, which remains a problem that challenges medium- and long-term follow up of stem cell-based therapy and/or tissue-engineered constructs.

The use of nano-scaled materials, particularly of magnetic nanoparticles (MNPs), has evolved as an increasing field of research and application for medicine and life sciences [10]. Iron oxide MNPs internalized by the cells enable cell maneuverability, making them remotely controllable under an applied magnetic field (MF) as well as being traceable in vivo using clinically available magnetic resonance imaging (MRI). MNPs' biocompatibility is reportedly excellent, as they can be degraded by already-existent cellular iron handling molecular pathways. MSCs that have incorporated MNPs were shown to retain their specific phenotype and to become remotely controllable using an applied external magnetic field [11] with large applicability for cell targeting and cellular imaging using MRI or magnetic particle imaging (MPI) [12]. ADSCs loaded with MNPs are shown to retain their main phenotypic features in terms of proliferative and differentiation capability [13]. Little is known, however, about the immunomodulatory potential of ADSCs preconditioned with MNPs. MNPs' interaction with living matter is known to be determined by a their constituent physical parameters such as size, shape and coating materials but also by cell phenotype and functions. As a consequence, every MNP variety and cell type interaction needs to be carefully characterized before considering them as potential therapeutic agents. Several reports indicate that antioxidant drugs are capable of increasing the anti-inflammatory and regenerative potential of ADSCs both in vitro and in vivo [14,15]. To date, MNPs' mediation of the delivery of antioxidant compounds to stem cells is underexplored but has important potential in increasing the therapeutic efficiency of ADSCs. PCA is a compound found in some traditional Chinese herbs which was reported to exert good antioxidant properties [16]. Citric acid (CA) is an organic compound found in lots of fruits and vegetables and is also known for its antioxidant and regenerative capabilities [17]. In this study, we tested the interaction between iron oxide MNP coated with citric acid (CA) and functionalized with antioxidant-protocatechuic acid (PCA) and human primary ADSCs. The purpose was to detect if ADSCs retain their basic phenotypic features (viability, differentiation, surface markers) when exposed to MNP-CA-PCA as well as to test if conditioned media from MNP-CA-PCA-preconditioned cells elicit an immune response in vitro. The cell viability and retention of characteristic mesenchymal stem cell phenotype of ADSCs exposed to MNP-AC-PCA complexes were tested as well as the in vitro effect of MNP-AC-PCA preconditioning on ADSC cytokine release and interaction with the cellular immune system.

2. Materials and Methods

General information

Ferric chloride ($FeCl_3 \times 6H_2O$), ferrous chloride ($FeCl_2 \times 4H_2O$), 25% ammonium solution, citric acid (CA) and protocatechuic acid (PCA) were purchased from Sigma-Aldrich (USA). The Minimum Essential Medium composed of a mixture of Alpha Eagle 1% Penicillin, Streptomycin and Amphotericin B (10K/10K/25 µg in 100 mL), OsteoImage™ Mineralization Assay and AdipoRed™ Assay Reagent were from Lonza (Verviers, Belgium); the fetal bovine serum (FBS), Tryple, StemPro™ Adipogenesis Differentiation Kit and StemPro™ Osteogenesis Differentiation Kit were from Gibco (Langley, VA, USA); the phosphate-buffered saline (PBS) and Live/DeadTM Cell Imaging Kit were from Invitrogen (Eugene, OR, USA); the CellTiter-Glo 2.0 Assay was from Promega (Madison, WI, USA); the Max Discovery ELISA kits for human IL6 and IL8 were from Bioo Scientific (Austin, TX, USA) and the Pancoll was from Pan-Biotech (Aidenbach, Germany).

Mouse anti-human antibodies for flowcytometry: anti-CD14-PACIFIC BLUE, anti-CD19-ECD, anti-CD34-PC5, anti-CD90 (Thy-1)-APC-AlexaFluor 750 and anti-CD105-PC7 were purchased from Beckman Coulter (Marseille, France) and Alexa Fluor® 488 Anti-CD73 from Abcam.

Magnetic nanoparticle synthesis

MNP-CA was prepared using the pre-addition method as previously described [18]. Briefly, 20 mL each of $FeCl_2 \times 4H_2O$ and $FeCl_3 \times 6H_2O$ were mixed in a molar ratio of 1:2, 1 mL citric acid (0.5 g/mL) and pre-added to the ferrous and ferric solution followed by 40 mL of distilled water. After heating at 65 °C, 14 mL NH_4OH was added drop-wise into the mixture under vigorous mechanical stirring (650 rpm); the final product was centrifuged and washed 3 times with distilled water. Then, 1 mL solution PCA (10 mg/mL) was added to 1 mL MNP-CA (50 mg/mL) and submitted to mechanical stirring for 15 min before purification by magnetic decantation and washing 3 times with distilled water. The entrapment efficiency of PCA in a CA shell was calculated by absorbance reading at 287 nm of the supernatant solution using the following formula: Entrapment efficiency (%) = 100 (total drug-free amount of drug)/(total amount of drug), where free amount of drug and total amount of drug were determined using the calibration curves for PCA at 287 Nm vs. concentration of free PCA

MNP characterization

FT-IR

The Fourier transform infrared (FT-IR) spectra were recorded on a Bruker Vertex 70 FTIR instrument in a 400–4000 cm^{-1} range, in transmission mode, in KBr pellet.

DLS

The hydrodynamic diameter and zeta potential were recorded using a Delsa Nano C Submicron Particle Size Analyzer (Beckman Coulter, Inc., Fullerton, CA, USA) equipped with a laser diode operating at 658 nm.

STEM images

MNP morphology was analyzed in STEM mode with a Verios G4 UC Scanning electron microscope (Thermo Scientific, Brno, Czech Republic) equipped with an energy-dispersive X-ray spectroscopy analyzer (Octane Elect Super SDD detector, Pleasanton, CA, USA). The STEM studies were performed using the STEM 3+ detector (bright-field mode) at an accelerating voltage of 30 kV. For STEM analysis, the samples were dispersed in water and ultrasonicated, then placed on carbon-coated copper grids with 300 mesh sizes and dried in an oven until the solvent was removed.

Release of antioxidant agent

The release profile of PCA from the MNP-CA-PCA sample was studied in PBS with a pH of 7.4. First, 30 mg loaded magnetic nanoparticles were placed in a 12 kDa dialysis bag and introduced in 100 mL PBS at 37 °C, under gentle stirring. Then, 1 mL of supernatant was taken out at fixed intervals (30 min) and replaced with 1 mL fresh buffer. This 1 mL of supernatant was diluted with 1 mL PBS and then assayed by UV-VIS spectrophotometry at 250 nm. The concentration values of the released PCA were determined using the calibration curve of PCA and the following formula:

$$C_f' = C_f + v/V \sum C_{(f_{(i-1)})};$$

where: v = volume of the release media taken out every time; V = volume measured by UV-VIS; C_f' = concentration of the released drug and C_f = concentration in volume V at specific intervals.

Free radical scavenging activity by DPPH method

The DPPH method was used for measuring the antioxidant activity of functionalized magnetic nanoparticles. First, 3 mL ethanol solution of DPPH (0.1 mg/mL) was added in each 3 mL suspension of MNP-CA-PCA of different concentrations. After 30 min, the absorbance values were measured using 1 cm quartz cuvettes. The absorbance values were read at 517 nm and the radical scavenging activity was determined using the following equation:

$$\% \text{ of inhibition} = (A_c - A_s)/A_c \cdot 100$$

where: As is the absorbance of MNP-CA-PCA samples of different concentrations and Ac is the absorbance of the DPPH solution of 0.05 mg/mL.

Human primary adipose-derived mesenchymal cells (ADSC)

ADSCs were obtained from healthy donors undergoing liposuction procedures for cosmetic reasons after institutional board ethical approval and informed patient consent was obtained; transportation to the laboratory was carried out in sterile conditions. The resulting lipoaspirate was processed within 24 h as previously described [13]. The lipoaspirate was washed three times with PBS, digested with collagenase type I (0.01 mg/mL) for 2 h at 37.5 °C and centrifuged twice at 300 g for 5 min at RT. The supernatant consisting of tissue debris was removed and the remaining medium further centrifuged at 300 g for 5 min. Pelleted cells were re-suspended in complete culture media (CCM-αMEM with 10% fetal bovine serum and a 1% Penicillin–Streptomycin–Amphotericin B mixture) and counted. Cells were plated at 1×10^6 cells/cm^2 in appropriate tissue culture flasks (CellBIND surface, Corning). Cells in passage 3–4 were used for experiments, counted automatically and incubated at 37 °C and at 5% CO_2 in an incubator with the media replaced every 3 to 4 days.

Flow cytometry

For the flow cytometry experiment, ADSCs were cultured in a T25 flask, harvested by detachment with Tryple, washed with PBS twice and finally resuspended in microcentrifuge tubes in 300 μL PBS each, for the unlabeled and labeled samples. The following markers were tested for presence/absence: negative markers for stem cells CD14, CD 19 and CD 34 on the fluorescence channels PB450, ECD and PC5.5 respectively; positive markers for stem cells CD73, CD90 and CD105 on fluorescence channels FITC, APCA750 and PC7, respectively; 1 μL of each antibody was added. Samples were vortexed briefly and incubated for 15 min at 37 °C, centrifuged at 300 g and washed twice with PBS, resuspended in 300 μL and analyzed on a CytoFLEX benchtop flow cytometer (Beckman Coulter Life Sciences, Indianapolis, IN, USA).

In vitro toxicity of MNPs

In vitro MNP cytotoxicity was tested using the CellTiter-Glo kit. Cells were plated on 96-well white opaque tissue-culture-treated plates at densities of 5×10^3 cells/well in 100 μL/well complete medium and incubated for 24 h. The next day the media were replaced with serial dilutions of magnetite concentrations in complete cell culture medium and the plates were incubated for another 48 h. Before reading the results, the plates were removed from the incubator and kept at RT for 30 min followed by the addition of 100 μL/well of CelltTiter-Glo. Plates were shaken for 2 min and incubated for 15 min at

RT. Light emission was assessed by spectrophotometry using the FLUOstar®Omega plate reader (BMG, Offenberg Germany). The relative cell viability is expressed as a percentage of the viability of control (cells treated only with cell culture medium) according to the following formula:

$$\text{relative cell viability} = (RLup - RLub)/(RLuc - RLub) \times 100$$

where RLup, RLub and RLuc have relative light units recorded for samples, blank and control wells, respectively.

Live/dead viability assay

ADSCs were plated on 12-well tissue-culture-treated plates at densities of 40×10^3 cells/well in 1 mL/well complete medium and incubated for 24 h. The next day, the media were replaced with coated and non-coated MNPs at a concentration of 63 and 125 µm/mL, respectively; plates were incubated for another 7 days in CCM. At the end of the experiment, component A and component B from the kit were mixed as per the manufacturer's instructions; plates were incubated at RT for 20 min after which the images were collected using a Leica DMI 3000B inverted microscope (Wetzlar, Germany) using GFP and Texas Red filter cubes.

ADSC differentiation: adipogenesis and osteogenesis

Cells were cultured in 96-well black flat-bottom clear plates for quantitative evaluation and in 12-well plates to be photographed under a microscope. A density of 3200 cells/well was used for the 96-well plates, while 32,000 cells/well were seeded for the 12-well plates in complete αMEM medium. The next day, the medium was replaced with magnetite solutions in αMEM. After another 3 days, the medium was again replaced with commercially available adipocyte differentiation medium, respectively with osteogenic differentiation medium (see general information above). Adipogenesis assay was performed for 11 days while osteogenesis for 19 days as per the manufacturer's instructions.

Assessment of differentiation: adipogenesis

At 11 days, AdipoRed™ reagent was added according to the manufacturer's protocol. Briefly, the differentiation medium was removed and the cells were washed with PBS; AdipoRed™ dissolved in PBS was added and the plates were incubated 10 min at RT. Fluorescence (excitation 485 nm; emission 570) was read with a plate reader as described above. Similarly, the plates were qualitatively investigated with fluorescence microscopy.

Assessment of differentiation: osteogenesis

For the osteogenesis assay, cells were fixed with ethanol for 20 min. For qualitative and quantitative evaluation, Osteoimage™ was used as per the manufacturer's instructions. After staining, the samples were washed 3 times with wash buffer. To quantify the results, the 96-well plates were recorded with the plate reader (excitation 485 nm; emission 505), while the 12-well plates were analyzed with the fluorescence microscope.

Cytokine release

ELISA

ADSCs with or without MNP-AC-PCA were cultured in T25 flasks in αMEM medium with 0.2% FBS and 1% antibiotics for 11 days without changing the medium. After 11 days, the supernatant was removed and kept at $-80\,°C$ until the day of the ELISA test. For the ELISA test, steps were followed according to the manufacturer's protocol. Briefly, 100 µL of $1\times$ assay diluent was added in the negative control wells, 100 µL of interleukin standards in separate wells, as well as 100 µL of the sample in other separate wells and the assay plates were incubated 2 h at RT. After incubation, the liquid was removed, washed 3 times with 250 µL wash solution, 100 µL detection antibody was added to the plates and incubated 1 h at RT, the liquid was aspirated, washed 3 times with 250 µL wash solution, 100 µL $1\times$ avidin-HRP was added and the plates were incubated for 3 h at RT. The wells were washed 3 times with 250 µL wash solution, 100 µL TMB substrate was added and the plates were incubated for 15 min. Then, 100 µL stop buffer was added and absorbance was detected immediately at 450 nm using a plate reader (same as above).

Mixed lymphocyte reaction (MLR)

For MLR, we used the modified protocol by Herzig et al. [19]. First, 5 mL complete blood was collected in a vacutainer containing citrate as anticoagulant. Then, 15 mL Pancoll was placed in a 50 mL tube; 5 mL of blood was mixed with 5 mL PBS and allowed to settle, followed by centrifugation at 900 g for 30 min at 18 °C without the brake. PBMCs were extracted and resuspended, diluted with CCM and counted. The number of replicates for each of the 16 conditions was 3 with 6 × 10 × 5 cells per sample (sample set = 18; there were 16 treated and two controls (one positive and one negative) for lectin (Figure S1, Supplementary Materials). The sample set included conditioned media (CM) from ADSCs with or without MNP-CA-PCA at a 50% concentration (ADSC 50% (50 µL/100 µL) 50 µL concentrated CM and 50 µL medium = 100 µL) and at a 25% concentration (ADSC 25% (25 µL/100 µL) 25 uL concentrated CM and 75 µL medium = 100 µL) in the presence and absence of lectin; 96-well plates were used for this assay. Then, 100 µL per sample was left to incubate for 72 h at 37 °C. PBMC viability/proliferation was determined using 100 µL celltiter-Glo/well; data were processed in GraphPad.

3. Results

3.1. MNP Characterization

3.1.1. FTIR

PCA has its characteristic peaks at 1676 cm and 1299 cm (C=O stretching vibration) and at 1467 cm and 1528 cm (C-C aromatic ring stretching mode). Citric acid has its characteristic peaks at 1753 cm (C=O stretch in the carboxylic groups) and in the 1500–1000 domain (C-O, C-OH, C-C vibrations). MNP has a characteristic peak at 572 cm (Fe-O bond). In the spectrum of MNP-CA, we found the characteristic peaks for the Fe-O bond (611 cm) and citric acid (1612 cm C=O stretch). In the spectrum of MNP-CA-PCA we found the characteristic peaks for Fe-O (611 cm), CA (1622 cm) and PCA (1485 cm) (Figure 1).

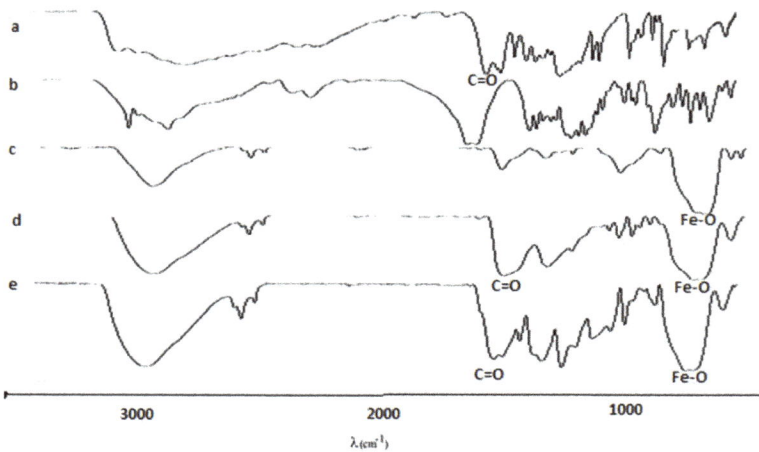

Figure 1. Fourier transformed infrared (FTIR) spectra of magnetic nanocomposites (**a**) protocatechuic acid (**b**) citric acid (**c**) magnetic nanoparticles (**d**) magnetic nanoparticles covered with citric acid (**e**) magnetic nanoparticles covered with citric acid and loaded with protocatechuic acid.

3.1.2. DLS for the Uncoated MNPs

DLS measurements showed a hydrodynamic diameter of 325.6 nm and a zeta Potential of −2.88 mV. After coating with citric acid, the hydrodynamic diameter increased to 478 nm and zeta potential decreased to −17, 25 mV, which confirms the successful coating with CA. For MNP-CA-PCA, the hydrodynamic diameter was 397.9 nm and the zeta potential was −20.24 mV, which confirmed the adsorption of PCA in the CA shell (Table 1).

Table 1. DLS measurements for MNP, MNP-CA and MNP-CA-PCA.

Sample	Hydrodynamic Diameter (nm)	Zeta Potential (mV)
MNP	325.6	−2.88
MNP-CA	478	−17.25
MNP-CA-PCA	397.9	−20.24
Title 1	Title 2	Title 3
entry 1	data	data
entry 2	data	data

3.1.3. STEM

The STEM measurements of MNPs showed spherical particles of 7–10 nm with a tendency to agglomerate. For MNP-CA, the STEM images showed the CA coating around the bare MNPs. The difference between DLS measurements and the TEM ones consisted of the fact that in TEM, the solvent evaporated slowly, but in DLS the nanoparticles moved in an aqueous medium, resulting in bigger structures (Figure 2a,b).

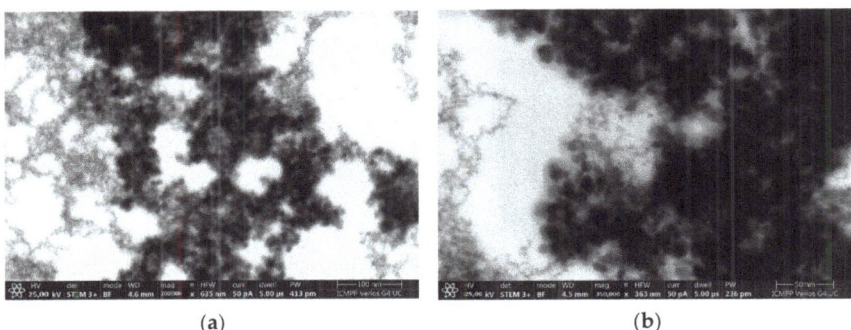

Figure 2. STEM images for MNP (**a**) and MNP-CA (**b**).

3.1.4. EDX

The EDX spectra of MNPs confirmed the presence of magnetite nanoparticles (Table 2) For MNP-CA and MNP-CA-PCA, the EDX spectra showed the presence of carbon because of the coating with citric acid. For MNP-CA-PCA, the oxygen content was the highest because of the presence of PCA (Table 2).

Table 2. EDX measurements for MNP, MNP-CA and MNP-CA-PCA.

Sample	Fe%	O%	C%
MNP	84.9	15.1	0
MNP-CA	95.8	0.3	3.9
MNP-CA-PCA	67.1	24.4	8.5

3.1.5. DPPH

For MNP-CA-PCA, the DPPH tests indicated an IC50 value of 600 µg/mL. This confirmed good antioxidant activity. Not only did the magnetic core of MNPs not decrease the antioxidant activity of simple PCA but also had an overall contribution in the final antioxidant activity of the MNP-CA-PCA samples (Figure 3a,b).

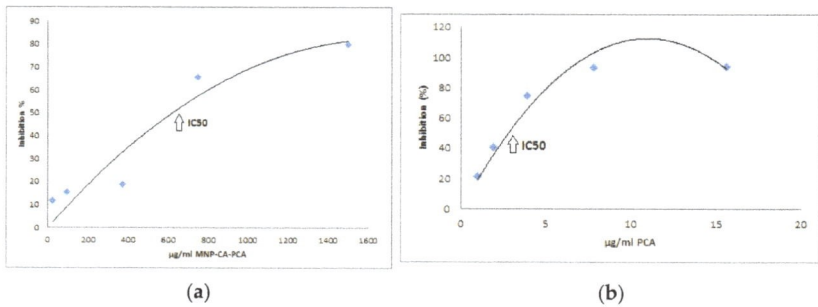

Figure 3. (**a**) MNP-CA-PCA antioxidant activity; (**b**) PCA antioxidant activity.

3.2. Drug Release

The drug release profile of MNP-CA loaded with PCA showed a rapid and continuous release of the antioxidant PCA over the course of three days (Figure 4).

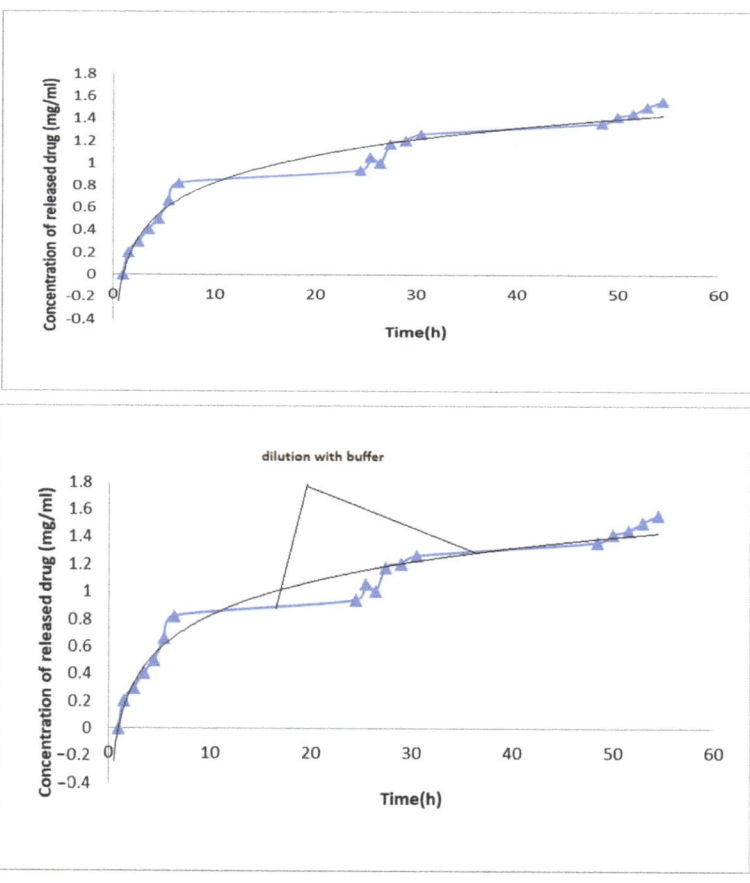

Figure 4. PCA release profile of MNP-CA functionalized with antioxidant PCA. The blue dots represent the number of measurements eash time the release media was taken out ant the straight portion of lines represent the overnight stopping of stirring and temperature over the course of three days.

3.2.1. In Vitro MNP Cytotoxicity/ADSC Viability

We used two methods to determine cell viability in the presence of MNPs and MNP-CA-PC, respectively. For the quantitative Celltite-Glo test, we firstly tested ADSC viability at 48 h with increasing concentrations of non-coated MNPs in order to determine the particle working concentration. We found that LC 50% was situated between the concentrations of 62.5 and 125 µg/mL (Figure 5a). Next, dextran and citric acid-coated MNPs containing PCA in concentrations of 62.5–125 µg/m were tested for long-term viability against ADSCs. Since MNP-CA-PCA exposure yielded higher viability at 7 days, this coating was chosen to proceed with further experiments (Figure 5b).

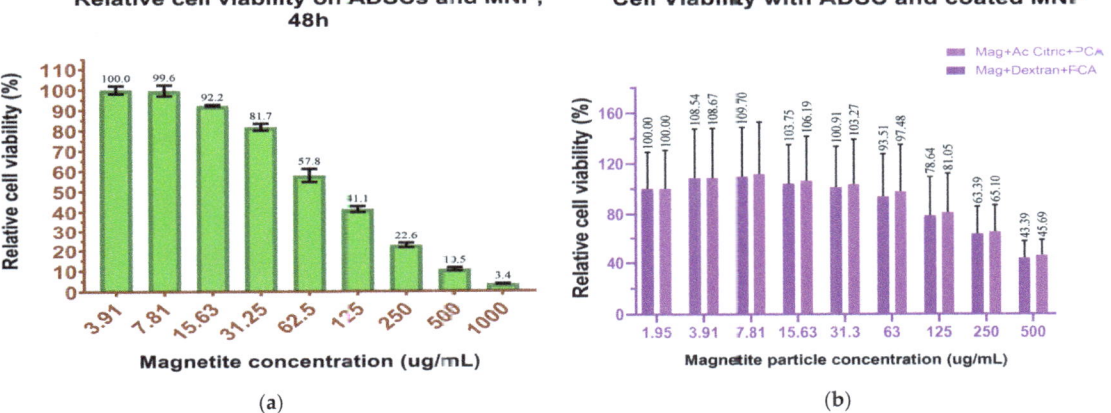

Figure 5. (a) ADSC viability with increasing concentrations of as-prepared MNP; (b) ADSC viability with MNP coated with dextran and protocatechuic acid D-PCA and citric acid and protocatechuic acid CA-PCA in 63 mg/mL and 125 mg/mL concentrations added in the culture, respectively.

Qualitatively, ADSC viability was tested using the LIVE/DEAD assay. The method is based on the use of two fluorescent dyes for cell staining: a membrane-permeable dye for living cells and an impermeable dye to mark dead cells. The two dyes can be observed microscopically. The living cells display an intense fluorescence in the green domain (ex/em 488 nm/515 nm), while dead cells emit in the red domain (ex/em 570 nm/602 nm). We found that ADSCs in the presence of MNP-CA-PCA and MNP-D-PCA, 63 and 125 µg/mL, displayed an increased number of dead cells for both types of coatings for 125 µg/mL as compared with 63 µg/mL (Figure 6).

3.2.2. ADSC Differentiation

We tested the differentiation potential of ADSCs cultured in specific, commercially available adipogenic and osteogenic differentiation media in the presence and absence of magnetic nanoparticles. The aim was to assess if the presence of MNP interferes with one of the definitory traits of mesenchymal progenitors: mesenchymal lineage differentiation. For the qualitative assessment of adipogenesis, we used AdipoRed®. The AdipoRed® reagent is a commercially available fluorescent dye used to color intracellular fat droplets because it is associated with triglycerides and in this way provides an image of the stage of adipocytic differentiation. It is a more sensitive assay than other methods such as the Oil Red O assay. ADSCs exposed and not exposed to as-prepared MNPs, MNPs loaded with citric acid or dextran, respectively and functionalized with PCA displayed positive AdipoRed® staining after 10 days in culture, signifying the successful conversion to preadipocytes. This was true for both concentrations of MNPs at 63 and 125 µg, respectively (Figure 7).

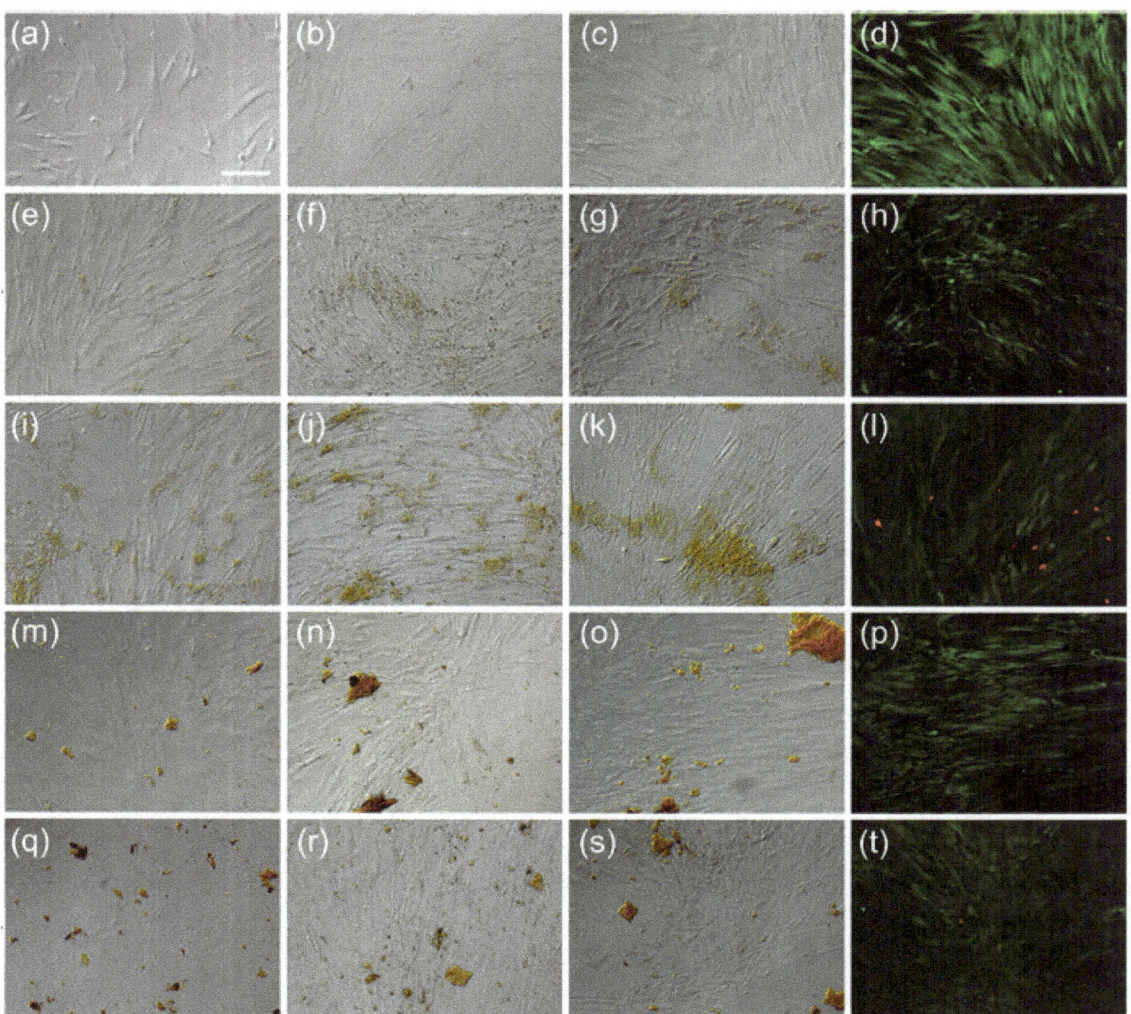

Figure 6. LIVE/DEAD qualitative evaluation of ADSC viability in the presence of MNP. (**a–d**) ADSC from day 0 to day 7 (in that order), bright field (BF) d 10×. (**e**) LIVE/DEAD staining at day 7 after LIVE/DEAD fluorescence, 10×. (**f–h**) ADSC-MNP-CA-PCA 63 µg/mL at days 3, 5 and 7, respectively BF 10×; (**i**) ADSC-MNP-CA-PCA LIVE/DEAD 7 day fluorescence. (**j–l**) ADSC-MNPs of 125 µg/mL at days 3, 5 and 7 BF 10×; (**m**) ADSC-MNP LIVE/DEAD day 7 fluorescence at BF 10×. (**n–p**) ADSC-MNP-D-PCA 63 µg/mL, BF 10×; (**q**) ADSC-MNP-D-PCA 7 day LIVE/DEAD fluorescence BF 10×; (**r,s**) ADSC-MNP-D-PCA 125 µg/mL, BF 10×; (**t**) ADSC-MNP-D-PCA 125 µg LIVE/DEAD, fluorescence, BF 10×; ADSC = cells non exposed to magnetic nanoparticles; ADSC-MNP = cells exposed to as-prepared magnetic nanoparticles; ADSC-MNP-CA-PCA = ADSC exposed to magnetic nanoparticles coated with citric acid and functionalized with protocatechuic acid; ADSC-MNP-D-PCA = ADSC exposed to magnetic nanoparticles coated with dextran and functionalized with protocatechuic acid.

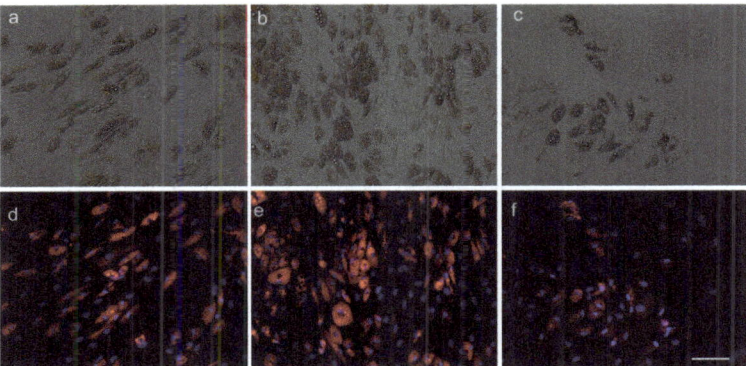

Figure 7. Adipogenic differentiation of ADSCs exposed and not exposed to magnetic nanoparticles: (**a**) ADSC-MNP-CA-PCA 63 µg/mL adipogenic differentiation after 10 days, BF 20×.; (**b**) ADSC-MNP-CA-PCA 125 µg/mL; (**c**) ADSCs not exposed to MNF ((**a**–**c**) bright field); (**d**) ADSC-MNP-CA-PCA 63 µg/mL fluorescence (Adipored). The lipids are reddish-orange and the nuclei are blue (Hoechst); (**e**) ADSC-MNP-CA-PCA 125 µg/mL fluorescence (AdipoRed); (**f**) ADSCs not exposed to MNP (**d**–**f**) fluorescence (Adipored). The scale bar is 100 µm. Representative results are from one donor.

For assessing osteogenic conversion, we used fluorescent OsteoImage® dye (Lonza) that specifically binds to mineralized extracellular matrices deposited by pre-osteoblasts and osteoblasts if osteogenic conversion is successful. We found that ADSCs exposed and not exposed to as-prepared MNPs, MNPs loaded with citric acid or dextran, respectively and those functionalized with PCA displayed positive OsteoImage® staining after 19 days in culture, signaling osteogenic conversion. This was true for both concentrations of MNPs, i.e., 63 and 125 µg/mL, respectively (Figure 8).

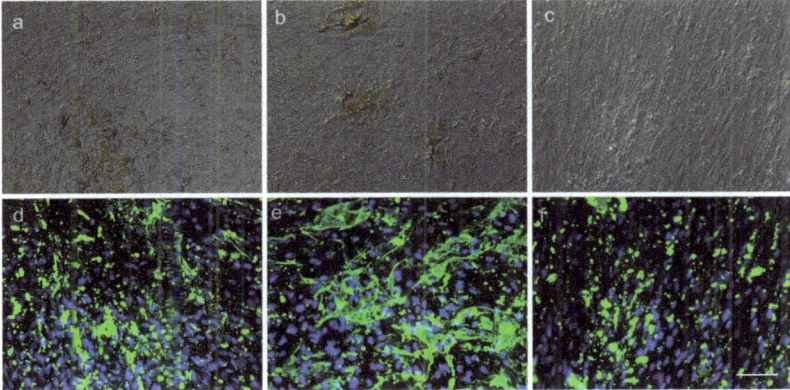

Figure 8. Osteogenic differentiation of ADSCs exposed and not exposed to MNP after 19 days in culture: (**a**) ADSC-MNP-CA-PCA 63 µg/mL osteogenic differentiation after 19 days, BF 20×; (**b**) ADSC-MNP-CA-PCA 125 µg/mL; (**c**) ADSCs not exposed to MNP ((**a**–**c**) bright field); (**d**) ADSC-MNP-CA-PCA 63 µg/mL fluorescence (OsteoImage®). The deposited mineralized extracellular matrix is green and the nuclei are blue (Hoechst); (**e**) ADSC-MNP-CA-PCA 125 µg/mL fluorescence OsteoImage® (**f**) ADSCs not exposed to MNP (**d**–**f**) fluorescence OsteoImage® 20×. The scale bar is 100 µm. Representative results are from one donor; ADSC-MNP = cells exposed to non-coated magnetic nanoparticles; ADSC-MNP-CA-PCA = ADSC exposed to magnetic nanoparticles coated with citric acid and functionalized with protocatechuic acid; ADSC-MNP-D-PCA = ADSC exposed to magnetic nanoparticles coated with dextran and functionalized with protocatechuic acid.

Quantitative evaluation of adipogenesis, respectively, osteogenesis using a spectofotometric assesment of fluorescent AdipoRed® and OsteoImage® revealed that MNP-CA-PCA-loaded cells in both concentrations displayed increased differentiation potential compared with non-MNP-loaded controls (Figure 9).

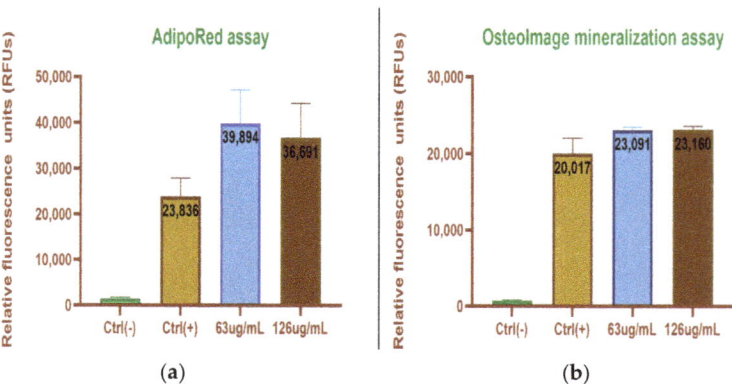

Figure 9. Quantitative differentiation assay. (**a**) Adipogenic differentiation of ADSCs exposed and not exposed to magnetic nanoparticles MNP-CA-PCA; (**b**) osteogenic differentiation of ADSCs exposed and not exposed to MNP-CA-PCA.

3.2.3. Mesenchymal Stem-Cell-Specific Surface Markers

Flow cytometry was used to identify positive and negative cell markers that define the phenotype of mesenchymal stem cells and identify the cells tested as being ADSCs. The positive markers for these cells are CD 73, CD 90 and CD 105. The negative markers or the markers that should not be present on ADSCs are CD 14, CD 19 and CD 34. Figure 9 depicts the presence of the positive markers and the absence of the negative markers for ADSCs representative of one donor (Figure 10).

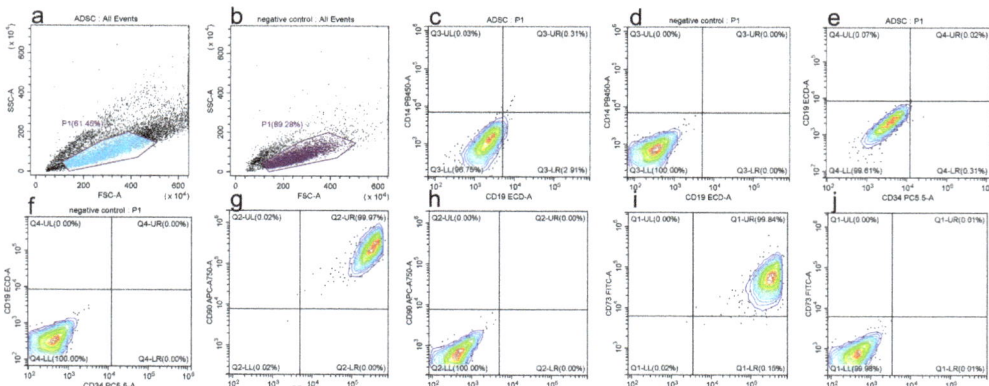

Figure 10. Flow cytometry evaluation of surface markers. (**a**) gating around all significant events, (**b**) gating around the events in the negative control, (**c**) CD 14 and CD 19 where a cluster can be observed in the negative quadrants signifying the absence of CD 14 and CD 19, (**d**) negative control for CD 14 and CD 19, (**e**) Cell cluster CD 19 and CD 34 found in the negative quadrants, (**f**) negative control for CD 19 and CD 34, (**g**) CD 90 and CD 105 cell clusters found in the positive quadrants signifying the presence of these markers in the ADSCs, (**h**) negative control CD 90 and CD 105 in the negative quadrants, (**i**) Cell clusters CD 90 and CD 73 in the positive quadrants and (**j**) negative control CD 73 and CD 105 in the negative quadrants.

3.2.4. Cytokine Release

The alteration of the anti-inflammatory profile of ADSCs in the presence of MNPs was investigated by measuring the level of interleukins IL-6 and IL-8 released in serum-free culture media using the ELISA technique. We found that after 11 days in culture, ADSCs and ADSC-MNP-AC-PCA release had strikingly comparable levels of IL-6, averaging 590/609 pg/m, while non-significant increases of IL-8 could be detected in ADSC-MNP-AC-PCA (averaging 171/2 compared with 213/6 pg/m (Figure 11a,b).

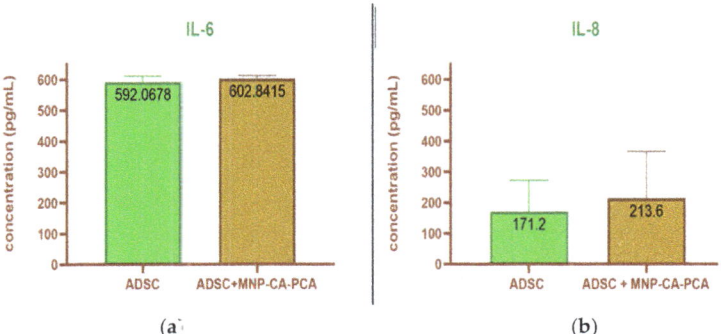

Figure 11. Cytokine release in CM from ADSCs preconditioned with MNP-CA-PCA: (a) IL-6; (b) IL-8. In green adipose derived stem cells (ADSC) cytokine release in brown adipose derived stem cells treated with MNP-CA-Pca cytokine release.

3.2.5. MLR

We tested the ability of conditioned media from ADSCs and ADSC-MNP to influence peripheral blood monocyte reactivity to induce stimulation with a common allergen (lectin). As expected, fresh isolated human PBMCs in the presence of lectin displayed higher viability than non-stimulated PBMCs, showing their reactivity and induced cellular immune response. We found that conditioned media from ADSCs inhibited the proliferation of non-stimulated PBMCs by 10%, while conditioned media from ADSC-MNP resulted in inhibition of proliferation by 3%. A similar profile was recorded in the case of lectin-stimulated PBMC-conditioned media from ADSCs, which decreased lectin-stimulated PBMC proliferation by 7.7%, while conditioned media from ADSC-MNP decreased stimulated PBMC only by 0.3% (Figure 3). While ADSCs have the ability to decrease proliferation of allergen-stimulated PBMCs, albeit non-significantly, MNP treatment decreases this ability. Lectin-stimulated as well as naïve PBMCs, however, did not increase proliferations in the presence of ADSC-MNP-conditioned media in this model in vitro (Figure 12).

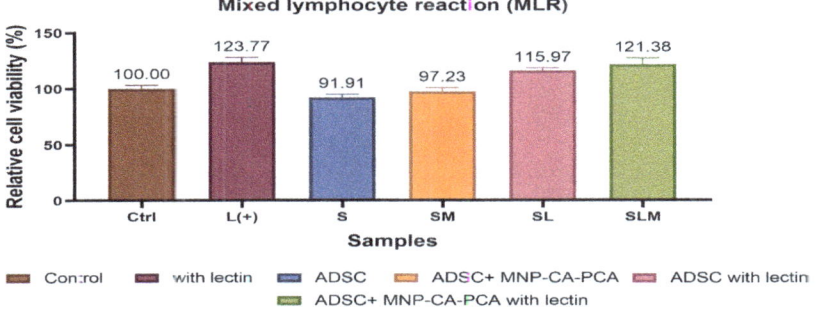

Figure 12. The effect of CM from ADSC-CA-MNP on the proliferative reaction of lectin-stimulated allogeneic peripheral blood monocytes (PBMC) tested using CellTiter-Glo viability assay.

4. Discussion

Recently, the use of nanoparticles and especially MNPs has elicited constant interest for the development of potentially novel breakthrough therapies. MNPs' relevance as drug delivery systems constitutes a special field of research and their relevance for regenerative medicine is increasingly recognized. Given the significance of immune reactivity in regenerative processes, the design of therapeutic agents that have the ability to modulate soluble and cellular immune responses is of the utmost importance [20]. The use of stem-cell-based therapies as regenerative and immune-modulatory agents has already been tested in clinical trials for a large variety of therapeutic applications [21]. Stem-cell-based regenerative strategies for congenital or acquired hearing loss are expected to offer improved therapies [22]. However, the complexity of producing and marketing products that are based on living cells in terms of manufacturing, costs and ethical and regulatory approval has consistently impaired their advancement to clinical settings. Serum-free conditioned media (CM) from ADSCs has been sought out as a modality to avoid the hurdles involved in the therapeutic delivery of living cells [23]. CM from ADSCs preconditioned with various molecules has proven efficient in rescuing hair cell loss due to paracrine regenerative and immunomodulatory activity [24].

In this study, CM from human primary ADSCs preconditioned with MNPs coated with citric acid and antioxidant protocatechuic acid were tested for their effects on immunomodulatory cytokine release and in limiting cellular responses initiated in allogeneic human PBMC by a known allergen (lectin) using a modified protocol [19].

In-house-synthetized MNP-CA-PCA proved to have regular geometry, excellent dispersibility and good colloidal stability (zeta potential -24, 2 compared with as-prepared MNPs (-2), certifying the method used for coating and functionalization results in MNPs with superior characteristics related to their interaction with living matter.

Herein, we reported the synthesis and characterization of a novel formulation of core-shell iron oxide MNPs coated with CA and functionalized with antioxidant molecule PCA as well as their interaction with ADSCs.

The adsorption of an organic shell on the surface of MNPs allows the stabilization of MNPs, decreasing their tendency to agglomerate. Additionally, the zeta potential of coated MNPs tends to increase (positive or negative), making them more suitable for biomedical applications [25].

Furthermore, the core-shell nanoparticles can be used for loading therapeutic agents (drugs, redox substances) which can release the molecules at the site of interest [26].

We tested cell viability using two distinct methods, i.e., a qualitative (LIVE/DEAD) and a quantitative one (CellTiter-Glo) as a modality to investigate a larger panel of enzymatic equipment that is mandatory for cell viability and/or proliferation. The CellTiter-Glo test is based on the reaction between the luciferase enzyme and its substrate (luciferin), a reaction catalyzed by cellular ATP that results in the formation of oxyluciferin and the emission of photons. Since the efficiency of the reaction depends on the amount of ATP, and the latter depends on the number of living cells, the CellTiter-Glo test indirectly measures cell viability as well as cell proliferation. The CellTiter-Glo test is much more reliable than the colorimetric tests in which the absorbance of the chemicals to be tested can be difficult to subtract from the calculations and where the chemicals can produce reactions with the reagents of the test kits, leading to interference [27]. LIVE/DEAD detects the presence of intact cellular membranes as well as the presence of enzyme esterase activity characteristic of viable cells. Both tests performed indicated the excellent viability of ADSCs in the presence of MNP-CA-PCA added in the culture media and allowed to establishment of a working concentration for further experiments (i.e., 63 and 125 µg/mL, respectively). Previous studies reported good to excellent biocompatibility of MNPs with different coatings interacting with ADSCs in vitro as well as in vivo [28,29]. Good viability was reported in different mesenchymal stem cell types upon internalization of commercially available MNPs with different coatings [30]. Herein, we reported that human primary ADSCs interacting with as-prepared custom-made magnetite (Fe_3O_4) MNP as well as MNPs coated with citric acid and antioxidant PCA display excellent short- and medium-term viability up to 7 days in culture. Compared with MNP-D-PCA, we found cell viability to be increased when exposed to MNP-CA-PCA, albeit non-significantly, at every concentration, therefore used we used the latter for further experiments. This effect was found to be, however, dose dependent since cell viability dropped below 50% at 50 µg/mL added in culture media (Figure 3). A particularity of MNPs that governs their interaction with cells and is distinctive from other nanoparticles is the existence of an intrinsic mechanism for iron storage and metabolism. Ferritin-dependent iron metabolism is an endogenous mechanism ubiquitous and evolutionarily conserved in all mammalian cells. Ferritin protein cages were shown to store degradation products of MNP cores, concomitantly slowing down the process due to their colloidal behavior in the acidic medium of the lysosomes [31]. A possible biosynthesis of bio magnetite by human mesenchymal stem cells after MNP degradation has been proposed as well, a process that might be cell-state-dependent [32].

We next tested if human primary cell interaction with MNP-AC-PCA interferes with their basic phenotypic features. The defining characteristics of ADSCs consist of their ability to adhere to a plastic surface of a culture dish, expression of CD73, CD90 and CD105, and lack of CD11b or CD34, CD19 or CD79, CD45 and HLA-DR as well as trilineage mesenchymal differentiation [33,34]. We found that after being exposed to different concentrations of as-prepared MNPs and CA-PCA-coated MNPs, ADSCs retained their adherence to a plastic culture dish for up to 7 days in culture. Cells retained their characteristic surface marker profile (Figure 10) and were capable of undergoing adipogenesis as well as osteogenesis in the presence of MNP-CA-PCA at 63 µg/mL as well as 125 µg/mL (Figures 7–9). Moreover both adipogenesis as well as osteogenesis were increased in the presence of MNP-CA-PCA, a fact that suggests cells not only preserve but increase their differentiation potential. Similar reports using commercially available [35] or proprietary MNPs with various coatings [27] indicate that ADSCs retain their differentiation potential to mesenchymal lineages in the presence of MNPs with various coatings. Enhanced cell metabolism produced by the presence or iron as well as changes in cell shape and cytoskeletal rearrangement were proposed to explain this finding. Several groups reported the increased osteogenic potential of bone marrow mesenchymal stem cells (BMSCs) loaded with MNPs [36,37]. Adipogenesis and increased osteogenesis were previously reported in ADSCs incorporating MNPs [27,38], a process that appears to, however, decrease with increasing concentrations of MNPs [39,40]. Herein, we found that both 63.5 as well as 125 µg/mL MNP-CA-PCA support ADSC adipogenesis and osteogenesis in vitro in the experimental conditions created.

We then tested the effect of MNP-CA-PCA presence on inflammatory cytokine expression by ADSCs. Serum-free CM from ADSCs treated with 125 µg/mL MNP-CA-PCA were found to release comparable levels of IL-6 and slightly non-significant increased levels of IL-8. IL-6 is a common denominator of acute inflammation and member of the pro-inflammatory cytokine family [41]. Since the presence of MNPs does not increase its release, it is possible ADSCs do not acquire an inflammatory phenotype in their presence. A slight increase in IL-8, another pro-inflammatory cytokine which can, however, act as an anti-inflammatory myokine [42], can possibly indicate ADSC reactivity. This process is very likely to be donor-dependent since very different values were obtained in CM media from different donors.

MSCs and especially ADSC cell suspension, CM or CM-derived extracellular vesicles are known to inhibit proliferation of allergen-stimulated allogeneic monocytes [43,44]. Herein, we found that CM from ADSCs but also from ADSC-CA-PCA reduce allogeneic blood monocyte proliferation under non-allergen stimulation, which indicates their ability to modulate cellular immune responses in vitro. This is a very important finding that has not been reported before which promotes the use of cell-free regenerative solutions. Hearing loss of various degenerative, traumatic congenital abnormalities [45] could benefit from such therapeutic approaches. Previous reports indicate that free iron ions are potentially capable of promoting immune modulation by stem cells [46] in a process that could potentially be similar to macrophage polarization. This process is very likely fine-tuned with many factors involved (including ferric/ferrous iron balance, transferrin and hepcidin protein activity) [47]; therefore, our findings need to be further tested in vivo. Further tests are warranted to detect the potential of MNP-CA-PCA-preconditioned allogeneic ADSCs both in vitro and in vivo and to discriminate donor-related differences regarding ADSC immune profile. The present findings lay the foundation for and justify further investigation of the use of CM from preconditioned ADSCs as regenerative therapies for rescuing auditory hair cells and for treating hearing loss, with the important potential to translate the aforementioned to clinically available therapies.

5. Conclusions

This is,to our knowledge, the first report on the effect of MNP-CA-PCA preconditioning on ADSC phenotype retention and immune profile. We found that ADSC pretreatment with 63.5 and 125 μg/mL did not interfere with stem cell phenotype and supported cells' immune modulatory activity. Further tests are needed to validate the use of CM from MNP-CA-PCA-preconditioned ADSCs to rescue auditory hair cells and potentially in other sensory epithelia. These findings are important for the design of regenerative approaches to address hearing loss with important potential to translate them to clinically available therapies.

Supplementary Materials: The following supporting information can be downloaded at: https://www.mdpi.com/article/10.3390/medicina59030587/s1, Figure S1: MLR experiment set up details.

Author Contributions: Conceptualization, L.L. and L.R.; data curation, D.P. and L.L.; formal analysis, A.J.C., D.P. and A.-L.L.; funding acquisition, M.P. and L.R.; investigation, A.J.C., D.P. and A.-L.L.; project administration, L.R.; supervision, M.P. and L.R.; writing—original draft, A.J.C. and D.P.; writing—review and editing, L.L., M.P. and L.R. All authors have read and agreed to the published version of the manuscript.

Funding: This scientific research is financed by the University of Medicine and Pharmacy "Grigore T. Popa" Iasi-grant no.4711/25:02:2021.

Institutional Review Board Statement: The study was conducted in accordance with the Declaration of Helsinki, and donor sample collection was approved by the Institutional Review Board (or Ethics Committee) of County Emergency Hospital Saint Spiridon Iasi Romania Nr 31567/1507/2015 and Ethical Committee of County Emergency Hospital Saint Spiridon Iasi Nr 23/01/08/201.

Informed Consent Statement: Informed consent was obtained from all adipose tissue donors.

Data Availability Statement: Data are available from authors at reasonable request.

Acknowledgments: Authors wish to thank Florin Zugun-Eloae for critical referral of the manuscript.

Conflicts of Interest: The authors declare no conflict of interest.

References

1. Daar, A.S.; Greenwood, H.L. A proposed definition of regenerative medicine. *J. Tissue Eng. Regen. Med.* **2007**, *1*, 179–184. [CrossRef] [PubMed]
2. Trounson, A.; McDonald, C. Stem Cell Therapies in Clinical Trials: Progress and Challenges. *Cell Stem Cell* **2015**, *17*, 11–22. [CrossRef] [PubMed]
3. Li, Z.; Xiang, S.; Li, E.N.; Fritch, M.R.; Alexander, P.G.; Lin, H.; Tuan, R.S. Tissue Engineering for Musculoskeletal Regeneration and Disease Modeling. *Organotypic Model. Drug Dev.* **2020**, *265*, 235–268. [CrossRef]
4. Dzobo, K.; Thomford, N.E.; Senthebane, D.A.; Shipanga, H.; Rowe, A.; Dandara, C.; Pillay, M.; Motaung, K.S.C.M. Advances in regenerative medicine and tissue engineering: Innovation and transformation of medicine. *Stem Cells Int.* **2018**, *2018*, 2495848. [CrossRef] [PubMed]
5. Oshima, K.; Shin, K.; Diensthuber, M.; Peng, A.W.; Ricci, A.J.; Heller, S. Mechanosensitive hair cell-like cells from embryonic and in-ducedpluripotent stem cells. *Cell* **2010**, *141*, 704–716. [CrossRef]
6. Reyes, J.H.; O'Shea, K.S.; Wys, N.L.; Velkey, J.M.; Prieskorn, D.M.; Wesolowski, K.; Miller, J.M.; Altschuler, R.A. Glutamatergic neuronal differentiation of mouse embryonic stem cells after transient expression of neurogenin 1 and treatmentwith BDNF and GDNF: In vitro and in vivo studies. *J. Neurosci.* **2008**, *28*, 12622–12631. [CrossRef]

7. Erdö, F.; Bührle, C.; Blunk, J.; Hoehn, M.; Xia, Y.; Fleischmann, B.; Föcking, M.; Küstermann, E.; Kolossov, E.; Hescheler, J.; et al. Host dependent tumorigenesis of embryonic stem cell trans-plantation in experimental stroke. *J. Cereb. Blood Flow Metab.* **2003**, *23*, 780–785. [CrossRef]
8. Labusca, L. Adipose tissue in bone regeneration—Stem cell source and beyond. *World J. Stem Cells* **2022**, *14*, 372–392. [CrossRef]
9. Lin, Z.; Perez, P.; Sun, Z.; Liu, J.-J.; Shin, J.H.; Hyrc, K.L.; Samways, D.; Egan, T.; Holley, M.C.; Bao, J. Reprogramming of Single-Cell–Derived Mesenchymal Stem Cells into Hair Cell-like Cells. *Otol. Neurotol.* **2012**, *33*, 1648–1655. [CrossRef]
10. Chen, Y.; Hou, S. Application of magnetic nanoparticles in cell therapy. *Stem Cell Res. Ther.* **2022**, *13*, 135. [CrossRef]
11. Hauser, A.K.; Wydra, R.J.; Stocke, N.A.; Anderson, K.W.; Hilt, J.Z. Magnetic nanoparticles and nanocomposites for remote controlled therapies. *J. Control. Release* **2015**, *219*, 76–94. [CrossRef] [PubMed]
12. Billings, C.; Langley, M.; Warrington, G.; Mashali, F.; Johnson, J. Magnetic Particle Imaging: Current and Future Applications, Magnetic Nanoparticle Synthesis Methods and Safety Measures. *Int. J. Mol. Sci.* **2021**, *22*, 7651. [CrossRef] [PubMed]
13. Labusca, L.S.; Herea, D.-D.; Radu, E.; Danceanu, C.; Chiriac, H.; Lupu, N. Human Adipose Derived Stem Cells and Osteoblasts Interaction with Fe–Cr–Nb–B Magnetic Nanoparticles. *J. Nanosci. Nanotechnol.* **2018**, *18*, 5143–5153. [CrossRef]
14. Liao, N.; Shi, Y.; Wang, Y.; Liao, F.; Zhao, B.; Zheng, Y.; Zeng, Y.; Liu, X.; Liu, J. Antioxidant preconditioning improves therapeutic outcomes of adipose tissue-derived mesenchymal stem cells through enhancing intrahepatic engraftment efficiency in a mouse liver fibrosis model. *Stem Cell Res. Ther.* **2020**, *11*, 237. [CrossRef]
15. Abu-Shahba, N.; Mahmoud, M.; Abdel-Rasheed, M.; Darwish, Y.; AbdelKhaliq, A.; Mohammed, E.; ElHefnawi, M.; Azmy, O. Immunomodulatory and Antioxicative potentials of adipose-derived Mesenchymal stem cells isolated from breast versus abdominal tissue: A comparative study. *Cell Regen.* **2020**, *9*, 18. [CrossRef] [PubMed]
16. Song, J.; He, Y.; Luo, C.; Feng, B.; Ran, F.; Xu, H.; Ci, Z.; Xu, R.; Han, L.; Zhang, D. New progress in the pharmacology of protocatechuic acid: A compound ingested in daily foods and herbs frequently and heavily. *Pharmacol. Res.* **2020**, *161*, 105109. [CrossRef] [PubMed]
17. Salihu, R.; Razak, S.I.A.; Zawawi, N.A.; Kadir, M.R.A.; Ismail, N.I.; Jusoh, N.; Mohamad, M.R.; Nayan, N.H.M. Citric acid: A green cross-linker of biomaterials for biomedical applications. *Eur. Polym. J.* **2021**, *146*, 110271. [CrossRef]
18. Li, L.; Mak, K.Y.; Leung, C.W.; Chan, K.Y.; Chan, W.K.; Zhong, W.; Pong, P.W.T. Effect of synthesis conditions on the properties of citric acid coated iron oxide nanoparticles. *Microelectron. Eng.* **2013**, *110*, 329–334. [CrossRef]
19. Herzig, M.C.; Delavan, C.P.; Jensen, K.J.; Cantu, C.; Montgomery, R.K.; Christy, B.A.; Cap, A.P.; Bynum, J.A. A streamlined proliferation assay using mixed lymphocytes for evaluation of human mesenchymal stem cell immunomodulation activity. *J. Immunol. Methods* **2020**, *488*, 112915. [CrossRef]
20. Abnave, P.; Ghigo, E. Role of the immune system in regeneration and its dynamic interplay with adult stem cells. *Semin. Cell Dev. Biol.* **2019**, *87*, 160–168. [CrossRef]
21. Hoang, D.M.; Pham, P.T.; Bach, T.Q.; Ngo, A.T.L.; Nguyen, Q.T.; Phan, T.T.K.; Nguyen, G.H.; Le, P.T.T.; Hoang, V.T.; Forsyth, N.R.; et al. Stem cell-based therapy for human diseases. *Signal Transduct. Target. Ther.* **2022**, *7*, 272. [CrossRef] [PubMed]
22. He, Z.; Ding, Y.; Mu, Y.; Xu, X.; Kong, W.; Chai, R.; Chen, X. Stem Cell-Based Therapies in Hearing Loss. *Front. Cell Dev. Biol.* **2021**, *9*, 730042. [CrossRef] [PubMed]
23. Guo, X.; Schaudinn, C.; Blume-Peytavi, U.; Vogt, A.; Rancan, F. Effects of Adipose-Derived Stem Cells and Their Conditioned Medium in a Human Ex Vivo Wound Model. *Cells* **2022**, *11*, 1198. [CrossRef]
24. Yoo, T.; Du, X.; Zhou, B. The paracrine effect of mesenchymal human stem cells restored hearing in β-tubulin induced autoimmune sensorineural hearing loss. *Hear. Res.* **2015**, *330*, 57–61. [CrossRef] [PubMed]
25. Serrano-Lotina, A.; Portela, R.; Baeza, P.; Alcolea-Rodriguez, V.; Villarroel, M.; Ávila, P. Zeta potential as a tool for functional materials development. *Catal. Today*, 2022, in press. [CrossRef]
26. Liu, S.; Yu, B.; Wang, S.; Shen, Y.; Cong, H. Preparation, surface functionalization and application of Fe_3O_4 magnetic nanoparticles. *Adv. Colloid Interface Sci.* **2020**, *281*, 102165. [CrossRef] [PubMed]
27. Śliwka, L.; Wiktorska, K.; Suchocki, P.; Milczarek, M.; Mielczarek, S.; Lubelska, K.; Cierpiał, T.; Łyżwa, P.; Kiełbasiński, P.; Jaromin, A.; et al. The Comparison of MTT and CVS Assays for the Assessment of Anticancer Agent Interactions. *PLoS ONE* **2016**, *11*, e0155772. [CrossRef] [PubMed]
28. Cardoso, V.F.; Francesko, A.; Ribeiro, C.; Bañobre-López, M.; Martins, P.; Lanceros-Mendez, S. Advances in Magnetic Nanoparticles for Biomedical Applications. *Adv. Healthc. Mater.* **2018**, *7*, 1700845. [CrossRef]
29. Chu, D.-T.; Nguyen Thi Phuong, T.; Tien, N.L.B.; Tran, D.K.; Minh, L.B.; Thanh, V.V.; Gia Anh, P.; Pham, V.H.; Thi Nga, V. Adipose Tissue Stem Cells for Therapy: An Update on the Progress of Isolation, Culture, Storage, and Clinical Application. *J. Clin. Med.* **2019**, *8*, 917. [CrossRef] [PubMed]
30. Kolosnjaj-Tabi, J.; Wilhelm, C.; Clément, O.; Gazeau, F. Cell labeling with magnetic nanoparticles: Opportunity for magnetic cell imaging and cell manipulation. *J. Nanobiotechnol.* **2013**, *11* (Suppl. S1), S7. [CrossRef]
31. Volatron, J.; Carn, F.; Kolosnjaj-Tabi, J.; Javed, Y.; Vuong, Q.L.; Gossuin, Y.; Ménager, C.; Luciani, N.; Charron, G.; Hémadi, M.; et al. Ferritin Protein Regulates the Degradation of Iron Oxide Nanoparticles. *Small* **2016**, *13*, 1602030. [CrossRef]
32. Van de Walle, A.; Sangnier, A.P.; Abou-Hassan, A.; Curcio, A.; Hémadi, M.; Menguy, N.; Lalatonne, Y.; Luciani, N.; Wilhelm, C. Biosynthesis of magnetic nanoparticles from nano-degradation products revealed in human stem cells. *Proc. Natl. Acad. Sci. USA* **2019**, *116*, 4044–4053. [CrossRef] [PubMed]

33. Dominici, M.; Le Blanc, K.; Mueller, I.; Slaper-Cortenbach, I.; Marini, F.C.; Krause, D.S.; Deans, R.J.; Keating, A.; Prockop, D.J.; Horwitz, E.M. Minimal criteria for defining multipotent mesenchymal stromal cells. The International Society for Cellular Therapy position statement. *Cytotherapy* **2006**, *8*, 315–317. [CrossRef] [PubMed]
34. Horwitz, E.M.; Le Blanc, K.; Dominici, M.; Mueller, I.; Slaper-Cortenbach, I.; Marini, F.C.; Deans, R.J.; Krause, D.S.; Keating, A.; International Society for Cellular, T. Clarification of the nomenclature for MSC: The International Society for Cellular Therapy position statement. *Cytotherapy* **2005**, *7*, 393–395. [CrossRef]
35. Zhou, S.; Yin, T.; Zou, Q.; Zhang, K.; Gao, G.; Shapter, J.G.; Huang, P.; Fu, Q. Labeling adipose derived stem cell sheet by ultrasmall super-paramagnetic Fe_3O_4 nanoparticles and magnetic resonance tracking in vivo. *Sci. Rep.* **2017**, *7*, srep42793. [CrossRef]
36. Zhang, H.; Li, S.; Liu, Y.; Yu, Y.; Lin, S.; Wang, Q.; Miao, L.; Wei, H.; Sun, W. Fe_3O_4@GO magnetic nanocomposites protect mesenchymal stem cells and promote osteogenic differentiation of rat bone marrow mesenchymal stem cells. *Biomater. Sci.* **2020**, *8*, 5984–5993. [CrossRef]
37. Di Wu, D.; Chang, X.; Tian, J.; Kang, L.; Wu, Y.; Liu, J.; Wu, X.; Huang, Y.; Gao, B.; Wang, H.; et al. Bone mesenchymal stem cells stimulation by magnetic nanoparticles and a static magnetic field: Release of exosomal miR-1260a improves osteogenesis and angiogenesis. *J. Nanobiotechnol.* **2021**, *19*, 209. [CrossRef]
38. Fan, J.; Tan, Y.; Jie, L.; Wu, X.; Yu, R.; Zhang, M. Biological activity and magnetic resonance imaging of superparamagnetic iron oxide nanoparticles-labeled adipose-derived stem cells. *Stem Cell Res. Ther.* **2013**, *4*, 44. [CrossRef] [PubMed]
39. He, F.; Cao, J.; Qi, J.; Liu, Z.; Liu, G.; Deng, W. Regulation of Stem Cell Differentiation by Inorganic Nanomaterials: Recent Advances in Regenerative Medicine. *Front. Bioeng. Biotechnol.* **2021**, *9*, 898. [CrossRef]
40. Kostura, L.; Kraitchman, D.L.; Mackay, A.M.; Pittenger, M.F.; Bulte, J.W.M. Feridex labeling of mesenchymal stem cells inhibits chondrogenesis but not adipogenesis or osteogenesis. *NMR Biomed.* **2004**, *17*, 513–517. [CrossRef]
41. Uciechowski, P.; Dempke, W.C. Interleukin-6: A Masterplayer in the Cytokine Network. *Oncology* **2020**, *98*, 131–137. [CrossRef] [PubMed]
42. Nara, H.; Watanabe, R. Anti-Inflammatory Effect of Muscle-Derived Interleukin-6 and Its Involvement in Lipid Metabolism. *Int. J. Mol. Sci.* **2021**, *22*, 9889. [CrossRef]
43. Cui, L.; Yin, S.; Liu, W.; Li, N.; Zhang, W.; Cao, Y. Expanded Adipose-Derived Stem Cells Suppress Mixed Lymphocyte Reaction by Secretion of Prostaglandin E2. *Tissue Eng.* **2007**, *13*, 1185–1195. [CrossRef]
44. Fiori, A.; Uhlig, S.; Klüter, H.; Bieback, K. Human Adipose Tissue-Derived Mesenchymal Stromal Cells Inhibit CD4+ T Cell Proliferation and Induce Regulatory T Cells as Well as CD127 Expression on CD4+CD25+ T Cells. *Cells* **2021**, *10*, 58. [CrossRef]
45. Gheorghe, D.C.; Epure, V.; Oprea, D.; Zamfir-Chiru-Anton, A. Persistent Stapedial Artery, Oval Window Atresia and Congenital Stapes Agenesis—Case Report. *Medicina* **2023**, *59*, 461. [CrossRef]
46. Baldari, S.; Di Rocco, G.; Piccoli, M.; Pozzobon, M.; Muraca, M.; Toietta, G. Challenges and Strategies for Improving the Regenerative Effects of Mesenchymal Stromal Cell-Based Therapies. *Int. J. Mol. Sci.* **2017**, *18*, 2087. [CrossRef]
47. Xia, Y.; Li, Y.; Wu, X.; Zhang, Q.; Chen, S.; Ma, X.; Yu, M. Ironing Out the Details: How Iron Orchestrates Macrophage Polarization. *Front. Immunol.* **2021**, *12*, 669566. [CrossRef]

Disclaimer/Publisher's Note: The statements, opinions and data contained in all publications are solely those of the individual author(s) and contributor(s) and not of MDPI and/or the editor(s). MDPI and/or the editor(s) disclaim responsibility for any injury to people or property resulting from any ideas, methods, instructions or products referred to in the content.

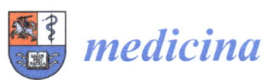

Review

Vertigo Associated with Otosclerosis and Stapes Surgery—A Narrative Review

Violeta Necula, Alma Aurelia Maniu, László-Péter Ujváry *, Maximilian-George Dindelegan *, Mara Tănase, Mihai Tănase and Cristina Maria Blebea

Otorhinolaryngology Department, "Iuliu Hațieganu" University of Medicine and Pharmacy, 400347 Cluj-Napoca, Romania
* Correspondence: ujvarypeter@outlook.com (L.-P.U.); maximilian.dindelegan@gmail.com (M.-G.D.)

Abstract: Otosclerosis is a pathological condition affecting the temporal bone, and is characterized by remodelling of the labyrinthine bone tissue through a dynamic process of osteolysis and osteogenesis. This condition progressively leads to hearing loss, tinnitus, and vertigo. Stapedotomy, a surgical procedure involving the removal of the stapes superstructure and its replacement with a prosthesis, is the treatment of choice to improve hearing in individuals with otosclerosis. However, vestibular dysfunction is a significant complication associated with this procedure, which can occur intraoperatively or postoperatively, ranging from the immediate postoperative period to weeks, months, or even years after surgery. This paper aims to provide a comprehensive review of the most important causes of vertigo associated with otosclerosis and stapes surgery with the goal of minimizing the incidence of this complication. Understanding the underlying factors contributing to vertigo in this context is crucial for the prevention and effective management of vertigo in patients undergoing stapecotomy.

Keywords: otosclerosis; vertigo; dizziness; stapes surgery

1. Introduction

Otosclerosis, also known as otospongiosis, is a progressive primary bone disorder of the otic capsule. It is characterized by abnormal focal resorption and recalcification of the endochondral layer of the temporal bone. This results in progressive conductive hearing loss, evolving in severe cases to a combination of conductive and sensorineural hearing loss. The otosclerotic process starts in the anterior part of the oval window, near the fissula ante fenestram resulting in fenestral otosclerosis. The disease can progress beyond the fissula ante fenestram and extend to the pericochlear otic capsule in cochlear otosclerosis or retrofenestral otosclerosis. The advanced stages can affect structures such as round window, semicircular canals, labyrinth, or vestibular nerve endings [1].

While progressive hearing loss is the main complaint in otosclerosis, other symptoms such as tinnitus and balance disorders are frequently associated with the condition. Up to 30% of patients with otosclerosis may experience vestibular symptoms, including instability, dizziness, and vertigo [2]. These symptoms can occur before or after treatment, and may arise as immediate or delayed complications of stapes surgery.

Surgical intervention is the preferred treatment for otosclerosis, with the aim of restoring the mechanism of sound transmission from the ossicular chain to the inner ear receptors, resulting in an air–bone gap closure of less than 10 dB in over 80% of cases [3,4]. Stapedotomy has become the most commonly performed surgical technique, replacing stapedectomy. For patients who are not suitable for or decline surgery, hearing aids can be recommended to improve hearing [5].

Considering the significant impact of vertigo on quality of life, this study aims to evaluate the presence of vertigo in otosclerosis and assess the risk of developing vestibular disorders following stapes surgery. By understanding the relationship between otosclerosis,

Citation: Necula, V.; Maniu, A.A.; Ujváry, L.-P.; Dindelegan, M.-G.; Tănase, M.; Tănase, M.; Blebea, C.M. Vertigo Associated with Otosclerosis and Stapes Surgery—A Narrative Review. *Medicina* **2023**, *59*, 1485. https://doi.org/10.3390/medicina59081485

Academic Editor: Silviu Albu

Received: 16 July 2023
Revised: 13 August 2023
Accepted: 15 August 2023
Published: 18 August 2023

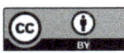

Copyright: © 2023 by the authors. Licensee MDPI, Basel, Switzerland. This article is an open access article distributed under the terms and conditions of the Creative Commons Attribution (CC BY) license (https://creativecommons.org/licenses/by/4.0/).

vertigo, and stapes surgery, clinicians can better manage and minimize the incidence of this distressing complication.

2. The Otosclerotic Process

The otosclerotic process consists of abnormal replacement of enchondral bone with cancellous bone and subsequently with sclerotic bone. The process occurs in waves of osteolysis followed by osteogenesis. During the active phase of otospongiosis, the resorption process consists of replacing the normal bone around the blood vessels, which has cellular fibrous connective tissue, with mononuclear histiocytes, osteocytes, and osteoclasts [6]. A number of studies have shown that the enzymes secreted by the cells from the otospongiotic foci play a role in bone decalcification [7,8], while other studies have investigated the level of alkaline phosphates in the decalcification process of the otic capsule [9]. The final stage of the process is the otosclerosis stage, when the bone becomes mineralized and presents a mosaic appearance [10].

Lim et al. [11] described three types of otosclerotic lesions: cellular or spongiotic, characterized by the activation of monocytes, macrophages, osteoblasts, and osteoclasts; fibrotic, in which extensive bone fibrosis occurs; and sclerotic, characterized by a marked reduction of bone cells. Chevance et al. [12] reported the presence of osteolytic enzymes in the perilymph of patients who underwent surgery for otosclerosis, and suggested that these enzymes may have an important role in the development of otosclerotic lesions in the inner ear.

Stapes fixation occurs due to calcification of the annular ligament and the invasion of otosclerotic lesions at the oval window [13]. Otosclerotic lesions in the cochlear endosteum can lead to atrophic and hyalinization changes of the spiral ligament [14]. Damage to the spiral ligament can disrupt the chemical balance of ion-fluid recycling [15] and obstruct the endolymphatic duct and sac, resulting in biochemical changes [16,17]. Gros et al. [18] observed that vestibular disorders are frequently associated with sclerotic lesions. Saim and Nadol [19] reported that patients with vestibular symptoms have elevated bone-conduction thresholds and suggested that the degeneration of the vestibular nerve and Scarpa ganglion cells could be responsible for these symptoms, regardless of otosclerotic damage to the vestibular end organs.

Otosclerosis is associated with inflammation, disturbed collagen expression, and the presence of viral receptors and antigens in the otosclerotic foci [20]. At the molecular level, the bone remodelling process is regulated by a series of cytokines, signalling molecules that play a crucial role in regulating various cellular processes including bone remodelling. In otosclerosis, cytokines such as osteoprotegerin (OPG), receptor activator of nuclear factor kB (RANK), and RANK liand (RANKL), as well as transforming growth factor ß1 (TGF-ß1), are involved in controlling the balance between bone resorption and bone formation [20,21]. The presence of the measles virus and concurrent inflammation may trigger the abnormal bone remodeling that is a characteristic of otosclerosis. In the active phase, there is an increase in inflammation, detectable measles virus particle, local expression of tumor necrosis factor alpha (TNF-α), and negativity for OPG expression. During this phase, the balance between bone resorption and formation may be disrupted. In the inactive phase of otosclerosis, OPG positivity and TNF-α negativity are observed, along with absence of inflammation [22,23]. The increased level of TNF-α can stimulate osteoclast activation, induce RANKL expression, and reduce osteoclast apoptosis. This sequence of events ultimately leads to osteolysis and contributes to the process of otospongiosis [22,24]. TNF-α overexpression stimulates osteoclast formation both by inhibiting OPG secretion and by stimulating RANKL formation [23,24].

3. Anatomy of the Membranous Labyrinth

The anatomy of the membranous labyrinth is essential to understanding certain pathological processes; in surgical procedures involving the inner ear, these particularly relate to otosclerosis and stapes surgery. The middle ear communicates with the inner ear through the oval and round windows. The footplate articulates with the oval window through the annular ligament. Beyond the oval window is the vestibule, which is filled with perilymph. The membranous labyrinth is supported by periotic connective tissue within the perilymphatic space, which is medial and superior to the utricle and saccule and absent lateral to them [25].

The otolith organs of the vestibule are the macula of the utricle and saccule, located medially in the vestibule. Their role is to detect the position and direction of the head as well as the linear and gravitational acceleration [26].

The utricle has an elongated shape and communicates with the semicircular canals. On the inferior wall, the more lateral is the macula of the utricle, oriented horizontally. It is localized next to the upper edge of the oval window at 0.5–1 mm distance [27]. In surgical procedures, the macula of the utricle can be observed as a white plaque within the vestibule [28].

The saccule is situated in the spherical recess, and its macula has a vertical orientation perpendicular to the macula of the utricle. The anterior wall of the saccule is adjacent to the footplate. Between these two structures is found a connective tissue, named the reinforced area of the saccular membrane [29]. The macula of the saccule projects below the horizontal line passing through the arm of the stapes [30]. The distance between the saccule and the anterior edge of the oval window is between 1 and 1.5 mm [27]. The saccule communicates with the utricle through the utriculo-saccular duct, with the cochlea through the reuniens duct, and with the endolymphatic duct through the sinus of the duct.

The membrana limitans is a membranous structure, similar to a network, which delimits the superior vestibular labyrinth from the inferior part, laying below the utricle and supporting its macula [31]. In certain cases, the membrana limitans can present thin fibrillary attachments to the footplate, especially in the posterior third [25]. Its role is more of a support than a barrier, as it has a discontinuous structure that allows the passage of perilymph. Its insertion is in the superior part of the vestibule, superior to the oval window, immediately above the stapes footplate. In certain cases, the membrana limitans can be directly inserted in the footplate [25]. Pauw et al. [32] reported that the distance between the footplate and the utricle is smaller in patients with otosclerosis than in normal subjects. These rapports and adhesions of the labyrinthine structures to the footplate may partially explain the vertigo experienced during stapes surgery.

Vestibular symptoms can be part of the clinical manifestations of otosclerosis or can occur during or after stapes surgery, either immediately or with delayed onset.

4. Preoperative Vertigo

The incidence of preoperative vestibular symptoms in otosclerosis patients varies greatly from one study to another. Different studies have reported incidence ranging from 8.6 to 30% [33–35]. While the exact cause of vertigo in patients with otosclerosis is not fully understood, several factors have been proposed (Table 1).

One factor is the presence of otosclerotic foci, which can affect the endolymphatic duct and sac, leading to hydrops [15]. This abnormal accumulation of fluid in the inner ear can contribute to vertigo. Temporal bone studies have shown the presence of endolymphatic hydrops (EH) in specimens with extensive otosclerotic lesions in the cochlear endosteum or in the vestibular aqueduct, obstructing the flow of endolymph and disrupting labyrinthine fluid homeostasis [15,16]. The presence of endolimphatic hydrops can be visualized on delayed three-dimensional (3D) fluid-attenuated inversion recovery (FLAIR) MRI images obtained after intravenous administration of gadolinium. Sone et al. [36] suggested that the presence of preoperative asymptomatic vestibular EH could serve as a predictive factor for postoperative complications following stapes surgery. EH located adjacent to the oval window could be a contraindication for stapes surgery. The proximity of EH to the surgical site may increase the risk of vestibular complications after the procedure, including vertigo.

Table 1. Summarised data on vertigo associated with otosclerosis.

	Preoperative	Intraoperative	Immediate Postoperative	Late Postoperative
Incidence	8.6–30%	2.1%	3.4–70%	0.5–17%
Causes	-endolymphatic hydrops -detachment of the otoconia–cupular deposits -vestibular endorgan and/or neural degeneration -hydrolytic enzymes, cytokines	-manipulation of the footplate -suctioning in the middle ear/oval window -floating footplate	-serous and chemical labyrinthitis -suction of perilymph -penetration of instrument or prosthesis into the vestibule -traumatization of the utricle or saccule -release of proteolytic enzymes -antigen-antibody reaction -changes in labyrinthine fluids pressure -reduction of blood supply to the labyrinth -stapes surgery in the opposite ear	-perilymphatic fistula -secondary endolymphatic hydrops -irritation by prolonged prosthesis -reparative granuloma -bone fragments entering the vestibule -pneumolabyrinth, barotrauma -stapes surgery in the opposite ear
Progress	-Fluctuating -Permanent	Usually temporary	Usually temporary	-Temporary -Fluctuating -Permanent
Treatment	-Sodium fluoride -Bisphosphonates	-Vertiginous drugs -Bed rest	-Vertiginous drugs -Bed rest	-Sodium fluoride -Bisphosphonates -Vestibular rehabilitation exercises

Detachment of the otoconia from the macula of the utricle is another factor that could contribute to positional vertigo, and may explain anomalies observed in the ocular and cervical vestibular-evoked myogenic potentials (oVEMP and cVEMP), which are used to assess the status of the utricle and saccule, respectively [37–39].

The third factor is vestibular end organ and/or neural degeneration due to otosclerotic foci involving the utricular or ampullary nerve. These changes could be related to the utricular deficit and oVEMP anomalies in patients with vertigo and otosclerosis [40].

Additionally, hydrolytic enzymes originating in the otosclerotic foci have been identified in the perilymph of otosclerosis patients; these can produce vascular and neuroepithelial lesions. Moreover, the cytokines produced in these foci can cause changes in labyrinthine fluids' chemical composition and homeostasis [41].

Degeneration of receptor cells in the vestibule and changes in the nonsensory epithelium have been observed in temporal bone studies of otosclerosis patients. Kaya et al. [42] studied temporal bones harvested from patients diagnosed with otosclerosis and found a decrease in the population of vestibular dark cells and vestibular transitional cells in temporal bone specimens with endosteal involvement. The role of these cells is to maintain the homeostasis of the labyrinthine fluid by controlling the transport of ions and water in order to prevent vestibular dysfunction. Another study by Hizli et al. [43] found that the mean density of type I hair cells in the saccule was significantly reduced in cases with endosteal involvement, suggesting that the extension of the otosclerotic foci towards the endosteum may be an important factor in the occurrence of vestibular symptoms in patients with otosclerosis. They suggested that this might explain the abnormal oVEMP and cVEMP response in patients with otosclerosis and vestibular symptoms.

Saka et al. [44] studied the vestibular-evoked myogenic potential in response to bone-conducted sound (BC-VEMP) in a group of 25 patients and showed that 9 of 10 patients with vestibular dysfunction presented abnormal BC-VEMPs. This suggests that saccular dysfunction may be involved in these patients, possibly due to saccular hydrops or the extension of otosclerotic foci to the saccular macula or saccular afferent, considering the anatomical proximity of the saccule to the oval window.

On the other hand, another study involving 27 patients with otosclerosis and vertigo reported abnormal oVEMPs in response to impulsive stimulation, suggesting pathological abnormalities related to the utricle [40]. Hayasi et al. [37] studied 35 temporal bones with otosclerosis, reporting a higher incidence of cupular deposits compared to temporal bone without otosclerosis. They suggested that the origin of these deposits was probably the otoconia from the utricle, from where they detached and migrated to the cupula of semicircular canals.

The specific manifestation of vestibular symptoms can vary from person to person, and may be influenced by factors such as the extent of otosclerotic involvement and individual differences in anatomy and physiology. A study conducted by Eza-Nuñez et al. [45] highlighted the diversity of vestibular symptoms experienced by patients with otosclerosis. Patients with otosclerosis mention vertigo or imbalance, which can manifest in different ways, including a single episode or recurrent attacks either triggered by positional changes or occurring spontaneously. In their study, positional vertigo was associated with otosclerosis in 32.5% of patients and Ménière syndrome was reported in 30% of patients. Around 27.5% of patients experienced spontaneous recurrent vertigo, approximately 7.5% of patients presented with chronic unrelapsing imbalance, and a small percentage of patients (2.5%) had acute unilateral vestibulopathy [45].

These findings suggest that multiple factors, including endolymphatic hydrops, detachment of otoconia, degeneration of receptor cells, and cupular deposits, may lead to vertigo in otosclerosis patients. Further research is needed in order to fully understand the underlying mechanisms and develop targeted interventions for vestibular symptoms in this population.

5. Immediate Postoperative Vertigo

Treatment of otosclerosis is mainly surgical, generally with good results. The most common technique is stapedotomy, a minimally invasive technique that has largely replaced stapedectomy due to having fewer complications, including vestibular disorder [33]. The surgical approach can be either classical, using a microscope, or endoscopic, and the stapedotomy can be carried out by a conventional or laser-assisted technique.

Vertigo is reported to occur intraoperatively in 2.1% of patients, mainly due to the manipulation of the footplate. It may occur due to frequent suctioning in the middle ear, and less often to a floating footplate. This is treated by reassurance of the patient and vertiginous drugs [46] (Table 1).

After surgical treatment, immediate postoperative vertigo can occur in a significant percentage of patients. The reported incidence of vestibular symptoms varies among studies, ranging from 3.4% to 70% [47–49] (Table 1).

Early postoperative vertigo is usually temporary, and authors report remission of symptoms in most cases after 5 to 7 days with conservative management, including medication and bed rest [50,51].

The use of a CO_2 Laser in footplate perforation has been suggested to reduce the prevalence of postoperative vertigo due to minimal mechanical trauma to the inner ear through lesser footplate manipulation [47,52].

Several factors contribute to the occurrence of immediate postoperative vertigo. A possible cause of premature vertigo could be serous and chemical labyrinthitis, which involves irritation of the membranous labyrinth, particularly the macula of the utricle located near the oval window [53]. Suction of the perilymph from the vestibule or contact of the instrument with the membranous labyrinth can trigger vertigo [54]. According to measurements taken Pauw et al., penetration of instruments or the prosthesis into the vestibule is considered less risky in the centre and lower third of the oval window [32].

Nystagmus is observed postoperatively in approximately 65.7% of patients, and may persist for over one month, as shown by Fukuda et al. [55] in a study conducted in 2021

Singh et al. [52] used posturography to evaluate patients, and found that patients experienced vestibular deficits and increased subjective symptom scores at one week after surgery, with remission occurring after four weeks.

Assessment of cVEMP with air conducted stimuli before surgery and three months after stapedotomy showed a significant reduction in the amplitude of P1/N2 waves in patients who complained of dizziness and vertigo, suggesting a saccular lesion in these patients [56]. The reduction of air conduction (AC) and bone conduction (BC) VEMPs in patients with otosclerosis was reported by Trivelli et al. [57], with the observation that although the air conduction thresholds improved after surgery in all patients, AC-VEMP and BC-VEMP did not significantly improve in operated patients. Akazawa et al. [58] evaluated the cervical and ocular VEMPs through bone-conducted vibration before and after surgery, finding no significant changes in VEMPs in the operated ear after stapes surgery.

Postoperative vertigo following stapedotomy may be attributed to traumatization of the utricle, release of proteolytic enzymes, antigen–antibody reactions, pressure changes in labyrinthine fluids, and reduction of blood supply to the labyrinth caused by a floating footplate during the operation [53,59].

Among the three semicircular canals (SCC), the lateral SCC appears to be the most affected in both otosclerosis and after stapes surgery. SCC function can be evaluated by vHIT. Postoperative vHIT results have indicated subclinical damage to the lateral and posterior SCC. This is further supported by studies on temporal bones which revealed degeneration of the sensory epithelium in the cristae of the SCC [60,61]. Kujala et al. [62] evaluated patients after stapes surgery and found latent spontaneus horizontal-torsional nystagmus in 33% of patients on the day of surgery. The presence of this nystagmus suggests minimal impairment of the SCC.

Overall, immediate postoperative vertigo is a common occurrence following surgery for otosclerosis, though it is usually temporary and resolves with conservative management. Monitoring vestibular function through VEMPs and other tests can provide insights into the underlaying mechanisms and help to evaluate the impact of surgery on vestibular function.

6. Late Postoperative Vertigo

Late postoperative vertigo can occur following stapes surgery for otosclerosis, with a reported incidence ranging from 0.5% to 17% [54]. The persistence of vertigo beyond four weeks is observed in approximately 4% of patients, as shown by Birch et al. [63] in a study of 722 patients, while in Albera's study 17% (58/347) [54] showed changes in the caloric test even up to 15 years after surgery. A small percentage of patients (2.6%) may experience vertigo lasting over 12 months, indicating permanent postoperative vestibular hypofunction [64] (Table 1).

One potential cause of late postoperative vertigo is the perilymphatic fistula, which occurs due to inadequate sealing around the prosthesis at the oval window. Its incidence is variable from one study to another, ranging from 1.3% to 10% [65–68]. Pedersen et al. [65] suggested that the cause may be inadequate sealing around the prosthesis in the oval window. A systematic review of the results and complications of stapes surgery confirms that perilymphatic fistula is a rare complication of stapes surgery and represents approximately one third of surgical revision cases [69]. Although its existence has been highlighted intraoperatively in only a few cases, the correlation between filling with tissue or fibrin glue and remission of symptoms suggests that the perilymphatic fistula is often underestimated [70].

The perilymphatic fistula can persist postoperatively if the hole around the prosthesis has not been closed, or may appear later if the graft or prosthesis moves as a consequence of increased pressure due to coughing or sneezing. Usually, complaints involve fluctuating hearing loss and vertigo, and the audiogram indicates deterioration of cochlear function [71]. Incidence can be reduced in the case of stapedectomy by placing a graft over the oval window [72].

Due to the risk of meningitis and hearing loss, the presence of perilymphatic fistula represents a serious complication. If a perilymphatic fistula is suspected and the symptoms do not improve with treatment, surgical exploration of the ear is necessary in order to close the fistula with a soft tissue graft. Persistence of the fistula can lead to irreversible hearing loss and persistence of vertigo [2].

According to Nakashima et al., the incidence of perilymphatic fistula can reach 22% in patients in whom the obliteration was performed with gelfoam and 4% in those in whom the obliteration was performed with tissue [73]. An older study comparing gelfoam, fat tissue, and fascia showed an incidence of perilymphatic fistula of 3.5% in case of gelfoam, 1.9% in case of fat tissue, and 0.6% in the case of fascia [74]. According to Lim et al. [75], from an auditory point of view fatty tissue is to be preferred in stapedotomy and fascia in stapedectomies.

Other causes of postoperative vertigo include irritation produced by a protracted prosthesis or a displaced one. Symptoms intensify when moving the head or during the Valsalva manoeuvre. The patient may experience dizziness related to hiccupping, burping, yawning, popping of the ears, and specific acoustic stimuli [76].

Reparative granuloma, which is a pyogenic inflammatory reaction, autoimmune or allergic reaction, or exuberant healing response, can occur in approximately 0.1% to 18% of cases after stapedectomy or stapedotomy [77–80]. Reparative granulomas occur more frequently after stapedectomy, and are characterized by sensorineural hearing loss along with vertigo. Typically, reparative granuloma manifests 7 to 15 days after surgery [81].

Persistent late vertigo can be due to bone fragments entering the vestibule during surgery; additional causes include direct compression of the saccule due to adhesion between the prosthesis and the tympanic membrane, Eustachian tube dysfunction, and Tullio phenomenon [82–84]. Stapes surgery can damage the inner ear and eventually leads to endolymphatic hydrops without decreasing the hearing threshold at low frequencies [85]. Endolymphatic hydrops (EH) can be associated with otosclerosis as a secondary condition following stapes surgery, when EH can occur immediately after the surgery or at a later time. Clinical manifestations include low-frequency fluctuating sensorineural hearing loss, episodic vertigo, tinnitus, and aural fullness. However, according to Halpin et al. [85] these symptoms are much more rare compared to the presence of histopathological findings or TB specimens of patients who underwent otosclerosis surgery.

Rarely, late-onset vertigo can be associated with pneumolabyrinth or barotrauma, a condition presented by Mandala et al. in a patient who started to have vertigo years after surgery [86]. Additionally, Gomes et al. [87] published a case report about a patient who came back 4 weeks after stapedectomy for displacement of the prosthesis and the graft. In most cases, this complication occurred a few weeks or months after the surgery. The diagnosis is based on HRCT scan showing the presence of air bubbles in the vestibule in patients with vertigo and a positive fistula test.

Several factors can contribute to prolonged vertigo, including age, sex, stapes surgery in the opposite ear, the seal around the prosthesis in the footplate, and postoperative hearing outcomes. A history of stapes surgery in the opposite ear has been identified as a significant predictive factor for prolonged nystagmus and subjective vestibular symptoms [55].

Intractable vertigo may be an indicator for revision surgery in otosclerosis cases [54]. Prompt diagnosis and appropriate management are crucial in addressing the underlying causes of late postoperative vertigo and improving patient outcomes.

7. Treatment of Vertigo

The treatment of vertigo in patients with otosclerosis depends on the underlying cause and the severity of symptoms.

The immediate postoperative vertigo during the surgical procedure and in the first few days resolves mostly with bed rest and symptomatic treatment within approximately 5 to 7 days, rarely lasting more than 4 weeks.

If vertigo symptoms persist or are caused by specific complications such as a perilymphatic fistula or malposition of the prosthesis, surgical intervention can be considered to obliterate a possible perilymphatic fistula, reposition the prosthesis, or take other corrective measures to address the underlying cause of vertigo.

Postoperative or late vertigo can be improved by treatment with the latest generation of bisphosphonates or by physical therapy, including vestibular rehabilitation exercises. These exercises aim to improve balance, reduce dizziness, and promote central compensation of the vestibular system.

Medical treatment of otosclerosis includes drugs that can directly influence bone metabolism, anti-inflammatory agents that address the inflammatory etiology, targeted (biological) therapies, and, last but not least, anti-measles vaccination [88].

Bone metabolism inhibitors aim to preserve hearing thresholds and alleviate symptoms such as tinnitus and vertigo associated with otosclerosis. Sodium fluoride, often combined with calcium carbonate and vitamin D, is used to slow down the progression of otosclerosis. It has been shown to reduce the deterioration of hearing loss and help to control tinnitus and vestibular symptoms. However, there are differing opinions as to its overall effectiveness in treating otosclerosis. Studies have stated that sodium fluoride can slow down the evolution of the disease in more than 50% of cases [89], while others have shown reduced efficiency in the treatment of otosclerosis [88].

Studies have shown that bisphosphonates can influence vestibular symptoms in patients with otosclerosis before or after surgery. Brookler and Tanyeri have reported that 54% of patients presented an improvement in vestibular symptoms after treatment with bisphosphonates, while 39% reported disappearance of dizziness and 35% presented improvement in the results of tests performed with a rotatory chair [90]. The newer generations of bisphosphonates (e.g., risedronate, zoledronate) have more favorable tolerability and are more powerful bone resorption inhibitors [91].

Bioflavonoids can reduce bone resorption by inhibiting the phosphodiesterase enzyme. While they might not significantly affect hearing loss, they have been found to significantly reduce tinnitus [92].

Vitamin D's anti-inflammatory effects and vitamin A's ability to inhibit osteoclast differentiation could potentially have a beneficial impact on otosclerosis [88,93].

Regarding anti-inflammatory agents, corticosteroids are often used in inner ear diseases, including otosclerosis. Transtympanic administration can be a solution to minimize systemic side effects. Nonsteroidal anti-inflammatory drugs have been considered for their inhibitory effect on bone resorption; however, there is a lack of long-term clinical data in otosclerosis [88,92].

From the class of immunosuppressive agents, only cyclosporine A has been studied, and there is limited data on the use of other immunosuppressive drugs in treating otosclerosis [94].

Emerging treatments such as anti-TNF-α agents (e.g., infliximab), recombinant human OPG (rhOPG), and other anti-osteoporotic targeted therapies (e.g., denosumab, odanacatib) hold potential for otosclerosis treatment, however, more long-term studies are needed [92].

Fluoride-based medications and bisphosphonates are among the treatments considered for medical management of otosclerosis-related hearing loss and associated symptoms such as tinnitus and vertigo.

8. Limitations of the Study

The reported percentages of balance disorders in otosclerosis patients both pre- and postoperatively varies significantly in the literature due to differences in study design and patient assessments. The main complaint in otosclerosis is typically hearing loss, with balance disorders often being secondary, which can lead to variations in the assessment and reporting of vestibular symptoms. Postoperative vertigo can vary depending on factors such as the individual patient, surgeon's experience, surgical technique, and type of prosthesis used.

Advancements in technology have provided new tools for assessing vestibular deficits, allowing for more objective evaluation of vertigo. Objective measures can provide valuable information about vestibular function before and after surgery.

Multicentre studies with larger patient populations and standardized evaluation protocols would be beneficial in providing more comprehensive and reliable data on balance disorders in otosclerosis patients before and after surgery.

9. Conclusions

Vertigo is a common manifestation in otosclerosis both before and after surgical treatment. It can present as benign paroxysmal positional vertigo, vertigo attacks, or hydrops, as well as dizziness or light-headedness. While vertigo quite frequently appears immediately after surgery, the symptoms typically subside quickly with medical treatment, and only persist for longer periods of time in a very few cases.

When vertigo occurs months or years after the surgery, this can be an alarming signal of a complication that may require surgical reintervention. In such cases, careful evaluation and appropriate management are crucial in order to address the underlying cause and alleviate the vertigo symptoms.

Overall, understanding the occurrence and characteristics of vertigo in otosclerosis both pre- and postoperatively is essential for effective diagnosis, treatment, and patient management. Further research and standardized assessment protocols are needed in order to provide more comprehensive data and improve the management of balance disorders in otosclerosis patients.

Author Contributions: Conceptualization, V.N., A.A.M., L.-P.U., M.-G.D., M.T. (Mara Tănase), M.T. (Mihai Tănase) and C.M.B.; writing—original draft preparation, V.N., A.A.M., L.-P.U., M.-G.D., M.T. (Mara Tănase), M.T. (Mihai Tănase) and C.M.B.; writing—review and editing, V.N., A.A.M., L.-P.U., M.-G.D., M.T. (Mara Tănase), M.T. (Mihai Tănase) and C.M.B. All authors have read and agreed to the published version of the manuscript.

Funding: This research received no external funding.

Institutional Review Board Statement: Not applicable.

Informed Consent Statement: Not applicable.

Data Availability Statement: Data sharing not applicable.

Conflicts of Interest: The authors declare no conflict of interest.

References

1. Schuknecht, H.F. Otosclerosis. In *Pathology of the Ear*, 2nd ed.; Lea & Febiger: New York, NY, USA, 1993; pp. 365–379.
2. Merchant, S.N.; McKenna, M.J.; Browning, G.G.; Rea, P.A.; Tange, R.A. Otosclerosis. In *Scott-Brown's Otorhinolaryngology, Head and Neck Surgery*; Michael, G., Browning, G.G., Burton, M.J., Eds.; Edward Arnold Ltd.: London, UK, 2008; pp. 3453–3485.
3. Karimi Yazdi, A.; Sazgar, A.A.; Motiee, M.; Ashtiani, M.K. Improvement of bone conduction after stapes surgery in otosclerosis patients with mixed hearing loss depending from surgical technique. *Eur. Arch. Otorhinolaryngol.* **2009**, *266*, 1225–1228. [CrossRef] [PubMed]
4. Justicz, N.; Strickland, K.F.; Motamedi, K.K.; Mattox, D.E. Review of a single surgeon's stapedotomy cases performed with a nickel titanium prosthesis over a 14-year period. *Acta Otolaryngol.* **2017**, *137*, 442–446. [CrossRef] [PubMed]
5. Batson, L.; Rizzolo, D. Otosclerosis: An update on diagnosis and treatment. *JAAPA* **2017**, *30*, 17–22. [CrossRef]
6. Rudic, M.; Keogh, I.; Wagner, R.; Wilkinson, E.; Kiros, N.; Ferrary, E.; Sterkers, O.; Bozord Grayeli, A.; Zarkovic, K.; Zarkovic, N. The pathophysiology of otosclerosis: Review of current research. *Hear. Res.* **2015**, *330*, 51–56. [CrossRef]
7. Ziff, J.L. A Molecular and Genetic Analysis of Otosclerosis. Doctoral Dissertation, University College London, University of London, London, UK, 2014.
8. Purohit, B.; Hermans, R. Imaging in otosclerosis: A pictorial review. *Insights Imaging* **2014**, *5*, 245–252. [CrossRef] [PubMed]
9. Huang, C.C. Bone resorption in experimental otosclerosis in rats. *Am. J. Otolaryngol.* **1987**, *8*, 332–341. [CrossRef]
10. Quesnel, A.M.; Moonis, G.; Appel, J.; O'malley, J.T.; McKenna, M.J.; Curtin, H.D.; Merchant, S.N. Correlation of computed tomography with histopathology in otosclerosis. *Otol. Neurotol.* **2013**, *34*, 22–28. [CrossRef]
11. Lim, D.J.; Robinson, M.; Saunders, W.H. Morphologic and immunohistochemical observation of otosclerotic stapes: A preliminary study. *Am. J. Otolaryngol.* **1987**, *8*, 282–295. [CrossRef] [PubMed]
12. Chevance, L.G.; Causse, J.; Bretlau, P.; Jorgensen, M.B.; Berges, J. Hydrolytic activity of the perilymph in otosclerosis. A preliminary report. *Acta Otolaryngol.* **1972**, *74*, 23–28. [CrossRef] [PubMed]
13. Linthicum, F.H., Jr. Histopathology of otosclerosis. *Otolaryngol. Clin. N. Am.* **1993**, *26*, 335–352. [CrossRef]
14. Schuknecht, H.F. (Ed.) Disorders of bone. In *Pathology of the Ear*, 2nd ed.; Lea & Febiger: Philadelphia, PA, USA, 1993; pp. 365–414.
15. Liston, S.L.; Paparella, M.M.; Mancini, F.; Anderson, J.H. Otosclerosis and endolymphatic hydrops. *Laryngoscope* **1984**, *94*, 1003–1007. [CrossRef] [PubMed]
16. Yoon, T.H.; Paparella, M.M.; Schachern, P.A. Otosclerosis involving the vestibular aqueduct and Meniere's disease. *Otolaryngol. Head Neck Surg.* **1990**, *103*, 107–112. [CrossRef] [PubMed]

17. Ghorayeb, B.Y.; Linthicum, F.H., Jr. Otosclerotic inner ear syndrome. *Ann. Otol.* **1978**, *87 Pt 1*, 85–90. [CrossRef]
18. Gros, A.; Vatovec, J.; Sereg-Bahar, M. Histologic changes on stapedial footplate in otosclerosis. Correlations between histologic activity and clinical findings. *Otol. Neurotol.* **2003**, *24*, 43–47. [CrossRef]
19. Saim, L.; Nadol, J.B., Jr. Vestibular symptoms in otosclerosis—Correlation of otosclerotic involvement of vestibular apparatus and Scarpa's ganglion cell count. *Am. J. Otol.* **1996**, *17*, 263–270. [PubMed]
20. Stankovic, K.M.; McKenna, M.J. Current research in oto sclerosis. *Curr. Opin. Otolaryngol. Head Neck Surg.* **2006**, *14*, 347–351. [CrossRef] [PubMed]
21. Thys, M.; Van Camp, G. Genetics of otosclerosis. *Otol. Neurotol.* **2009**, *30*, 1021–1032. [CrossRef] [PubMed]
22. Karosi, T.; Jokay, I.; Konya, J.; Szabo, L.Z.; Pytel, J.; Jori, J.; Szalmas, A.; Sziklai, I. Detection of osteoprotegerin and TNF-alpha mRNA in ankylotic Stapes footplates in connection with measles virus positivity. *Laryngoscope* **2006**, *116*, 1427–1433. [CrossRef]
23. Karosi, T.; Csomor, P.; Szalmas, A.; Konya, J.; Petko, M.; Sziklai, I. Osteoprotegerin expression and sensitivity in otosclerosis with different histological activity. *Eur. Arch Otorhinolaryngol.* **2011**, *268*, 357–365. [CrossRef]
24. Takayanagi, H. Osteoimmunology: Shared mechanisms and crosstalk between the immune and bone systems. *Nat. Rev. Immunol.* **2007**, *7*, 292–304. [CrossRef]
25. Mukherjee, P.; Cheng, K.; Curthoys, I. Three-dimensional study of vestibular anatomy as it relates to the stapes footplate and its clinical implications: An augmented reality development. *J. Laryngol. Otol.* **2019**, *133*, 187–191. [CrossRef]
26. Naganuma, H.; Tokumasu, K.; Okamoto, M.; Hashimoto, S.; Yamashina, S. Three-Dimensional Analysis of Morphological Aspects of the Human Saccular Macula. *Ann. Otol. Rhinol. Laryngol.* **2001**, *110*, 1017–1024. [CrossRef]
27. Rask-Andersen, H.; Schart-Morén, N.; Strömbäck, K.; Linthicum, F.; Li, H. Special Anatomic Considerations in Otosclerosis Surgery. *Otolaryngol. Clin. N. Am.* **2018**, *51*, 357–374. [CrossRef]
28. Nomura, Y. Structure of inner ear. In *Morphological Aspects of Inner Ear Disease*; Springer: Tokyo, Japan, 2014; pp. 1–22.
29. Igarashi, M. *Comparative Histological Study of the Reinforced Area of the Saccular Wall in Mammals*; NASA Order No. R-93; NASA: Washington, DC, USA, 1964.
30. Lindeman, H.H. Studies on the morphology of the sensory regions of the vestibular apparatus with 45 figures. *Ergeb. Anat. Entwicklungsgesch.* **1969**, *4*, 1–113.
31. Smith, C.M.; Curthoys, I.S.; Mukherjee, P.; Wong, C.; Laitman, J.T. Three-dimensional visualisation of the human membranous labyrinth: The membrana limitans and its role in vestibular form. *Anatomical. Record.* **2022**, *305*, 1033–1293. [CrossRef] [PubMed]
32. Pauw, B.K.; Pollak, A.M.; Fisch, U. Utricle, saccule, and cochlear duct in relation to stapedotomy. A histologic human temporal bone study. *Ann. Otol. Rhinol. Laryngol.* **1991**, *100*, 966–970. [CrossRef] [PubMed]
33. de Vilhena, D.; Gambôa, I.; Duarte, D.; Lopes, G. Vestibular Disorders after Stapedial Surgery in Patients with Otosclerosis. *Int. J. Otolaryngol.* **2016**, *2016*, 6830648. [CrossRef]
34. Shiao, A.S.; Kuo, C.L.; Cheng, H.L.; Wang, M.C.; Chu, C.H. Controversial issues of optimal surgical timing and patient selection in the treatment planning of otosclerosis. *Eur. Arch. Otorhinolaryngol.* **2014**, *271*, 1007–1014. [CrossRef]
35. Mansour, S.; Magnan, J.; Nicolas, K.; Haidar, H. Otosclerosis. In *Middle Ear Diseases*; Springer: Berlin/Heidelberg, Germany, 2018; pp. 1–83.
36. Sone, M.; Yoshida, T.; Sugimoto, S.; Morimoto, K.; Okazaki, Y.; Teranishi, M.; Naganawa, S.; Nakashima, T. Magnetic resonance imaging evaluation of endolymphatic hydrops andpost-operative findings in cases with otosclerosis. *Acta Otolaryngol.* **2017**, *137*, 242–245. [CrossRef]
37. Hayashi, H.; Cureoglu, S.; Schachern, P.A.; Oktay, M.F.; Fukushima, H.; Sone, M.; Paparella, M.M. Association between cupular deposits and otosclerosis. *Arch. Otolaryngol. Head Neck Surg.* **2006**, *132*, 1331–1334. [CrossRef]
38. Wang, S.J.; Tseng, C.C.; Young, Y.H. Selective effects of head posture on ocular vestibular-evoked myogenic potential (oVEMP) by bone-conducted vibration. *Clin. Neurophysiol.* **2014**, *125*, 612–616. [CrossRef]
39. Cozma, R.S.; Cristina, M.C.; Cobzeanu, M.D.; Olariu, R.; Bitere, O.R.; Mârțu, C.; Dima-Cozma, L.C.; Dascălu, C.G.; Georgescu, M.G.; Necula, V.; et al. Saccular function evolution related to cochlear implantation in hearing impaired children. *Rom. J. Morphol. Embryol.* **2020**, *61*, 113–119. [CrossRef] [PubMed]
40. Lin, K.Y.; Young, Y.H. Role of ocular VEMP test in assessing the occurrence of vertigo in otosclerosis patients. *Clin. Neurophysiol.* **2015**, *126*, 187–193. [CrossRef]
41. Adams, J.C. Clinical implications of inflammatory cytokines in the cochlea: A technical note. *Otol. Neurotol.* **2002**, *23*, 316–322. [CrossRef] [PubMed]
42. Kaya, S.; Paparella, M.M.; Cureoglu, S. Does Otosclerosis Affect Dark and Transitional Cells in the Human Vestibular Labyrinth? *Otol. Neurotol.* **2017**, *38*, 234–238. [CrossRef]
43. Hızlı, Ö.; Kaya, S.; Schachern, P.A.; Kwon, G.; Paparella, M.M.; Cureoglu, S. Quantitative assessment of vestibular otopathology in otosclerosis: A temporal bone study. *Laryngoscope* **2016**, *126*, E118–E122. [CrossRef] [PubMed]
44. Saka, N.; Seo, T.; Fujimori, K.; Mishiro, Y.; Sakagami, M. Vestibular-evoked myogenic potential in response to bone-conducted sound in patients with otosclerosis. *Acta Otolaryngol.* **2012**, *132*, 1155–1159. [CrossRef] [PubMed]
45. Eza-Nuñez, P.; Manrique-Rodriguez, M.; Perez-Fernandez, N. Otosclerosis among patients with dizziness. *Rev. Laryngol. Otol. Rhinol.* **2010**, *131*, 199–206. [PubMed]
46. Kumar, D.; Kumaresan, S. Pitfalls and complications of stapedectomy: A prospective study. *Int. J. Sci. Study* **2016**, *4*, 70–78.

47. Wegner, I.; Kamalski, D.M.; Tange, R.A.; Vincent, R.; Stegeman, I.; van der Heijden, G.J.; Grolman, W. Laser versus conventional fenestration in stapedotomy for otosclerosis: A systematic review. *Laryngoscope* **2014**, *124*, 1687–1693. [CrossRef]
48. Danesh, A.A.; Shahnaz, N.; Hall, J.W., 3rd. The audiology of otosclerosis. *Otolaryngol. Clin. N. Am.* **2018**, *51*, 327–342. [CrossRef]
49. Harmat, K.; Thurén, G.; Simon, L.; Nepp, N.; Nemeth, A.; Gerlinger, I.; Bako, P. Comparative evaluation of vertigo in patients after stapedotomy and stapedectomy. *Orv. Hetil.* **2017**, *158*, 1503–1511. [CrossRef] [PubMed]
50. Magliulo, G.; Gagliardi, M.; Cuiuli, G.; Celebrini, A.; Parrotto, D.; D'Amico, R. Stapedotomy and postoperative benign paroxysmal positional vertigo. *J. Vestib. Res.* **2005**, *15*, 169–172. [CrossRef] [PubMed]
51. Wang, Z.M.; Chi, F.L.; Dai, C.F. Modified stapes prosthesis to limit postoperative vertigo. *Otolaryngol. Head Neck Surg.* **2005**, *132*, 50–54. [CrossRef] [PubMed]
52. Singh, A.; Datta, R.; Prasad, B.K.; Nilakantan, A.; Rajguru, R.; Kanzhuly, M.K.; Gupta, S.K.; Singh, I. Post stapedotomy vestibular deficit: Is CO_2 laser better than conventional technique? A non-randomized controlled trial. *Indian J. Otolaryngol. Head Neck Surg.* **2018**, *70*, 306–312. [CrossRef] [PubMed]
53. Causse, J.B.; Causse, J.R.; Cezard, R.; Briand, C.; Bretlau, P.; Wiet, R.; House, J.W. Vertigo in postoperative follow-up of otosclerosis. *Am. J. Otol.* **1988**, *9*, 246–255.
54. Albera, R.; Canale, A.; Lacilla, M.; Cavalot, A.L.; Ferrero, V. Delayed vertigo after stapes surgery. *Laryngoscope* **2004**, *114*, 860–362. [CrossRef]
55. Fukuda, A.; Fujiwara, K.; Morita, S.; Hoshino, K.; Yanagi, H.; Nakamaru, Y.; Homma, A. Prognostic factors for duration of vertigo after stapes surgery via a time-to-event analysis. *Acta Otolaryngol.* **2021**, *141*, 216–221. [CrossRef]
56. Catalano, N.; Cammaroto, G.; Galletti, B.; Freni, F.; Nicita, R.A.; Azielli, C.; Galletti, F. The role of cVEMPs and vHIT in the evaluation of otosclerosis and its eventual vestibular impairment: Preliminary findings. *B-ENT* **2017**, *13* (Suppl. S27), 31–36. [PubMed]
57. Trivelli, M.; D'Ascanio, L.; Pappacena, M.; Greco, F.; Salvinelli, F. Air- and bone-conducted vestibular evoked myogenic potentials (VEMPs) in otosclerosis: Recordings before and after stapes surgery. *Acta Otorhinolaryngol. Ital.* **2010**, *30*, 5–10.
58. Akazawa, K.; Ohta, S.; Tsuzuki, K.; Sakagami, M. Bone-conducted vestibular-evoked myogenic potentials before and after stapes surgery. *Otol. Neurotol.* **2018**, *39*, 6–11 [CrossRef] [PubMed]
59. Sakamoto, T.; Kikuta, S.; Kikkawa, Y.S.; Tsutsumiuchi, K.; Kanaya, K.; Fujimaki, Y.; Ueha, R.; Saito, Y.; Yamasoba, T. Differences in postoperative hearing outcomes and vertigo in patients with otosclerosis treated with laser-assisted stapedotomy versus stapedectomy. *ORL J. Otorhinolaryngol. Relat. Spec.* **2015**, *77*, 287–293. [CrossRef] [PubMed]
60. Sando, I.; Hemenway, W.G.; Miller, D.R.; Black, F.O. Vestibular pathology in otosclerosis temporal bone histopathological report. *Laryngoscope* **1974**, *84*, 593–605. [CrossRef] [PubMed]
61. Satar, B.; Karaçaylı, C.; Çoban, V.K.; Özdemir, S. Do otosclerosis and stapedotomy affect semicircular canal functions? Preliminary results of video head impulse test. *Acta Otolaryngol.* **2021**, *141*, 348–353. [CrossRef]
62. Kujala, J.; Aalto, H.; Hirvonen, T. Video-oculography findings and vestibular symptoms on the day of stapes surgery. *Eur. Arch. Otorhinolaryngol.* **2010**, *267*, 187–190. [CrossRef]
63. Birch, L.; Elbrønd, O. Stapedectomy and vertigo. *Clin. Otolaryngol. Allied Sci.* **1985**, *10*, 217–223. [CrossRef]
64. Plaza Mayor, G.; Herraiz Puchol, C.; Martínez Rodríguez, B.; de los Santos Granados, G. Delayed vertigo after stapedotomy with good hearing results. *Anales Otorrinolaringológicos Ibero-Americanos* **2007**, *34*, 447–457.
65. Pedersen, C.B. Revision surgery in otosclerosis—An investigation of the factors which influence the hearing result. *Clin. Otolaryngol. Allied Sci.* **1996**, *21*, 385–388. [CrossRef]
66. Shea, J. LXVIII Fenestration of the Oval Window. *Ann. Otol. Rhinol. Laryngol.* **1958**, *67*, 932–951. [CrossRef]
67. Bellucci, R.J. Footplate extraction in stapedotomy. *Laryngoscope* **1978**, *88*, 701–706 [CrossRef]
68. Hall, A.C.; Mandavia, R.; Selvadurai, D. Total endoscopic stapes surgery: Systematic review and pooled analysis of audiological outcomes. *Laryngoscope* **2019**, *130*, 1282–1286. [CrossRef] [PubMed]
69. Betsch, C.; Ayache, D.; Decat, M.; Elbaz, P.; Gersdorff, M. Revision stapedectomy for otosclerosis: Report of 73 cases. *J. Otolaryngol.* **2003**, *32*, 38–47. [CrossRef]
70. Lippy, W.H.; Battista, R.A.; Berenholz, L.; Schuring, A.G.; Burkey, J.M. Twenty-year review of revision stapedectomy. *Otol. Neurotol.* **2003**, *24*, 560–566. [CrossRef]
71. Toscano, M.L.; Shermetaro, C. Stapedectomy. [Updated 2022 Aug 19]. In *StatPearls [Internet]*; StatPearls Publishing: Treasure Island, FL, USA, 2022. Available online: https://www.ncbi.nlm.nih.gov/books/NBK562205/ (accessed on 5 June 2023).
72. Derlacki, E.L. Revision stapes surgery: Problems with some solutions. *Laryngoscope* **1985**, *95 Pt 1*, 1047–1053. [CrossRef] [PubMed]
73. Nakashima, T.; Sone, M.; Fujii, H.; Teranishi, M.; Yamamoto, H.; Otake, H.; Sugiura, M.; Naganawa, S. Blood flow to the promontory in cochlear otosclerosis. *Clin. Otolaryngol.* **2006**, *31*, 110–115. [CrossRef] [PubMed]
74. Gristwood, R.E.; Venables, W.N. Otosclerotic obliteration of oval window niche: An analysis of the results of surgery. *J. Laryngol. Otol.* **1975**, *89*, 1185–1217. [CrossRef]
75. Lim, J.; Goo, W.; Kang, D.W.; Oh, S.H.; Kim, N. Effect of closing material on hearing rehabilitation in stapedectomy and stapedotomy: A finite element analysis. *Front. Neurosci.* **2023**, *17*, 1064890. [CrossRef] [PubMed]
76. Yehudai, N.; Masoud, S.; Most, T.; Luntz, M. Depth of stapes prosthesis in the vestibule: Baseline values and correlation with stapedectomy outcome. *Acta Oto-Laryngol.* **2010**, *130*, 904–908. [CrossRef]

77. Seicshnaydre, M.A.; Sismanis, A.; Hughes, G.B. Update of reparative granuloma: Survey of the American Otological Society and the American Neurotology Society. *Am. J. Otol.* **1994**, *15*, 155–160.
78. Gacek, R.R. The diagnosis and treatment of poststapedectomy granuloma. *Ann. Otol. Rhinol. Laryngol.* **1970**, *79*, 970–975. [CrossRef]
79. Tange, R.A.; Schimanski, G.; van Lange, J.W.; Grolman, W.; Zuur, L.C. Reparative Granuloma Seen in Cases of Gold Piston Implantation after Stapes Surgery for Otosclerosis. *Auris Nasus Larynx* **2002**, *29*, 7–10. [CrossRef] [PubMed]
80. Burtner, D.; Goodman, M.L. Etiological Factors in Post-Stapedectomy Granulomas. *Arch. Otolaryngol.* **1974**, *100*, 171–173. [CrossRef]
81. Kaufman, R.S.; Schuknecht, H.F. Reparative granuloma following stapedectomy: A clinical entity. *Ann. Otol. Rhinol. Laryngol.* **1967**, *76*, 1008–1017. [CrossRef] [PubMed]
82. Pauli, N.; Strömbäck, K.; Lundman, L.; Dahlin-Redfors, Y. Surgical technique in stapedotomy hearing outcome and complications. *Laryngoscope* **2020**, *130*, 790–796. [CrossRef] [PubMed]
83. Dumas, G.; Lion, A.; Karkas, A.; Perrin, P.; Perottino, F.; Schmerber, S. Skull vibration-induced nystagmus test in unilateral superior canal dehiscence and otosclerosis: A vestibular Weber test. *Acta Otolaryngol.* **2014**, *134*, 588–600. [CrossRef]
84. Ramaswamy, A.T.; Lustig, L.R. Revision surgery for otosclerosis. *Otolaryngol. Clin. N. Am.* **2018**, *51*, 463–474. [CrossRef]
85. Ishai, R.; Halpin, C.F.; McKenna, M.J.; Quesnel, A.M. How Often Does Stapedectomy for Otosclerosis Result in Endolymphatic Hydrops? *Otol. Neurotol.* **2016**, *37*, 984–990. [CrossRef]
86. Mandalà, M.; Colletti, L.; Carner, M.; Barillari, M.; Cerini, R.; Mucelli, R.P.; Colletti, V. Pneumolabyrinth and positional vertigo after stapedectomy. *Auris Nasus Larynx* **2011**, *38*, 547–550. [CrossRef]
87. Gomes, P.S.; Caselhos, S.; Vide, A.T.; Fonseca, R. Pneumolabyrinth: A rare complication of stapes surgery. *BMJ Case Rep.* **2019**, *12*, e232190. [CrossRef]
88. Liktor, B.; Szekanecz, Z.; Batta, T.J.; Sziklai, I.; Karosi, T. Perspectives of pharmacological treatment in otosclerosis. *Eur. Arch. Otorhinolaryngol.* **2013**, *270*, 793–804. [CrossRef]
89. Colletti, V.; Fiorino, F.G. Effect of sodium fluoride on early stages of otosclerosis. *Am. J. Otol.* **1991**, *12*, 195–198.
90. Brookler, K.H.; Tanyeri, H. Etidronate for the neurotologic symptoms of otosclerosis: Preliminary study. *Ear Nose Throat J.* **1997**, *76*, 371–381. [CrossRef]
91. Brookler, K. Medical treatment of otosclerosis: Rationale for use of bisphosphonates. *Int. Tinnitus. J.* **2008**, *14*, 92–96. [PubMed]
92. Gogoulos, P.P.; Sideris, G.; Nikolopoulos, T.; Sevastatou, E.K.; Korres, G.; Delides, A. Conservative Otosclerosis Treatment With Sodium Fluoride and Other Modern Formulations: A Systematic Review. *Cureus* **2023**, *15*, e34850. [CrossRef] [PubMed]
93. Hu, L.; Lind, T.; Sundqvist, A.; Jacobson, A.; Melhus, H. Retinoic acid increases proliferation of human osteoclast progenitors and inhibits RANKL-stimulated osteoclast differentiation by suppressing RANK. *PLoS ONE* **2010**, *5*, e13305. [CrossRef]
94. Arnold, W.; Kau, R.; Schwaiger, M. Clinical aspects of the osteolytic (inflammatory) phase of cochlear otosclerosis. *Laryngorhinootologie* **1999**, *78*, 20–23. [CrossRef] [PubMed]

Disclaimer/Publisher's Note: The statements, opinions and data contained in all publications are solely those of the individual author(s) and contributor(s) and not of MDPI and/or the editor(s). MDPI and/or the editor(s) disclaim responsibility for any injury to people or property resulting from any ideas, methods, instructions or products referred to in the content.

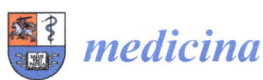

Review

Quality Standard for Rehabilitation of Young Deaf Children Receiving Cochlear Implants

Leo De Raeve [1], Marinela-Carmen Cumpăt [2,3,*], Aimée van Loo [4], Isabel Monteiro Costa [5,6], Maria Assunção Matos [5,6], João Canossa Dias [5,6], Cristian Mârțu [2,3], Bogdan Cavaleriu [2], Alois Ghergut [7], Alexandra Maftei [7], Ovidiu-Cristian Tudorean [7], Corina Butnaru [3,8], Roxana Șerban [3,8], Tatiana Meriacre [3,8] and Luminița Rădulescu [3,8]

1. Independent Information Center on CI's (ONICI), 3520 Zonhoven, Belgium; leo.de.raeve@onici.be
2. Clinical Rehabilitation Hospital, 700661 Iasi, Romania; cristimartu@gmail.com (C.M.); cavaleriu@yahoo.com (B.C.)
3. Department of Medical Specialties, University of Medicine and Pharmacy "Grigore T. Popa", 700115 Iasi, Romania; cmbutnaru@yahoo.com (C.B.); roxana_serban10@yahoo.com (R.Ș.); tatiana.meriacre.md@gmail.com (T.M.); lmradulescu@yahoo.com (L.R.)
4. Prevention Center Zuyd, Zuyd University of Applied Science, Nieuw Eyckholt 300, 6419 DJ Heerlen, The Netherlands; aimee.vanloo@zuyd.nl
5. School of Health Sciences (ESSUA), University of Aveiro, 3810-193 Aveiro, Portugal; imonteiro@ua.pt (I.M.C.); maria.matos@ua.pt (M.A.M.); joao.canossa@ua.pt (J.C.D.)
6. Center for Research in Health Technologies and Services (CINTESIS@RISE), Porto, 4200-450 Portugal
7. Faculty of Psychology and Education Sciences, Department of Education Sciences, "Alexandru Ioan Cuza" University of Iași, 11 Carol I Boulevard, 700506 Iasi, Romania; alois@uaic.ro (A.G.); psihologamaftei@gmail.com (A.M.); cristi.tudorean@gmail.com (O.-C.T.)
8. Society of Otology and Cochlear Implant (SOIC), Str. Pantelimon Halipa nr 14, 700661 Iasi, Romania
* Correspondence: marinela.cumpat@umfiasi.ro

Citation: De Raeve, L.; Cumpăt, M.-C.; van Loo, A.; Costa, I.M.; Matos, M.A.; Dias, J.C.; Mârțu, C.; Cavaleriu, B.; Ghergut, A.; Maftei, A.; et al. Quality Standard for Rehabilitation of Young Deaf Children Receiving Cochlear Implants. *Medicina* 2023, 59, 1354. https://doi.org/10.3390/medicina59071354

Academic Editor: Silviu Albu

Received: 4 June 2023
Revised: 10 July 2023
Accepted: 20 July 2023
Published: 24 July 2023

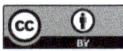

Copyright: © 2023 by the authors. Licensee MDPI, Basel, Switzerland. This article is an open access article distributed under the terms and conditions of the Creative Commons Attribution (CC BY) license (https://creativecommons.org/licenses/by/4.0/).

Abstract: *Background and objectives:* More and more children with severe-to-profound hearing loss are receiving cochlear implants (CIs) at an early age to improve their hearing and listening abilities, speech recognition, speech intelligibility, and other aspects of spoken language development. Despite this, the rehabilitation outcomes can be very heterogeneous in this population, not only because of issues related to surgery and fitting or the specific characteristics of the child with his/her additional disabilities but also because of huge differences in the quality of the support and rehabilitation offered by the therapist and the family. These quality standards for the rehabilitation of young deaf children receiving CIs are developed within the European KA202 Erasmus+ project "VOICE"—vocational education and training for speech and language therapists and parents for the rehabilitation of children with CIs, Ref. No.: 2020-1-RO01-KA202-080059. *Material and methods:* To develop these quality standards, we used the input from the face-to-face interviews of 11 local rehabilitation experts in CIs from the four partner countries of the project and the outcomes of the bibliographic analysis of 848 publications retrieved from six databases: Pub Med, Psych Info, CINAHL, Scopus, Eric, and Cochrane. Based on all this information, we created a first set of 32 quality standards over four domains: general, fitting, rehabilitation, and for professionals. Further on, the Delphi method was used by 18 international rehabilitation experts to discuss and agree on these standards. *Results:* The results from the literature analysis and the interviews show us that more than 90% of the consulted international experts agreed on 29 quality standards. They focus on different aspects of rehabilitation: the multidisciplinary team, their expertise and knowledge, important rehabilitation topics to focus on, and programming issues related to rehabilitation. *Conclusions:* These quality standards aim to optimize the activity of speech rehabilitation specialists so that they reach the optimal level of expertise. Also presented is the necessary equipment for the IC team to carry out the rehabilitation sessions in good conditions. This set of quality standards can be useful to ensure the appropriate postoperative care of these children. As a result, the rehabilitation process will be more relaxed, and therapists will have the opportunity to focus more on the specific needs of each child, with the provision of quality services, which will result in better results. This theme is particularly complex and dependent on multifactorial aspects of medicine, education, speech therapy, social work, and psychology that are very intricate and interdependent.

Keywords: cochlear implants; language therapists; speech recognition; speech intelligibility; quality standards

1. Introduction

The introduction of universal neonatal hearing screening made an earlier diagnosis of hearing loss in children possible. The benefits of early identification and intervention [1–6] are well known. Children fitted with hearing aids before the age of six months have a better outcome in terms of speech perception and speech production in the end, and they have a better chance to enter a mainstream educational setting [3,5,7].

Nowadays, more and more deaf children are receiving CIs, which results in a positive impact on their auditory perception [8,9] and language development [9–12]. These effects are even stronger in children who receive cochlear implantation early in life [10,11,13–17]. Yoshinago-Itano [3] concluded that the results of early cochlear implantation in deaf children, together with a high-quality rehabilitation program, may have similar results to those of children with mild-to-severe hearing loss wearing conventional hearing aids.

Furthermore, the WHO reports in the World Hearing Report [6] that timely intervention with cochlear implants leads to a better academic outcome and substantially improves the quality of life. In this World Hearing Report, the WHO also states that it is necessary that the rehabilitation of hearing loss is family-centered, and the approach to the deaf child is to answer to his individual and specific needs, of course, related to the resources available.

The importance of the content of the rehabilitation program and family support was also confirmed by Percy-Smith and colleagues [18], who found significant regional differences in the outcomes after CIs in Denmark. Although the cohorts that were studied and compared were matched in terms of age at implantation and hearing thresholds with CIs, the outcomes were significantly different in favor of those from East Denmark. They found that these differences arose mainly from the fact that the parents from West Denmark did not participate enough in the rehabilitation of their children and second from the fact that they used sign language to the detriment of spoken language. As a result of this study, a 3-year auditory verbal therapy (AVT) program has been set up since 2017 as part of the Danish healthcare system for children aged 0–5 years with severe bilateral hearing loss. The results of the program were significant: the majority of children acquired, after 3 years of AVT (which was less than 50%), age-equivalent spoken language, and through the process, 93% of parents were satisfied or very much satisfied with the program [19].

There are many studies on the benefits of CIs and the factors that influence the rehabilitation of these children. The factor recognized as the most important to obtain significant results is early implantation [20,21]. However, the diversity of the results obtained, even in conditions where all children are implanted early, must be considered. Children with CIs form a very diverse population with many variables to consider. Boons et al. [22] divided the predictive factors into three groups: child-related factors (aetiology, cognitive skills, and additional disabilities), auditory factors (age diagnosis, age of CI, unilateral or bilateral CI, and fitting), and environmental factors (multilingualism, communication mode, family environment, rehabilitation, and education). Rehabilitation appears as an essential factor in predicting the outcomes of these children [22–24], but it is not clear yet how to optimally involve parents and how much and what kind of support a child with one or two CIs needs.

Due to the huge differences in the service delivery models and intervention between countries, and even within the same country, between CI teams [18], we have created quality standards for the rehabilitation of children receiving CIs. The development of these standards is part of the European KA202 Erasmus+ project "VOICE", vocational education and training for speech and language therapists and parents for the rehabilitation of children with CIs, Ref. No.: 2020-1-RO01-KA202-080059. Seven partners from four European countries are involved in this project: the Clinical Rehabilitation Hospital, Iasi, Romania; the Society of Otology and Cochlear Implants (SOIC), Romania; the University Alexandru Ioan Cuza of Iasi, Romania; the EuroEd Foundation, Romania; the Independent Information Center on Cochlear Implants (ONICI), Belgium; the University de Aveiro, Portugal, and Zuyd University of Applied Sciences, the Netherlands.

The main objective of our project is to train speech and language pathologists (SLPs) and parents to teach children with CIs to understand speech and to speak. In the scope of this project, we also identified quality standards for good practice to help service providers maintain and improve their standards and quality service provision for young deaf children receiving CIs.

Rehabilitation, according to the WHO [25], represents all the actions carried out to optimize the functioning and reduce the disability of people with health conditions in their interactions with their environment. These activities are carried out by specialized health services that help people to acquire, maintain, or improve, partially or totally, skills related to communication and the activities of daily living. Rehabilitation refers to the gaining of skills, abilities, or knowledge that may have been lost or compromised as a result of illness, injury, or the acquisition of a disability [26].

2. Materials and Methods

2.1. Interview Local Experts

To develop the quality standards, the authors started by interviewing 12 local experts in rehabilitation of young CI children. Each of the 6 partners interviewed, in person or online, 2 local experts in the field of rehabilitation, resulting in 12 experts from 4 countries (Belgium, the Netherlands, Portugal, and Romania). For personal reasons, we could not make the interview with one expert from the Netherlands, so the final total number of experts was 11 (Appendix A). The method used to select the local experts was nonprobability sampling. To assure the representativeness of our sample, we only included people from our target audience (SLTs who are experienced in working with cochlear-implanted children), knowing that representativeness is much more important than the size.

To have a standardized interview across the partners, we created 8 open questions to focus on during the interview (Table S1 from Supplementary Materials):

- What is your experience in rehabilitation of young deaf children with CI's learning to speak and to develop spoken language?
- Who (what kind of professionals/parents) should be involved in the rehabilitation process after CI in young deaf children?
- What should be the role for the CI-team and what should we expect from local professionals? So, who is doing what?
- What are important domains to focus on during the rehabilitation of young CI-children?
- Should we involve the parents in the rehabilitation process? If so, Why + How + How often?
- Do you prefer a specific rehabilitation program or approach for therapy? Which resources (books, publications) do you suggest for other therapists to become an expert too?
- Do we have to monitor the listening, speech and spoken language development of these young CI-children? If so, Why and how often?
- What frequency of therapy sessions do you suggest for these young CI-children and their families? How often? For how many minutes? For how many months/years?

The content of all these interviews was analyzed and structured following the 8 open questions above. We focused especially on common answers between the local experts. All this was summarized in a report, which is available from the project website https://voice-erasmus.eu (accessed on 12 January 2023)

2.2. Standards—Bibliographic Context Analysis

The topic itself is emergent because of the recent technological history, with few professionals involved and with procedures that are not consolidated yet.

To have input from latest scientific research, we performed a review of literature on rehabilitation of young children receiving CIs. The present methodological framework is based on the Preferred Reporting Items for Systematic Reviews and Meta-Analyses (PRISMA) guidelines to ensure replicability and transparency [27].

All studies at all levels of evidence were included: best practice, case studies, prospective and retrospective studies, cross-sectional and longitudinal studies, and (non)randomized control studies (RCSs). The articles had to be published in peer-reviewed journals or books in the English language between 2000 and 31 May 2021. The articles had to focus on CI children under age of 6 with bilateral hearing loss.

2.2.1. Search Strategy

The literature search was conducted between 31 May 2021 and 31 August 2021 using a 4-word search (cochlear implant + children + rehabilitation + education) through the following 6 databases: PubMed, Eric, Cochrane, CINAHL, Scopus, and Psych Info.

Three authors (L.D.R., A.M., and T.M.) performed independent systematic title and abstract screening based on the predefined inclusion criteria. A.M. and T.M. first performed the same literature search using PubMed. Their outcomes were compared to each other (inter-reliability) and checked independently by the main author (L.D.R.). As the inter-reliability score was very high (>90%), A.M. further performed the search on Cochrane and Scopus, and T.M., together with L.D.R., performed the literature search using Eric, CINAHL, and Psych Info. Separate from the search through the 6 databases, PubMed (339), Psych info (203), CINAHL (189), Scopus (95), Eric (14), and Cochrane (8), there was also the possibility to add additional records identified through other sources (39). In total, we retrieved 848 publications.

2.2.2. Level of Evidence

A bibliographic analysis was performed after more than 150 papers were evaluated from the point of view of the level of evidence, as defined by Lebwohl and colleagues [28], i.e., in a very brief presentation: level A refers to double-blind study; level B to prospective clinical trial with more than 20 subjects; level C to clinical study with less than 20 subjects, possibly case reports, or retrospective data analyses; level D to clinical study with less than 5 subjects; and level E to brief case-by-case presentations or expert opinions.

The level of evidence from all full-text articles was scored by 5 coauthors (L.D.R., A.v.L., I.M.C., M.A.M., and C.M.). All scores were extra-checked by the main author L.D.R., and in case of a different score (which exceptionally happened), they had a short discussion to come to a final score.

2.3. Quality Standards

The development of the quality standards involved a modified Delphi consensus process that was informed by outcome of the interviews of the local experts and the extensive analysis of the literature. Based on all this information, we created a list of 32 quality standards over 4 domains related to rehabilitation: (1) general, (2) fitting, (3) rehabilitation per se, and (4) standards for professionals.

An international group of world-renowned clinical experts in the field of rehabilitation of young children with CIs and with significant experience joined a Delphi consensus panel. All 6 partners suggested 3 international experts on which they have based the rehabilitation in their center. The aim was to develop a series of quality standards for rehabilitation of children using CIs.

The Delphi method was modified to include 2 rounds of email questionnaires. In the first round, we asked the 18 international experts (Appendix B) in the field of rehabilitation to give their remarks and suggestions concerning the 32 quality standards. After adapting the quality standards, we asked the international experts in the second round to agree or not agree with each quality standard.

The proposed standards on rehabilitation of deaf children receiving CIs offer optimal level of expertise necessary for staff working in field of speech therapy and present the facilities CI teams should have. They cover different aspects of rehabilitation, such as multidisciplinary, the necessary knowledge, the domains to focus on, CI programming, and so on.

3. Results

3.1. Interview Local Experts

The group of local experts consisted of 10 speech and language pathologists and 1 otolaryngologist, with an average experience of 13 years in the field of pediatric cochlear implantation. All mentioned that the CI team should be a multidisciplinary team, which consists of an otolaryngologist, audiologist, and speech and language pathologist as a minimum. Preferably, also a psychologist, social worker, teacher of the deaf, and a physical or occupational therapist should be included in the team. Parents should be seen as equal partners too, and nearly all the experts (8/11) suggested to use a family-centered approach.

The local experts also suggested that the CI team should be the coordinator of the rehabilitation/aftercare and that there should be good liaison with the local support team. The most important domains to focus on during the rehabilitation process are audition/hearing/wearing devices; communication/speech/spoken language (11/11); parent (care) support/coaching (8/11); cognitive development (7/11); social–emotional development (6/11); reading/school performance (4/11); motor skills/planning (4/11); and self-advocacy/identity (3/11).

Auditory verbal therapy (AVT) was mentioned by 7 out of 11 experts as the approach which fits best most children and their families, but on the other hand, the same experts stated there is not one approach that fits all.

Most local experts (9/11) also mentioned that during the rehabilitation process, all steps in the development of the child should be monitored regularly, especially hearing and speech and language development. Concerning the frequency of therapy, there was huge variability between the experts, but ideally, most of the experts (6/11) suggested one session of 1 h on a weekly basis. But it was also mentioned that the frequency of rehabilitation will depend on the child, the family, the distance (although it can also take place online), and the availability of support services.

3.2. Bibliographic Analysis

In total, 848 individual publications were identified (Figure 1), but after removing the duplicates, 790 were left. In the next step, we excluded 618 records because they did not fall within the inclusion criteria: the content of 295 publications was not about rehabilitation, 214 were not about CI children with a bilateral hearing loss, 99 were not about young children (<6 years of age), and 10 were not in the English language. Therefore, we had 172 full-text articles to assess for eligibility and excluded another 22 publications based on population (15), the same study sample (6), and missing relevant information (1).

Finally, we could include 150 publications in the qualitative synthesis, and for this purpose, we only kept the 66 publications with an A or B level of evidence and excluded those that scored C, D, or E. Of these 66 publications, only 2 publications [29,30] received an A score on their level of evidence, which illustrates how weak the level of evidence is, in general, in studies related to the rehabilitation of children with CIs.

Within the field of the rehabilitation of children with CIs, it is exceptional to find research based on double-blind studies. A good level of evidence is mostly shown by publications on prospective clinical trials on more than 20 subjects, lacking adequate peer group controls or another key facet of the design.

There is still no consensus on the most appropriate methodology for approaching the rehabilitation of children with CIs [31,32]. A recent systematic review still abounds in the same direction. Fitzpatrick and colleagues [32], Kaipa and Danser [33], and Demers and Bergeron [24] showed that more data are needed to decide on rehabilitation methodology. Most articles present a relatively low level of evidence. Therefore, there are not enough elements to rely on in choosing the approach for children receiving CIs, at least as far as we know.

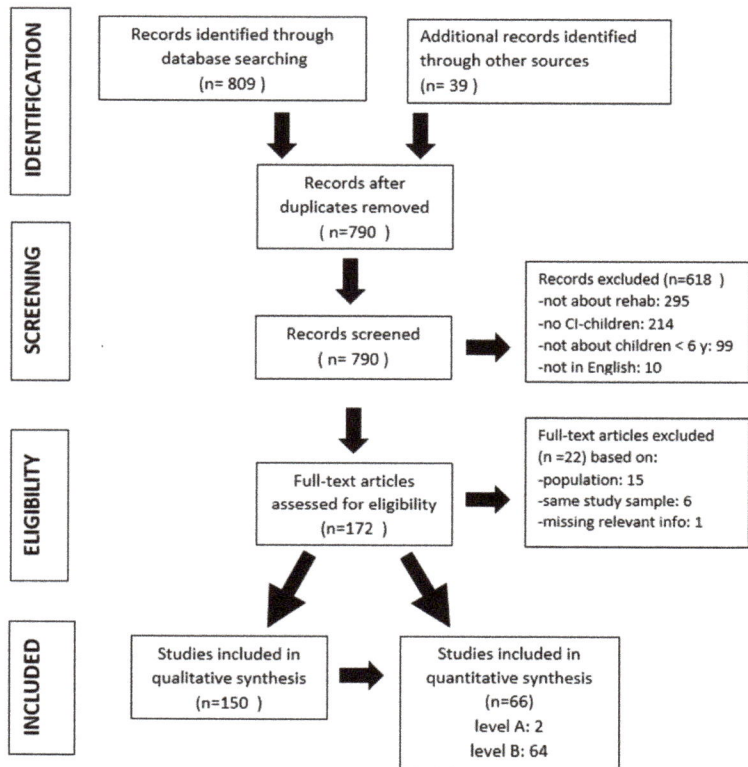

Figure 1. Flowchart of reviewed papers with exclusion and inclusion criteria.

3.3. Quality Standards

Based on the comments of the international experts during the first round, especially focusing on the overlap between some quality standards, we updated the quality standards and came to a new list of 29 quality standards. During the second round, we asked the same international experts to agree or not agree on the proposed standards. Finally, more than 90% of the international experts agreed on 29 quality standards over four domains: (1) general standards, (2) fitting, (3) rehabilitation, and (4) quality standards for staff, of which most of them contain several subcategories.

These standards for the rehabilitation of children with CIs can help health systems and, more specifically, CI teams and all those involved in the rehabilitation of children with CIs, to provide quality and State-of-the-Art care. We are absolutely convinced that by using these standards, they will improve the quality of their service delivery, and the result will be rehabilitation with better results.

4. Quality Standard for Rehabilitation of Young Children Receiving CIs (Table S2 from Supplementary Materials)

4.1. General Quality Standards for Pediatric Cochlear Implantation in Relation to Rehabilitation

- Providing a Child with a Cochlear Implant Requires a Dedicated Multi-Disciplinary Team Consisting at Minimum of an Otolaryngologist, Audiologist and a SLT Specialist
    - Ideally there should also be a psychologist and social worker included in the team.
    - The multidisciplinary team should work inter professionally (not next to each other but together) and in close cooperation with the parents/carers.
    - The multidisciplinary team will liaise and work with the child's local support team.
- The CI-Team of the Hospital Should Coordinate the Selection, Surgery, Fitting, Rehabilitation and after Care (Equipment Maintenance, Spare Materials)
- Parents/Educators/Professionals Need Balanced and Unbiased Up-to-Date Information about CI's and the Fitting/Rehabilitation Process
    - Ideally in their language.
    - Parents/educators/professionals should get appropriate counselling from the CI team and other professionals to have appropriate expectations from the cochlear implant, depending on several variables such as age at implantation or additional disabilities.
    - Parents/educators/professionals should have the opportunity to meet other families with CI children.
    - Parents/educators/professionals also need psychological support: taking care of their emotions and stress.
- Rehabilitation should Be Delivered by the CI-Team in Close Cooperation with A Local Expert (Team) in Listening and Spoken Language Development. (See Quality Standard # 29)
- Rehabilitation Is Not Possible without Parent/Family/Caregiver Involvement
    - In case of parents or legal guardians are not able to be actively engaged in the child's rehabilitation due to very low Social Economical Status, mental health matters, or cognitive delays, other family members or carers should be involved.
    - Professionals should use a child/family cantered approach.
- The Cochlear Implant Surgery Should Take Place as Soon as a Child Is Identified as a Candidate and Should Ideally Be Done by the Age of 12 Months or Sooner, Preferably under the Age of 36 Months, without Excluding Those Older Than 37 Months
- A Child with Bilateral Deafness Should Be Fitted Bilaterally with CI's, Preferably before the Age of 18 Months
    - We expect all countries to follow the principles and guidelines of the Joint Committee on Infant Hearing to have early hearing screening (before age 1 month), diagnosis (before 3 months) and start with rehabilitation (fitting hearing aids and early intervention) before 6 months of age.
- The CI-Team will Issue or Dispatch Replacements for Faulty External Equipment within Two Working Days
    - There should be a written policy regarding who is responsible in the event of loss/damage and what spares can be provided as a matter of routine.
- Each Child's Sound Processor Must Be up Graded Every 5 Years
- The National CI Program should Conduct and Publish Annual Audits and Comply with the Requirements of the Responsible National Authorities. Audits should Cover All Aspects Related to CI: Clinical Activity, Staff Expertise, Child Outcomes, Surgical Complications, Device Failures, and Child and Family/Caregiver Feedback on the Service Provided
    - The audits should become freely available to interested parties.

4.2. Quality Standards on Fitting/Programming in Relation to Rehabilitation

- The Fitting of the Sound Processor should Be Carried out by Qualified Paediatric Audiologist Preferably in Clinic, Face-to-Face Rather Than Remotely
- There should Be a Liaison between the Audiologist of the CI-Team and the Local Rehabilitation Expert/Local Support Team (and Vice Versa) to Exchange Information about the Progress of the Child's Auditory Skills
    - It is recommended that local professionals receives writen reports on the child's auditory function
    - It is recommended that local professionals received written reports on the child's auditory performance.
- Instructions on the Use of the Sound Processor Must Be Given to the Parent/Caregiver on or before the Day of Activation and should Be Repeated at Least Twice within the Six Months Following Activation
    - This is within the role of the audiologist and the rehabilitation therapist.
    - Supporting materials on the handling, operating and care of the sound processor should be issued to the parent/carer.
    - The recommended use of assistive listening accessories (e.g.,: AudioStream, Mini mic, Roger) should be explained to the parent/carer by the CI team (see Quality standard # 1) before the CI surgery and the information reviewed after the activation.
- Appropriate Audiological, Standardized Speech Perception Tests and Functional Hearing Assessment (by Family/Other Professionals' Questionnaire) should Be Performed at 6 Months Intervals to Enable Hearing to Be Monitored
    - It is recommended to assess speech perception with standardized tests and a functional hearing questionnaire. Ideally: every 6 months in the first 2 years after the cochlear implant activation and then every year minimum of once a year.
    - Measuring speech perception of soft speech and speech in noise should begin after two years of CI use.
    - The results should be shared with the child's parents/educators and local professionals.

4.3. Quality Standards on Rehabilitation of Young Children Receiving CI's

- Rehabilitation should Begin before Implantation and at the Latest Immediately after Initial Fitting, According to the Individual Needs of the Child
    - Even if rehabilitation does not start until initial fitting, written material about the content of rehabilitation should be shared with the parent/carer well before initial fitting, so that they have a good idea of what is needed to promote an appropriate child's listening and spoken language development.
- Parents/Educators/Professionals Are Considered and Valued as Equal Partners in the Rehabilitation Process of Their Child
    - Parents/educators/professionals must have equal access to information on CI in their preferred language.
    - CI companies should make their brochures available in the preferred language of the parents/caregivers.
- Appropriate Measures should Be Performed Yearly (Ideally Every 6 Months) to Monitor Progress in Language, Communicational and Educational Outcomes the First 3 Years after Implantation
    - Standardized assessments for typical hearing children should be used for comparisons.
    - Additional rehabilitation and/or referrals should take place where progress is slower than expected.

- A Diagnostic Coaching Approach to CI Rehabilitation Yields the Most Efficient and Best Benefit, Both to Children and to Parents/Educators/Professionals
  - Additional needs should be identified as soon as possible, so rehabilitation and expectations can be adapted to the special needs. Additional specialists in other fields can be incorporated into the team to share their expertise.
- The Audiologist and Speech and Language Therapist Together with the Parents should Decide on the Frequency of Specialist Contact Sessions for Fitting and for Rehabilitation Based on the Individual Needs of the Child and Their Family
- As the Recommended Approach of Services Is Family-Centered, It Is Understood That Rehabilitation Therapy Sessions can Take Place Weekly or Fortnightly, Considering That Most Listening and Spoken Language Experience Will Occur at Home between the Sessions
- Children with CI's should have Annually the Opportunity to Trial and Assess Assistive Listening Devices (FM-Systems, Bluetooth Accessories)
- Rehabilitation of Young CI-Children should Involve Collaboration between the CI Centre, Local Professionals, and Parents/Educators to Cover the Following Areas:
  - Listening skills/functional listening/speech perception.
  - Speech intelligibility, voice quality and prosody.
  - Communication skills including repair strategies.
  - All aspects of language development.
  - Theory of Mind development.
  - Ability to troubleshoot and maintain external equipment.
  - Using assistive listening devices.
  - Music.
  - Literacy (reading).
  - Cognitive skills (Executive Functions).
  - Mainstream education (inclusion).
  - Advocacy.
- It Is Recommended That All Children to Receive, Based on Their Need, Listening and Spoken Language Therapy after Implantation, Even Those Who Benefit Little from CI and Who Are Anticipated to Still Be Sign Reliant
  - Among all auditory-based early intervention approaches for children receiving CI, evidence-based practice has proven that an approach focusing on listening and spoken language has the most impact on the child's speech perception skills and expressive spoken language development.
  - The decision to add signed support or sign language in the rehabilitation therapy will be discussed among parents and professionals so parents can make an informed decision.
- Rehabilitation Therapists and Parents/Educators will Collaboratively Generate Measurable and Appropriate Goals in All Areas of the Child's Development (Auditory, Receptive, and Expressive Language, Speech, Cognition, and Social Skills), and Identify Ways to Integrate the Goals and Strategies to Achieve them in a Nurturing and Rich Language
- Music should Be Integrated in the Rehabilitation of Young Children Using CI's, Particularly as a Home-Based Fun Activity Rather Than in a Formal Setting

4.4. Quality Standards for Professionals in Relation to Rehabilitation

- Every Country should Have Training Opportunities for Professionals in the Various Communication Approaches (From Auditory Verbal to Sign Bilingualism) to Become An Expert in the Field of Rehabilitation and Education of CI-Children
- The Staff of the CI Team in the Hospital and Local Rehabilitation Therapists should Have the Knowledge and Expertise That Enables Them to Work Effectively with Children Wearing CI's, Including Those with Additional Needs Than Their Hearing Loss

- Some very complex children may need a very specialized service.
- Rehabilitation of Young CI-Children should Be Carried out by An Expert in Promoting Listening, Speech and Spoken Language Development, in Managing the Technology and the Environment
  - The therapist should also have expertise in coaching and counselling parents.
  - The therapist should also have expertise in a family-centered approach.
- The Expertise of the Rehabilitation Therapist/Rehabilitation Team should Include the Following Skills:
  - Expertise and skills working with infants and very young children (for pediatric services).
  - Expertise in auditory development and listening skills.
  - Knowledge on how to manage the technology.
  - Knowledge on how to manage the acoustics of the environment and on how to address challenging listening situations (e.g., assistive listening devices).
  - Gain insight into the impact of hearing loss on a child's overall development (eg mental health, language, speech, cognition, social and literacy) and how to support these skills.
  - Knowledge of communication support teams, i.e., speech to text or sign language interpreters.
  - Knowledge of audiology and assistive listening technology.
  - To get to know the culture and language of the deaf community.
  - Knowledge on how to coach/guide families.
  - Knowledge on inclusion of a CI-child (in education and in the local environment).

These standards for the rehabilitation of deaf children receiving CIs can be downloaded as a pdf file from the project website https://voice-erasmus.eu (accessed on 12 January 2023)

5. Discussion

Over the past two decades, there has been a great deal of research into the benefits of CIs and the search for the best way to support young CI children and their families. It is important to note that the overall level of evidence in the studies included in our literature analysis is low. Only two studies had a high level of evidence. Therefore, the level of available evidence does not seem to be sufficient to support the existence of differences in auditory and speech and language development between different rehabilitation approaches. This observation is consistent with the findings of recent systematic reviews, which concluded that more data are needed to be able to guide professionals and parents in their decision-making process [24,32,33].

The studies selected for the bibliographic analysis present some methodological limitations with the impact of the level of evidence. Due to the methodological design used in most studies, it is difficult to identify the rehabilitation factor and state that the approach led to an observed difference between groups.

Meanwhile, good prospective clinical trials with 20 or more subjects focusing on variables that predict good outcomes are needed. Ideally, but difficult from an ethical point of view, longitudinal prospective studies are needed, which include many subjects and a control group, in order to find the best rehabilitation techniques for the desired results. Parameters, such as the frequency and duration of the sessions, the content of the rehabilitation sessions, different neurobiological processes, sequential vs. simultaneous cochlear implantation, monaural versus binaural implantation, and various materials and listening conditions, must be evaluated.

There is an urgent need for quality standards on the rehabilitation of young children receiving CIs. To our knowledge, this is the first international consensus study to be published on quality standards for the rehabilitation of young CI children. Twenty-nine quality standards were developed and endorsed by the Delphi consensus panel. These quality standards will function best with an experienced team with knowledge and expertise in early implantation, fitting, rehabilitation, parent coaching, monitoring children, and the maintenance of the device and aftercare.

In addition, there is the challenge of ensuring the appropriate rehabilitation methods for each child with their individual needs. The results of recent and future neuroscience research on developmental critical periods, synaptic plasticity, auditory cortex changes after cochlear implantation, and auditory processing will help to better design the rehabilitation procedures after implantation. Better evaluations of therapy methods, applying the new developed tests that assess the progress of the implanted child (e.g., voice quality measurements when the test is standardized and available for all SLTs) as well as an increased availability of auditory support programs might help to deliver them more readily and widely in a variety of languages. These challenges reside amongst all professionals and parents dealing with implanted children on a daily basis.

The most discussed topics during our Delphi consensus panel were those related to standards of rehabilitation per se. For instance, one standard that was removed after heated debates was that "The paediatric CI may be only carried out if the parents are able to take responsibility for the child's rehabilitation". At a certain point, the standard became "Paediatric CI may be only carried out if there is rehabilitation available after CI", and finally, the standard was eliminated. Another standard that incited discussions was related to the recommendation to use sign language by the SLTs during the rehabilitation sessions. The majority of experts emphasized that "Rehabilitation approach that do not include signs language appear more frequent associated with a better auditory speech and language development". But there were voices who said that "For some children a signed supported approach to CI therapy yields the most benefit, both for children, parents and teacher". The standard was eliminated by itself but has been added to Standard 4.3.9. as a possible support method. The last eliminated standard was a reference to the "continuously diagnostic coaching approach to CI therapy yields the most benefit, both for children and to parents and teachers"; the idea of closely monitoring the progress of children has already been mentioned in Standard 4.3.3.

But there were some interesting talks related to some other standards; for instance, the reference to the frequency and quality of the therapy gave rise to numerous comments: "the frequency...of sessions for rehabilitation must be based on the individual need of the child", "it also depends on the needs of the local service professionals", "it is not frequency or the number of hours important but the quality of the therapy", "I think that it can depend on the number and the level of expertise of the local service professionals than on their (child's) needs", "I think both frequency and quality of the therapy are very important after paediatric CI", and so on. The result of this topic is illustrated by Standards 4.3.5. and 4.3.6.

A strength of this study on the quality standards for the rehabilitation of deaf children is that they were developed based on good practice from local experts, the evidence identified in a robust analysis of the medical literature on the topic of rehabilitation, and the expert opinion of an international Delphi consensus panel with experience in the rehabilitation of young children receiving CIs. This approach is in line with the American Academy of Otolaryngology–Head and Neck Surgery Foundation methods [34] for the development of clinical consensus statements, resulting in evidence-based consensus statements that are in line with clinical experience.

A limitation of the study is the minimal representation of Asia, Africa, and South America on the Delphi consensus panel and the preponderance of local experts from one country (Romania). However, the presence of two international experts from a Spanish speaking country and the fact that in most American Latin countries, the official language is Spanish, we expect that the standards may apply there too. The same applies for Afrikaans, a language that has its origin in German and Dutch languages, as long as we have international experts from Germany and Holland. We cannot tell if the consensus is true for SLTs from Asia, but we expect it is.

Another limit lies in the diversity of tests used to quantify the auditory and speech and language outcomes, which makes it difficult to compare results directly from the included studies. Furthermore, most studies did not clearly define the approach used or the intervention setting (frequency, length, and duration) that children were involved in.

Future research should try to avoid these limitations to bring more robust data to the field of rehabilitation. As many studies were based on retrospective data or cross-sectional designs, an important element that should be considered by future researchers is using a study design that has fewer methodological limits. Focusing on prospective and longitudinal data and using a bigger sample size would allow better control of the studied variables, enhance the level of evidence, and allow researchers to match the groups on key variables to reduce their influence on the results.

6. Conclusions

To develop quality standards for the rehabilitation of deaf children receiving CIs, we used the input from the interviews of 11 local rehabilitation experts on CIs from the four partner countries involved in the VOICE project and the outcome of the analysis of 848 publications related to the theme and retrieved from six databases. The Delphi method approach was used by 18 international rehabilitation specialists in CI intervention to discuss and agree on these quality standards. Finally, >90% of the international experts agreed on 29 quality standards, of which most of them contain some subcategories.

Further research is needed to address the issue of the rehabilitation of young deaf children receiving CIs. Studies involving larger samples, matched groups, and well-controlled interventions are essential to isolate the intervention factor and be able to generalize findings.

Meanwhile, we have to focus on good practice which takes into consideration the specific needs of the child, their family, and the contact they are evolving in [23].

We believe that the guidelines for good practices presented here can act as a lever for the necessary studies, as they already indicate the conceptual field where future studies should take place and, therefore, help in the creation of evidence-informed approaches.

Supplementary Materials: The following supporting information can be downloaded at: https://www.mdpi.com/article/10.3390/medicina59071354/s1. Table S1: Content of the standardized interview; Table S2: Quality standard for rehabilitation of young children receiving CI's. Supplementary_Final list of publications scored on level of evidence A and B.

Author Contributions: Conceptualization, L.D.R. and A.M.; methodology, C.M.; software, O.-C.T.; validation, A.v.L., L.R., and I.M.C.; formal analysis, M.A.M.; investigation, C.B. and R.Ș.; resources, B.C. and A.G.; data curation, J.C.D. and T.M. writing—original draft preparation, L.D.R.; writing—review and editing, M.-C.C.; visualization, L.R.; supervision, L.D.R. and L.R.; project administration, L.R.; funding acquisition, M.-C.C. All authors have read and agreed to the published version of the manuscript.

Funding: This research was funded by the National Agency for Community Programs in the Field of Education and Vocational Training, grant number 2020-1-RO01-KA202-080059.

Institutional Review Board Statement: Not applicable.

Informed Consent Statement: Not applicable.

Data Availability Statement: Not applicable.

Conflicts of Interest: The authors declare no conflict of interest. The funders had no role in the design of the study; in the collection, analyses, or interpretation of data; in the writing of the manuscript; or in the decision to publish the results.

Appendix A

Local experts: Martine de Smit (Belgium); Marlies Oyen (Belgium); Kirsten Gennotte (the Netherlands); Pedro Brás da Silva (Portugal); João Eloi Moura (Portugal); Camelia

Oana Radu (Romania); Ady Cristian Mihailov (Romania); Crăescu Adina (Romania); Elena Macovei (Romania); Mariana Pop (Romania); Theodor Sirbuletu (Romania)

Appendix B

International experts: Cheryl Dickson (Australia); Diana Zegg (Austria); Mila de Melo (Canada); Uwe Martin (Germany); Shirly Kaplan (Israel); Anneke Vermeulen (the Netherlands); Camelia Rusu (Romania); Mihaela Alexandru (Romania); Gal Katalina (Romania); Ion Mihaela (Romania); Theodor Sirbuletu (Romania); Mariana Pop (Romania); Luciana Frumos (Romania); Louise Ashton (South Africa); Manuel Manrique (Spain); Teresa Amat (Spain); Tricia Kemp (UK); Mihaela Fotescu Zamfir (UK).

References

1. Moeller, M.P. Early intervention and language development in children who are deaf and hard of hearing. *Pediatrics* **2000**, *106*, E43. [CrossRef] [PubMed]
2. Yoshinaga-Itano, C.; Sedey, A. Language, Speech and Social–Emotional Development of Children Who are Deaf or Hard of Hearing: The Early Years. *Volta Rev.* **2000**, *100*, 286–295.
3. Yoshinago-Itano, C. Early Identification, Communication Modality, and the Development of Speech an Spoken Language: Patterns and Considerations. In *Advances in the Spoken Language Development of Deaf and Hard-of-Hearing Children*; Spencer, P., Marschark, M., Eds.; Oxford University Press: New York, NJ, USA, 2006; pp. 298–327.
4. Watkin, P.; McCann, D.; Law, C.; Mullee, M.; Petrou, S.; Stevenso, J.; Worsfold, S.; Yuen, H.M.; Kennedy, C. Language ability in children with permanent hearing impairment: The influence of early management and family participation. *Pediatrics* **2007**, *120*, e694–e701. [CrossRef] [PubMed]
5. Verhaert, N.; Willems, M.; Van Kerschaver, E.; Desloovere, C. Impact of early hearing screening and treatment on language development and education level: Evaluation of 6 years of universal newborn hearing screening (ALGO) in Flanders, Belgium. *Int. J. Pediatr. Otorhinolaryngol.* **2008**, *72*, 599–608. [CrossRef] [PubMed]
6. World Health Organization. *World Report on Hearing*; Licence: CC, BY-NC-SA 3.0 IGO: Geneva, Switzerland, 2021.
7. De Raeve, L. Auditory Rehabilitation Therapy Guidelines for optimizing the benefits of Binaural Hearing, a Cochlear white paper. *Basel Cochlear Eur.* **2008**, 1–8.
8. Kirk, K.; Miyamoto, R.; Ying, E.; Perdew, A.; Zuganelis, H. Cochlear Implantation in Young Children: Effect of Age of Implantation and Communication Mode. *Volta Rev.* **2000**, *102*, 127–144.
9. De Raeve, L. A longitudinal study on auditory perception and speech intelligibility in deaf children implanted under the age of 18 months, in comparison to those implanted at later ages. *Otol. Neurotol.* **2010**, *31*, 1261–1267. [CrossRef]
10. Svirsky, M.A.; Teoh, S.W.; Neuburger, H. Development of language and speech perception in congenitally, profoundly deaf children as a function of age at cochlear implantation. *Audiol. Neurootol.* **2004**, *9*, 224–233. [CrossRef]
11. Schauwers, K.; Gillis, S.; Govaerts, P. Language acquisition in child-ren with a cochlear implant. In *Trends in Language Acquisition Research 4: Developmental Theory and Language Disorders*; Fletcher, P., Miller, J., Eds.; John Benjamins Press: Amsterdam, The Netherlands, 2005; pp. 324–329.
12. Vermeulen, A.; van Bon, W.; Schreuder, R.; Knoors, H.; Snik, A. Reading skills of deaf children with CI's. *J. Deaf. Stud. Deaf. Educ.* **2007**, *12*, 283–302. [CrossRef]
13. Anderson, I.; Weichbold, V.; D'Haese, P.; Szuchnik, J.; Quevedo, M.; Martin, J.; Dieler, W.S.; Phillips, L. Cochlear implantation in children under the age of two—What do the outcomes show us? *Int. J. Pediatr. Otorhinolaryngol.* **2004**, *68*, 425–431. [CrossRef]
14. Miyamoto, R.T.; Houston, D.M.; Kirk, K.I.; Perdew, A.E.; Svirsky, M.A. Language development in deaf infants following cochlear implantation. *Acta Otolaryngol.* **2003**, *123*, 241–244. [CrossRef]
15. Spencer, L.; Barker, B.; Tomblin, J. Exploring the language and literacy outcomes of pediatric cochlear implant users. *Ear Hear.* **2003**, *24*, 236–247. [CrossRef]
16. Tomblin, J.; Barker, B.; Hubbs, S. Developmental constraints on language development in children with CI's. *Int. J. Audiol.* **2007**, *46*, 512–523. [CrossRef]
17. Zwolan, T.A.; Ashbaugh, C.M.; Alarfaj, A.; Kileny, P.R.; Arts, H.A.; El-Kashlan, H.K.; Telian, S.A. Pediatric cochlear implant patient performance as a function of age at implantation. *Otol. Neurotol.* **2004**, *25*, 112–120. [CrossRef]
18. Percy-Smith, L.; Busch, G.W.; Sandahl, M.; Nissen, L.; Josvassen, J.L.; Bille, M.; Lange, T.; Cayé-Thomasen, P. Significant regional differences in Denmark in outcome after cochlear implants in children. *Dan. Med. J.* **2012**, *59*, A4435.
19. Dyrberg, S. The Auditory Verbal Therapy (AVT) program—Evaluation of the 3-year AVT-program 2017–2021. *EURO-CIU Newsl.* **2022**, 11–12. Available online: https://decibel.dk/files/media/document/Final2_Evalrapport_V.3.2_CalibriLight%20copy.pdf (accessed on 25 February 2023).
20. Dettman, S.; Pinder, D.; Briggs, R.; Dowell, R.; Leigh, J. Communication development in children who receive the cochlear implant younger than 12 months: Risks versus benefits. *Ear Hear.* **2007**, *28*, 11S–18S. [CrossRef]
21. Archbold, S.; Mayer, C. Deaf Education: The impact of cochlear implantation. *Deaf. Educ. Int.* **2012**, *14*, 2–15. [CrossRef]

22. Boons, T.; Brokx, J.P.; Frijns, J.H.; Peeraer, L.; Philips, B.; Vermeulen, A.; Wouters, J.; van Wieringen, A. Effect of pediatric bilateral cochlear implantation on language development. *Arch. Pediatr. Adolesc. Med.* **2012**, *166*, 28–34. [CrossRef]
23. Joint Committee on Infant Hearing. Position Statement: Principles and Guidelines for Early Hearing Detection and Intervention Programs. *J. Early Hear. Detect. Interv.* **2019**, *4*, 1–44.
24. Demers, D.; Bergeron, F. Effectiveness of rehabilitation approaches proposed to children with severe-to-profound prelinguistic deafness on the development of auditory, speech and language skills: A systematic review. *J. Speech Lang. Hear. Res.* **2019**, *62*, 4196–4230. [CrossRef]
25. World Health Organization. 2023. Available online: https://www.who.int/news-room/fact-sheets/detail/rehabilitation. (accessed on 17 February 2023).
26. New York State Speech, Language and Hearing Association. 2012, adapted from Fed. Reg. 52530; NAIC Glossary of Health Insurance and Medical Terms: 3. Available online: https://content.naic.org/sites/default/files/inline-files/committees_b_consumer_information_ppaca_glossary.pdf (accessed on 20 February 2023).
27. Moher, D.; Liberati, A.; Tetzlaff, J.; Altman, D.G.; PRISMA Group. Preferred reporting items for systematic reviews and meta-analyses: The PRISMA statement. *PLoS Med.* **2009**, *6*, e1000097. [CrossRef] [PubMed]
28. Lebwohl, M.; Heymann, W.R.; Berth-Jones, J.; Coulson, I. *Treatment of Skin Disease—Comprehensive Therapeutic Strategies*, 3rd ed.; Saunders-Elsevier: New York, NY, USA, 2010.
29. Monshizadeh, L.; Vameghi, R.; Rahimi, M.; Sajedi, F.; Yadegari, F.; Hashemi, S.B. The effectiveness of a specifically-designed language intervention protocol on the cochlear implanted children's communication development. *Int. J. Pediatr. Otorhinolaryngol.* **2019**, *126*, 109631. [CrossRef]
30. Qiao, X.F.; Ren, Q.; Li, X.; Li, T.L.; Mariano, R.S. Analysis of subjective perception and influencing factors of different inclusive education models among prelingually deaf children with a cochlear implant. *J. Int. Med. Res.* **2020**, *48*, 300060520929855. [CrossRef]
31. Hyde, M.L. Newborn hearing screening programs: Overview. *J. Otolaryngol.* **2005**, *34*, S70–S78.
32. Fitzpatrick, E.M.; Hamel, C.; Stevens, A.; Pratt, M.; Moher, D.; Doucet, S.P.; Na, E. Sign language and spoken language for children with hearing loss: A systematic review. *Pediatrics* **2016**, *137*, e20151974. [CrossRef]
33. Kaipa, R.; Danser, M.L. Efficacy of auditory–verbal therapy in children with hearing impairment: A systematic review from 1993 to 2015. *Int. J. Pediatr. Otorhinolaryngol.* **2016**, *86*, 124–134. [CrossRef]
34. Rosenfeld, R.M.; Nnacheta, L.C.; Corrigan, M.D. Clinical Consensus Statement Development Manual. *Otolaryngol. Head Neck Surg.* **2015**, *153*, S1–S14. [CrossRef]

Disclaimer/Publisher's Note: The statements, opinions and data contained in all publications are solely those of the individual author(s) and contributor(s) and not of MDPI and/or the editor(s). MDPI and/or the editor(s) disclaim responsibility for any injury to people or property resulting from any ideas, methods, instructions or products referred to in the content.

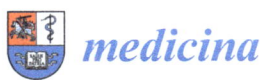

Review

Postoperative Outcomes of Endoscopic versus Microscopic Myringoplasty in Patients with Chronic Otitis Media—A Systematic Review

Iemima Stefan [1,2], Cristian Dragos Stefanescu [2,3,*], Ana Maria Vlad [2,3], Viorel Zainea [2,3] and Răzvan Hainarosie [2,3]

1. Medical Center of Special Telecommunications Service, 060044 Bucharest, Romania
2. ENT Department, Faculty of Medicine, "Carol Davila" University of Medicine and Pharmacy, 030167 Bucharest, Romania
3. "Prof. Dr. Dorin Hociota" Institute of Phonoaudiology and Functional ENT Surgery, 21st Mihail Cioranu Street, 061344 Bucharest, Romania
* Correspondence: dragos.stefanescu@umfcd.ro; Tel.: +40-730-047-455

Abstract: Endoscopes are increasingly being used in middle ear surgery as an adjunct to or replacement for the operative microscope. The superior visualization of hidden areas and a minimally invasive transcanal approach to the pathology are some of the endoscope's advantages. The aim of this review is to compare the surgical outcomes of a totally endoscopic transcanal approach with a conventional microscopic approach for type 1 tympanoplasty in patients with chronic otitis media (COM) in order to establish if endoscopic myringoplasty (EM) could be a better alternative to microscopic myringoplasty (MM). A literature review was performed using the Preferred Reporting Items for Systematic Reviews and Meta-Analysis recommendations. The selected articles were identified by searching PubMed Central, PubMed, MEDLINE and Embase databases for the relevant publications. Only studies where the same surgeon in the department performed both endoscopic and microscopic myringoplasty have been included in the review. The results suggest that with an endoscopic approach, minimally invasive myringoplasty can be achieved with a similar graft success rate and postoperative air–bone gap (ABG) improvement, a shorter operative time and less postoperative complications compared to a microscopic approach.

Keywords: endoscopic; microscopic; myringoplasty; chronic otitis media; review

1. Introduction

Chronic otitis media (COM) is a complex multifactorial inflammatory and infectious condition that is mainly characterized by middle ear mucosal inflammation with permanent tympanic membrane perforation and, in some cases, fixation or interruption of the ossicular chain.

The main objectives in treating chronic otitis media are to repair the tympanic membrane perforation, eradicate chronic infection and, if necessary, restore the integrity and mobility of the ossicular chain.

Microscopic myringoplasty (MM) has been the standard surgery for repairing perforated tympanic membranes since the 1950s, but since the late 1990s, endoscopic myringoplasty (EM) has been increasingly practiced.

The *MM approach* offers binocular vision along with an excellent stereoscopic surgical view and leaves both surgeons' hands free, but it is limited by the straight-line vision that makes the visualization of the middle ear through the ear canal relatively difficult [1]. Therefore, conventional MM is originally performed using a postauricular incision, with or without drilling of the bony ear canal, in order to obtain adequate visualization and illumination [2]. A postauricular incision may produce surgical scarring, temporary loss of cutaneous sensation [3] and malposition of the ear.

The *EM approach* has several advantages when compared to the conventional postauricular MM: it avoids unnecessary incisions and soft tissue dissections, ensures easy access to hidden areas, eliminates the potential need for canalplasty, provides a shorter operative time and has lower complication rates [4–7].

In the last years, there have been several comparative studies published regarding the efficacy of the two operative approaches [2,5,8–12], but few systematic reviews regarding the comparison between endoscopic and microscopic tympanoplasty [13].

Therefore, we decided to perform a systematic review to compare the postoperative outcomes of the totally endoscopic transcanal approach with a conventional microscopic approach for myringoplasty in patients with COM in order to analyze if the endoscopic approach can provide at least the same results as the microscopic approach or even better outcomes in terms of graft success rates, hearing improvement, operative time and postoperative complications, and to establish if EM could be a better alternative to MM.

2. Materials and Methods

This systematic review was conducted in accordance with the Preferred Reporting Items for Systematic Reviews and Meta-Analyses (PRISMA) guidelines [14]. No ethical approval was required as previously published studies were analyzed. The PICO framework was used to develop the specific research question:

1. Population: patients with chronic otitis media
2. Intervention: myringoplasty
3. Comparison: an endoscopic versus a microscopic approach
4. Outcome: graft success rate, air–bone gap (ABG) improvement, operative time, postoperative complications

2.1. Search Strategy

Two of the authors independently searched the PubMed Central, PubMed, MEDLINE and Embase databases for relevant publications on 8 March 2023. We searched for all available studies reporting comparisons between endoscopic type 1 tympanoplasty or myringoplasty and microscopic type 1 tympanoplasty or myringoplasty in patients with chronic otitis media. The following keywords were used for searching through the PubMed Central database: "((((endoscopic) AND microscopic)) AND (((myringoplasty) OR tympanoplasty) OR type 1 tympanoplasty)) AND ((chronic otitis media) OR COM)".

2.2. Selection of Studies

Only full-text English studies were selected, with no restriction regarding the date of publication. All duplicates were manually removed before the study titles and abstracts were screened. Lastly, the remaining studies had their full texts reviewed. The full texts of eligible articles were subsequently evaluated based on the inclusion and exclusion criteria (Figure 1).

The inclusion criteria consisted of: (1) patients with chronic suppurative otitis media with inactive disease and an intact ossicular chain; (2) studies comparing endoscopic with microscopic myringoplasty; (3) studies where the same surgeon carried out both endoscopic and microscopic myringoplasty; (4) studies providing outcome measures such as graft success rate, audiometric outcomes, or duration of surgery in both the endoscopic and microscopic groups.

The following exclusion criteria were applied: (1) studies including patients with cholesteatoma, ossicular chain disorders, adhesive/atelectatic otitis media, active/granulative COM; (2) studies performing simultaneous otologic procedures in addition to myringoplasty (e.g., ossicular chain reconstruction, mastoidectomy); (3) studies with non-available English full-text, duplicate publications, publications where original articles were inaccessible (e.g., only abstracts were available) and/or incomplete data were provided; (4) animal studies, in vitro studies; (5) review articles, case reports; (6) studies with only one approach assessed (only EM or only MM) or a mixture of the two (endoscope-assisted microscopic myringoplasty, microscopic-assisted endoscopic myringoplasty); and (7) subjects unrelated to the researched topic.

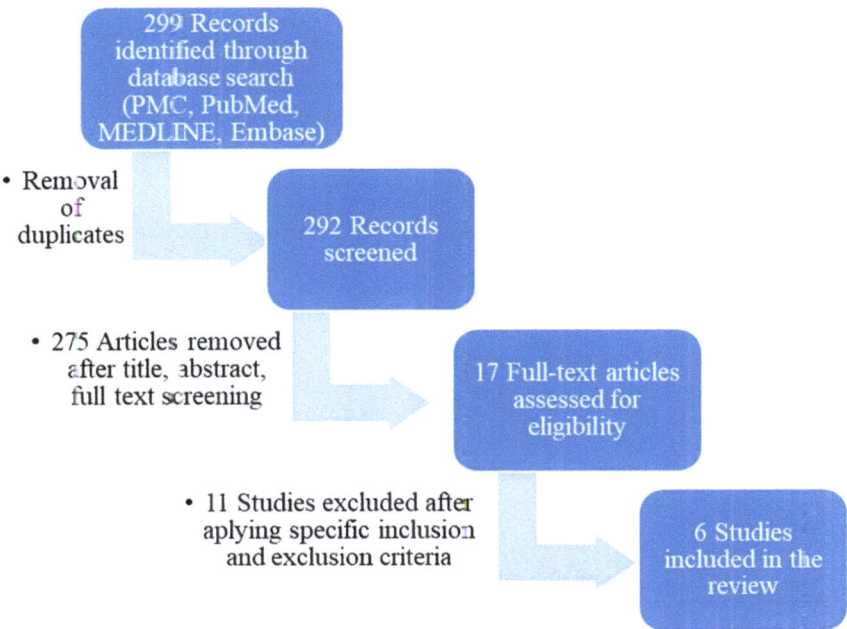

Figure 1. Preferred Reporting Items for Systematic Reviews and Meta-Analyses (PRISMA) flow diagram outlining the study design.

2.3. Data Extraction and Management

Two authors reviewed all the relevant studies and independently extracted the data; any discrepancies were resolved by consensus between the two authors.

For each selected article, the following information was noted in a template built for this study: the author, year of publication, period of the study, type of study, number of patients in total and in each comparative group, mean age of each comparative group, mean follow-up period in each group (Table 1), location and size of perforation, graft material, and graft technique in each comparative group (Table 2), graft success rate for each group, mean pre- and postoperative air–bone gap in each group, mean operative time for each approach (Table 3) and postoperative complications in each group.

Table 1. Baseline characteristics.

Author	Year of Publication	Study Period	Type of Study	Total Patients (n)	EM Patients (n)	MM Patients (n)	EM Age (Years)	MM Age (Years)	EM Follow-Up (Months)	MM Follow-Up (Months)
Secaattin Gulsen, Adem Baltac [15]	2019	2015–2018	RNRC	126 (149 ears)	67 (78 ears)	59 (71 ears)	45.4 (15–61)	54.8 (18–72)	8.2	9.3
Ahmad Daneshi et al. [16]	2020	2014–2016	RNRC	130	75	55	39.85 (18–68)	38.25 (16–77)	12	12
Qimei Yang et al. [17]	2022	2011–2016	RNRC	345	224	121	40.87 (18–67)	38.56 (18–66)	12.74 (6–48)	14.08 (5–35)
Chin-Kuo Chen et al. [18]	2022	2008–2018	RNRC	43	22	21	50.6	45.9	14	13.7
Tzu-Yen Huang et al. [19]	2018	2011–2014	RNRC	95 (100 ears)	47 (50 ears)	48 (50 ears)	54.2	49.9	6	6
A. C. Jyothi et al. [20]	2017	2011–2013	PRC	120	60	60	28.5	31.4	12	12

RNRC = Retrospective non-randomized comparative; PRC = Prospective randomized comparative; EM = Endoscopic myringoplasty; MM = Microscopic myringoplasty.

Table 2. Graft analysis.

Author	EM Graft Material	MM Graft Material	EM Graft Technique	MM Graft Technique
Secaattin Gulsen, Adem Baltacı [15]	Tragal chondroperichondrial	Tragal chondroperichondrial	Underlay	Underlay (postaural)
Ahmad Daneshi et al. [16]	0.5 mm thickness conchal chondroperichondrial	0.5 mm thickness conchal chondroperichondrial	Underlay	Underlay (postaural)
Qimei Yanget et al. [17]	Tragal chondroperichondrial	Temporalis fascia	Underlay	Underlay (postaural)
Chin-Kuo Chen et al. [18]	Postconchal perichondrium	Temporalis fascia	Over-underlay	Over–underlay (postaural)
Tzu-Yen Huang et al. [19]	Tragal perichondrium	Temporalis fascia	Underlay	Underlay (postaural)
A. C. Jyothi et al. [20]	Temporalis fascia	Temporalis fascia	Underlay	Underlay (postaural)

EM = Endoscopic myringoplasty; MM = Microscopic myringoplasty.

Table 3. Outcomes analysis.

Outcome Authors	Graft Success Rate		Pre-op. ABG (dB)		Post-op. ABG (dB)		Mean Operative Time (min)	
	EM	MM	EM	MM	EM	MM	EM	MM
Secaattin Gulsen, Adem Baltacı [15]	94.80%	92.90%	28.9	29.7	8.2	7.9	34.9	52.7
Ahmad Daneshi et al. [16]	97.30%	96.40%	25.2	24.9	15.7	14.4	76.7	161
Qimei Yanget et al. [17]	94.64%	90.90%	19.26	18.13	7.72	8.34	49.22	81.22
Chin-Kuo Chen et al. [18]	86.30%	85.70%	20.7	17.6	10.2	12.5	79.8	99.9
Tzu-Yen Huang et al. [19]	98%	98%	21.6	21.4	13.3	12.5	50.4	75.5
A. C. Jyothi et al. [20]	91.67%	93.30%	34.16	35.54	18	16	60	120

ABG = air–bone gap; EM = endoscopic myringoplasty; MM = microscopic myringoplasty.

3. Results

3.1. Results of the Literature Search

There were 299 articles identified in the databases. After the removal of duplicates, 292 studies remained. These studies were screened via the title, abstract and full-text, when needed, for relevance, leaving 17 studies for full-text review. Applying all the inclusion and exclusion criteria, there were another 11 studies excluded at this stage, leaving 6 eligible studies to be included in the present article [15–20].

The PRISMA flow diagram used to describe the flow of information throughout various phases of the systematic review is displayed in Figure 1.

3.2. Characteristics of the Included Studies

From the selected articles, five were retrospective non-randomized studies and one was a prospective randomized controlled trial.

The enrolled studies were conducted between 2008 and 2018. Four of the studies comprised over 100 patients each, and two of them had fewer than 100.

The total number of patients in the present review is 859 and the total number of ears analyzed is 887. Of these, 57.38% (n = 509) underwent EM and 42.62% (n = 378) MM.

The age of patients ranged from 15 to 77 years, with no significant difference in the mean age between the two comparative groups in each study.

Sex distribution. Overall, 47.26% (n = 406) of patients were male and 52.74% (n = 453) were female. In the EM groups, 50.5% (n = 250) of patients were male and 49.5% (n = 245) were female, whereas in the MM groups 42.86% (n = 156) of patients were male and 57.14% (n = 208) were female.

Perforation characteristics were assessed in four out of six studies with respect to its anatomic localization and size.

Regarding their anatomic localization, tympanic membrane perforations were grouped as central, marginal, anterior and posterior. In two studies, central perforations were more often described [16,18], whereas in one study, anterior perforations were more frequent, with no significant differences between the EM and MM groups [15]. With respect to the perforation size, they were classified as small, medium/moderate, large, subtotal or total, and the distribution of perforation size between the EM and MM groups was assessed. In one study [15], perforations of the tympanic membrane were classified as small (perforation of the tympanic membrane less than 25%), medium (between 25% and 75%) or large (more than 75%). The distribution of perforation size was similar between the EM and MM groups, with no statistically significant differences: 53.8% small, 29.5% medium and 16.7% large perforations in the EM group, and 54.9% small, 30.8% medium and 14.1% large perforations in the MM group. In the second study [16], the size of the perforation was assessed in the same way: small (<25%), moderate (25% to 75%) or large (>75%) of the surface of the tympanic membrane, although the distribution between the two groups was not described, but only general distribution, 18.5% small, 46.2% moderate and 35.4% large perforations. In the third study [17], all ears included in the study had subtotal perforation. Another study [18] included only large-sized perforations: 50–75% (large) or >75% (subtotal) of the pars tensa, with even distribution between the EM and MM groups: 72.7% large perforations and 27.3% subtotal perforations in the EM group and 76.2% large perforations and 23.8% subtotal perforations in the MM group.

Surgical approach. While for all subjects in the EM group the transcanal approach was utilized, those with MM were approached using the retroauricular technique. The surgeries in each study (both endoscopic and microscopic myringoplasties) were performed by the same surgeon.

EM surgical technique (Figure 2). Perforation edges were freshened. Transcanal incisions were made. The tympanomeatal flap was elevated. The fibrous annulus was separated from the tympanic sulcus with the preservation of the chorda tympani nerve, and the middle ear space was reached. The mobility and integrity of the ossicular chain were checked by gentle palpation of the ossicles. The graft was positioned using an underlay technique. The tympanomeatal flap was placed in its original position and tightly supported with Gelfoam.

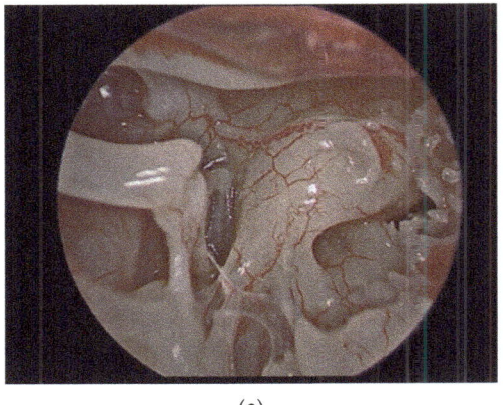 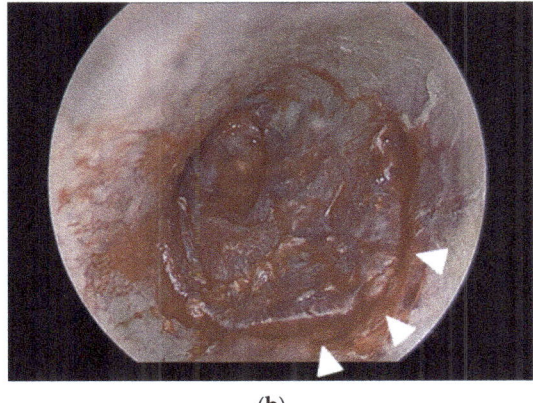

(a) (b)

Figure 2. (a) Endoscopic view of middle ear cavity during endoscopic myringoplasty; (b) view of transcanal incision (white arrow heads) in endoscopic myringoplasty. Final aspect of endoscopic myringoplasty. Adapted with the permission from Ref. [2]. Copyright © 2017 by Korean Society of Otorhinolaryngology-Head and Neck Surgery.

MM surgical technique (Figure 3). The perforation edges were freshened. A postauricular Wilde's incision was performed. The tympanomeatal flap was elevated under the guidance of the surgical microscope. A canalplasty was practiced, when needed, by drilling the bony ear canal. The mobility and the integrity of the ossicular chain were checked. The graft was positioned with the underlay technique. The tympanomeatal flap was placed in its original position and supported with Gelfoam. The postaural wound was sutured and a compressive dressing was applied over it.

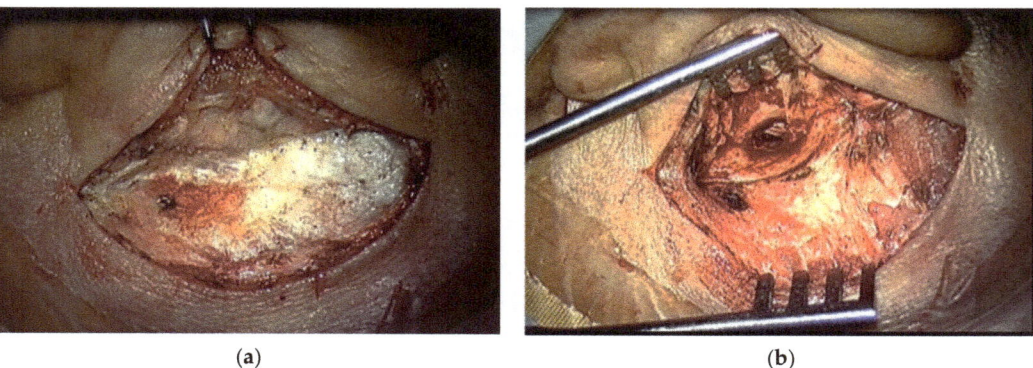

Figure 3. (**a**) Postauricular incision for microscopic postauricular myringoplasty. (**b**) Microscopic view of operation field of myringoplasty. Adapted with the permission from Ref. [2]. Copyright © 2017 by Korean Society of Otorhinolaryngology-Head and Neck Surgery.

The graft material consisted of temporalis fascia, postconchal or tragal perichondrium, full-thickness tragal chondroperichondial graft, or a 0.5 mm-thickness conchal chondroperichondrial graft (Table 2).

The graft technique. An underlay graft technique was the preferred method in five studies, while one study used the over–underlay technique [18].

The *follow-up period* extended between 6 and 12 months.

Outcomes assessed. All studies included data regarding the following outcomes: graft success rate, hearing outcome in terms of pre- and postoperative air–bone gap and the mean operative time, in both groups. All the studies, except one, provided information about the postoperative complications [15–18,20].

3.3. Outcomes Analysis (Table 3)

3.3.1. Graft Success Rate

The graft success rate ranged between 86.30% [18] and 98% [19] in the EM group and between 85.70% [18] and 98% [19] in the MM group. There were no statistically significant differences found between the graft success rates in the EM group and the MM group in each study (Table 2).

3.3.2. Pre-Op and Post-Op ABG

In all studies, Pure Tone Audiometry (PTA) was performed pre- and postoperatively at frequencies of 500, 1000, 2000 and 4000 Hz to determine the Air Conduction (AC) thresholds, Bone Conduction (BC) thresholds and air–bone gap (ABG) values.

Pre-op ABG values ranged from 20.7 dB [18] to 34.16 dB [20] in the EM group and from 17.6 dB [18] to 35.54 dB [20] in the MM group. On the other hand, post-op ABG values ranged from 7.72 dB [17] to 18 dB [20] in the EM group and from 7.9 dB [15] to 16 dB [20] in the MM group. One study found the difference between hearing improvement in the EM group and the MM group being statistically significant at 1 month follow-up in favor of the EM group ($p = 0.063$ [15]), but not at 12 months, and one study found the difference between ABG improvement in the EM group and the MM group being statistically significant at 12 months follow-up in favor of the MM group ($p = 0.0001$ [20]).

3.3.3. Mean Operative Time

All studies reported operation time data. The EM group had a shorter mean operative time than the MM group; this finding was consistent in all studies and statistically significant in five of six studies ($p < 0.05$ [15]; $p < 0.001$ [16]; $p < 0.0001$ [17]; $p = 0.006$ [18]; $p < 0.0001$ [19]). The mean operative time in the EM group varied between 34.9 [15] and 79.8 min [18] and between 52.7 [15] and 161 min [16] in the MM group.

3.3.4. Postoperative Complications

Four of the six studies [15–17,20] investigated postoperative complications that appeared in each group. The reported postoperative complications in the MM groups included: numbness around the ear [15,17], tinnitus [17], wet ear/granulation tissue [16,17,20], abnormal taste/dysgeusia [15,17], postauricular hematoma, wound infection, otitis externa, asymmetry of the auricle and wound dehiscence [15]. For the EM groups, the reported postoperative complications included: tinnitus [17], wet ear/granulation tissue [20], abnormal taste/dysgeusia [15,17] and otitis externa [15].

Postoperative pain was assessed in four studies [16–18,20]; one of them used the WILDA s pain assessment guide [20], two studies used the visual analog scaling (VAS) method (0 for no pain and 10 for the worst pain imaginable) [16,18] and one study only mentioned the percentage of patients that experienced ear pain postoperatively, irrespective of its intensity [17]. In the first case, the pain score was found to be 5 in the MM group as compared to 4 in the EM group [20]. In the studies using the VAS method, the pain scale scores did not differ significantly between the groups in one study [18], while postoperative pain was found to be significantly lower in patients who underwent endoscopic surgery ($p < 0.001$) in the other one [16].

3.4. Subgroup Analysis
3.4.1. Graft Material

Graft material varied between groups and between studies, consisting of either temporalis fascia, postconchal or tragal perichondrium, full-thickness tragal chondroperichondrial graft or a 0.5 mm-thickness conchal chondroperichondrial graft. Temporalis muscle fascia tended to be used more frequently in the MM group [17–20], as the approach was postaural and the graft place was close to the incision site. Tragal/conchal perichondrium as well as tragal/conchal chondroperichondial grafts were used in the EM group [15–18], the last being also used in the MM group in two studies [15,16].

Graft Success Rate

Groups with temporalis fascia grafts had a graft success rate varying from 85.70% [18] to 98% [20], with both the lowest and highest graft success rate values belonging to the MM group.

The graft success rate in groups with tragal chondroperichondrial grafts was between 92.90% in the MM group and 94.80% in the EM group [15], while for conchal chondroperichondrial grafts, success rates varied between 96.40% in the MM group and 97.30% in the EM group [16].

Postconchal perichondrium had a graft success rate of 86.30% [18] and tragal perichondrium of 98% [19], both being surgically placed using an endoscopic approach.

Post-Op AGB

For the temporalis muscle fascia graft, a post-op ABG of 8.34 to 18 dB was noted, with smaller post-op ABGs for MM groups [17–20].

For tragal chondroperichondrial grafts, the smallest post-op ABG was in an EM group (7.72 dB) [17], but similar to the MM group from another study (7.9 dB) [15].

Conchal chondroperichondrial grafts had a comparable mean post-op ABG between the EM and MM groups from the same study: 15.7 dB and 14.4 dB [16].

The smallest mean post-op ABG in the present review was achieved using a tragal chondroperichondrial graft (7.72 dB [17]) and the highest using temporalis fascia (18 dB [20]). Another study revealed very good results regarding post-op ABG using temporalis fascia grafts, of 8.34 dB [17]. Further studies are needed to compare the outcomes of myringoplasty in correlation with the graft material used.

Mean Operative Time

The shortest operative times were noted in both the EM and MM groups that used tragal chondroperichondrial grafts, 34.9 and 52.7 min [15], while the longest mean operative times were needed for myringoplasties that used temporalis fascia as graft material: 120 min, 99.9 min, 81.22 min and 75.5 min [17–20]; but also for 0.5 mm-thickness conchal chondroperichondrial graft, having the longest mean operative time in MM groups: 161 min [16] and almost the longest mean operative time in EM groups: 76.7 min [16].

Nonhomogenous data from the studies on postoperative complications did not allow us to conduct a subgroup analysis for this specific outcome.

3.4.2. Graft Technique

All studies included in the review used the underlay graft technique, except one study that used the over–underlay technique [18]. Looking at this specific study's outcomes in comparison with the other five studies included in the review, the following observations can be made: it has the lowest graft success rates in both the EM and MM groups, the highest mean operative time in EM groups, but satisfactory post-op ABGs in both groups. However, the results cannot be generalized because this study consisted of a small number of patients, collected over a long period of time, including patients from the beginning of the endoscopic era. Further studies are needed to elucidate which graft technique has better outcomes.

4. Discussion

The present review comprised a relatively large number of patients and it revealed a comparable graft success rate between endoscopic and microscopic approaches. The graft success rate via the EM ranged from 86.30% to 98%, which is consistent with that of the MM. There were no statistically significant differences found between graft success rates in the EM group and the MM group in each study.

Age is a factor previously associated with the graft success rate and it might influence the results [21]. In the present review, studies that had similar age distribution between the two groups (EM and MM) were included.

Previous studies suggested that the comparable graft success rate is more likely associated with the grafting technique than surgical approach [22]. In this review, all authors, except one, used the underlay graft technique. Additional studies comparing the different grafting techniques might clarify this aspect.

The graft material could also be considered a variable that might influence postoperative outcomes. Conceptually, one might anticipate significant conductive hearing loss in cartilage myringoplasty, especially in the lower tones, with a tympanic membrane that is rigid and thick. However, in several studies and meta-analyses, the subgroup of full-thickness cartilage grafts revealed a slight, but significantly superior, hearing outcome than the temporalis fascia graft group [23]. Moreover, Gerber et al. demonstrated that cartilage does not impede sound transmission [24]. Four meta-analyses [25–28] and one systemic review [29] showed no difference regarding audiometric results between the cartilage and temporalis fascia grafts. More research is needed in this direction as well. The hearing improvements of EM and MM were comparable, which supported previous studies, suggesting that an endoscopic approach can be a good alternative to microscopic technique for patients with COM that require myringoplasty. In our review, the EM was superior to the MM in terms of operation time and postoperative complications. The mean operative time in EM groups was significantly shorter than that in MM groups. Suturing the postauricular incision in the MM group might extend the operation time. Moreover, postoperative complications seemed to be more likely to appear in the MM group, and they were mostly related to the postaural incision. On the other hand, sometimes, bleeding may be an inconvenience and a time-consuming factor during the endoscopic approach, that could even lead, in some cases, to a conversion to the microscopic approach. Yet, we found the shortest average operative time in EM groups, which is consistent with relevant studies in the literature, and no study included in our review reported incomplete endoscopic surgery with a microscopic conversion due to bleeding. The management of bleeding in endoscopic ear surgery is feasible through widely available hemostatic agents such as the injection of diluted epinephrine, cottonoids soaked with epinephrine (1:1000), mono- or bipolar cautery, washing with hydrogen peroxide, and self-suctioning instruments, and even the highest bleeding scores could be managed in an exclusively endoscopic technique in a study conducted by Anschuetz L. et al. [30].

Looking beyond myringoplasty, the place of the endoscopic approach in middle ear surgery is yet to be established. Further research is needed to make it clear if an endoscopic approach could possibly be superior to a microscopic approach in solving various technical difficulties in more complex procedures than myringoplasty, such as cholesteatoma surgery or congenital anomalies [6,7,31].

Limitations of the Study

There are some limitations to our study that should be addressed in future studies. First, a lack of randomized controlled studies. The retrospective nature of all but one study included in our review is problematic in terms of controlling selection and allocation bias. For instance, in one study, it was suggested to the patients included in the EM group to use this specific approach in their cases in order to decrease postoperative pain [15]. Second, the risk factors that could influence surgical outcomes, such as age and size or site of the tympanic membrane perforation, were inconsistent among some of the included studies. Deviated outcomes are theoretically possible due to these uncontrolled factors. Finally, further larger cohort studies, ideally based on randomized controlled trials, are necessary to support our current interpretations.

5. Conclusions

The endoscopic approach allows the surgeon to perform a minimally invasive transcanal myringoplasty, avoiding surgical scarring, a temporary loss of cutaneous sensation and malposition of the ear, with comparable results to conventional MM in terms of the graft success rates and ABG gain, with a shorter operative time and fewer postoperative complications.

Since EM is an efficient minimally invasive technique, it should always be considered when performing myringoplasty in patients with COM.

Author Contributions: I.S. had equal contribution with C.D.S. in designing the research, data acquisition, analysis and interpretation of data, and wrote the manuscript. V.Z. and R.H. performed the experiments, data acquisition, analysis and interpretation of data and manuscript drafting. A.M.V., I.S. and C.D.S. contributed to statistical analysis, critical revision of the manuscript for important intellectual content. All authors have read and agreed to the published version of the manuscript.

Funding: This research received no external funding.

Institutional Review Board Statement: The study was conducted according to the guidelines of the Declaration of Helsinki, and approved by the Ethics Committee of Institute of Phonoaudiology and Functional ENT Surgery.

Informed Consent Statement: Informed consent was obtained from all subjects during each study included in the review.

Data Availability Statement: Data are available on request to the corresponding author.

Conflicts of Interest: The authors declare no conflict of interest.

References

1. Shakya, D.; Kc, A.; Nepal, A. A Comparative Study of Endoscopic versus Microscopic Cartilage Type I Tympanoplasty. *Int. Arch. Otorhinolaryngol.* **2020**, *24*, e80–e85. [CrossRef]

2. Choi, N.; Noh, Y.; Park, W.; Lee, J.J.; Yook, S.; Choi, J.E.; Chung, W.-H.; Cho, Y.-S.; Hong, S.H.; Moon, I.J. Comparison of endoscopic tympanoplasty to microscopic tympanoplasty. *Clin. Exp. Otorhinolaryngol.* **2017**, *10*, 44–49. [CrossRef] [PubMed]
3. Kang, H.S.; Ahn, S.K.; Jeon, S.Y.; Hur, D.G.; Kim, J.P.; Park, J.J.; Kim, D.W.; Woo, S.H. Sensation recovery of auricle following chronic ear surgery by retroauricular incision. *Eur. Arch. Otorhinolaryngol.* **2012**, *269*, 101–106. [CrossRef] [PubMed]
4. Kozin, E.D.; Gulati, S.; Kaplan, A.B.; Lehmann, A.E.; Remenschneider, A.K.; Alyson Kaplan, B.A.; Landegger, L.D.; Cohen, M.S.; Lee, D.J. Systematic Review of Endoscopic Middle Ear Surgery Outcomes. *Laryngoscope* **2015**, *125*, 1205–1214. [CrossRef] [PubMed]
5. Lee, S.; Cho, H.-H. Transcanal Endoscopic Tympanoplasty for Pediatric Patients Under 15 Years of Age with Chronic Otitis Media. *Clin. Exp. Otorhinolaryngol.* **2020**, *13*, 41–46. [CrossRef]
6. Badr-el-Dine, M. Value of ear endoscopy in cholesteatoma surgery. *Otol. Neurotol.* **2002**, *23*, 631–635. [CrossRef]
7. Thomassin, J.M.; Korchia, D.; Doris, J.M. Endoscopic-guided otosurgery in the prevention of residual cholesteatomas. *Laryngoscope* **1993**, *103*, 939–943. [CrossRef]
8. Zakir, I.; Ahmad, A.N.; Pasha, H.A.; Aqil, S.; Akhtar, S. Comparison of Endoscopic versus Microscopic Tympanoplasty. *Iran J. Otorhinolaryngol.* **2022**, *34*, 139. [CrossRef]
9. Mahawerawat, K.; Kasemsiri, P. Comparison of the clinical outcome of endoscopic push-through myringoplasty and microscopic overlay myringoplasty: Matching co-variated designs. *BMC Surg.* **2022**, *22*, 44. [CrossRef]
10. Pal, R.; Surana, P. Comparative Study between Microscopic and Endoscopic Tympanoplasty Type I. *Indian J. Otorhinolaryngol. Head Neck Surg.* **2019**, *71* (Suppl. S2), 1467–1473. [CrossRef]
11. Zhang, Y.; Wang, W.; Xu, K.; Hu, M.; Ma, Y.; Lin, P. Comparison of clinical outcome between endoscopic and postauricular incision microscopic type-1 tympanoplasty. *Acta Otolaryngol.* **2021**, *141*, 29–33. [CrossRef] [PubMed]
12. Cheng, X.; Wu, S.; Wang, W. Efficacy of Otomicroscopy Combined with Otoendoscopy Double-Lens Technology-Assisted Tympanic Membrane Repair on Elderly Patients with Chronic Suppurative Otitis Media. *Evid. Based Complement. Altern. Med.* **2021**, *2021*, 5164907. [CrossRef] [PubMed]
13. Lee, S.-Y.; Lee, D.Y.; Seo, Y.; Kim, Y.H. Can Endoscopic Tympanoplasty Be a Good Alternative to Microscopic Tympanoplasty? A Systematic Review and Meta-Analysis. *Clin. Exp. Otorhinolaryngol.* **2019**, *12*, 145–155. [CrossRef]
14. Moher, D.; Liberati, A.; Tetzlaff, J.; Altman, D.G.; PRISMA Group. Preferred reporting items for systematic reviews and meta-analyses: The PRISMA statement. *BMJ* **2009**, *339*, b2535. [CrossRef]
15. Gulsen, S.; Baltacı, A. Comparison of endoscopic transcanal and microscopic approach in Type 1 tympanoplasty. *J. Otorhinolaryngol.* **2021**, *87*, 157–163. [CrossRef]
16. Daneshi, A.; Daneshvar, A.; Asghari, A.; Farhadi, M.; Mohebbi, S.; Mohseni, M.; Yazdani, N.; Mohammadi, S.; Hosseinzadeh, F. Endoscopic versus Microscopic Cartilage Myringoplasty in Chronic Otitis Media. *Iran J. Otorhinolaryngol.* **2020**, *32*, 263–269. [CrossRef] [PubMed]
17. Yang, Q.; Wang, B.; Zhang, J.; Liu, H.; Xu, M.; Zhang, W. Comparison of endoscopic and microscopic tympanoplasty in patients with chronic otitis media. *Eur. Arch. Otorhinolaryngol.* **2022**, *279*, 4801–4807. [CrossRef] [PubMed]
18. Chen, C.-K.; Hsu, H.-C.; Wang, M. Endoscopic tympanoplasty with post-conchal perichondrium in repairing large-sized eardrum perforations. *Eur. Arch. Otorhinolaryngol.* **2022**, *279*, 5667–5674. [CrossRef]
19. Huang, T.-Y.; Ho, K.-Y.; Wang, L.-F.; Chien, C.-Y.; Wang, H.-M. A Comparative Study of Endoscopic and Microscopic Approach Type 1 Tympanoplasty for Simple Chronic Otitis Media. *J. Int. Adv. Otol.* **2016**, *12*, 28–31. [CrossRef]
20. Jyothi, A.C.; Shrikrishna, B.H.; Kulkarni, N.H.; Kumar, A. Endoscopic Myringoplasty versus Microscopic Myringoplasty in Tubotympanic CSOM: A Comparative Study of 120 Cases. *Indian J. Otolaryngol. Head Neck Surg.* **2017**, *69*, 357–362. [CrossRef]
21. Tseng, C.C.; Lai, M.T.; Wu, C.C.; Yuan, S.P.; Ding, Y.F. Endoscopic transcanal myringoplasty for anterior perforations of the tympanic membrane. *JAMA Otolaryngol. Head Neck Surg.* **2016**, *142*, 1088–1093. [CrossRef]
22. Tseng, C.C.; Lai, M.T.; Wu, C.C.; Yuan, S.P.; Ding, Y.F. Comparison of the efficacy of endoscopic tympanoplasty and microscopic tympanoplasty: A systematic review and meta-analysis. *Laryngoscope* **2017**, *127*, 1890–1896. [CrossRef]
23. Yang, T.; Wu, X.; Peng, X.; Zhang, Y.; Xie, S.; Sun, H. Comparison of cartilage graft and fascia in type 1 tympanoplasty: Systematic review andmeta-analysis. *Acta Otolaryngol.* **2016**, *136*, 1085–1090. [CrossRef] [PubMed]
24. Gerber, M.J.; Mason, J.C.; Lambert, P.R. Hearing results after primary cartilage tympanoplasty. *Laryngoscope* **2000**, *110*, 1994–1999. [CrossRef] [PubMed]
25. Iacovou, E.; Vlastarakos, P.V.; Papacharalampous, G.; Kyrodimos, E.; Nikolopoulos, T.P. Is cartilage better than temporalis muscle fascia in type I tympanoplasty? Implications for current surgical practice. *Eur. Arch. Otorhinolaryngol.* **2013**, *270*, 2803–2813. [CrossRef] [PubMed]
26. Jalali, M.M.; Motasaddi, M.; Kouhi, A.; Dabiri, S.; Robabeh Soleimani, R. Comparison of cartilage with temporalis fascia tympanoplasty: A meta-analysis of comparative studies. *Laryngoscope* **2017**, *127*, 2139–2148. [CrossRef]
27. Jeffery, C.C.; Shillington, C.; Andrews, C.; Ho, A. The palisade cartilage tympanoplasty technique: A systematic review and metaanalysis. *Otolaryngol. Head Neck Surg.* **2017**, *46*, 48–51. [CrossRef]
28. Lyons, S.A.; Su, T.; Vissers, L.E.; Peters, J.P.; Smit, A.L.; Grolman, W. Fascia compared to one-piece composite cartilage-perichondrium grafting for tympanoplasty. *Laryngoscope* **2016**, *126*, 1662–1670. [CrossRef]
29. Mohamad, S.; Khan, I.; Hussain, S.M. Is cartilage tympanoplasty more effective than fascia tympanoplasty? A systematic review. *Otol. Neurotol.* **2012**, *33*, 699–705. [CrossRef]

30. Anschuetz, L.; Bonali, M.; Guarino, P.; Fabbri, F.B.; Alicandri-Ciufelli, M.; Villari, D.; Caversaccio, M.; Presutti, L. Management of Bleeding in Exclusive Endoscopic Ear Surgery: Pilot Clinical Experience. *Otolaryngol. Head Neck Surg.* **2017**, *157*, 700–706. [CrossRef]
31. Gheorghe, D.C.; Epure, V.; Oprea, D.; Zamfir-Chiru-Anton, A. Persistent Stapedial Artery, Oval Window Atresia and Congenital Stapes Agenesis—Case Report. *Medicina* **2023**, *59*, 461. [CrossRef] [PubMed]

Disclaimer/Publisher's Note: The statements, opinions and data contained in all publications are solely those of the individual author(s) and contributor(s) and not of MDPI and/or the editor(s). MDPI and/or the editor(s) disclaim responsibility for any injury to people or property resulting from any ideas, methods, instructions or products referred to in the content.

Case Report

Persistent Stapedial Artery, Oval Window Atresia and Congenital Stapes Agenesis—Case Report

Dan Cristian Gheorghe [1,2], Veronica Epure [1,2,*], Doru Oprea [2] and Adina Zamfir-Chiru-Anton [3]

1. ENT Department, University of Medicine and Pharmacy Carol Davila Bucharest, 050474 Bucharest, Romania
2. ENT Department, MS Curie Hospital, 077120 Bucharest, Romania
3. ENT Department, Grigore Alexandrescu Emergency Hospital for Children, 011743 Bucharest, Romania
* Correspondence: veronica_epure@yahoo.co.uk; Tel.: +40-214-604-260

Abstract: *Background*: The persistent stapedial artery (PSA) is a rare congenital vascular malformation involving the middle ear. It is usually associated with pulsatile tinnitus and/or conductive hearing loss and can account for multiple risks during middle ear surgery. *Case Report*: we present a case of a 9-year-old male child with conductive hearing loss and persistent stapedial artery in his right ear, who was admitted to our ENT Department for hearing loss. During surgery, we discovered PSA along with congenital stapes agenesis and oval window atresia, as well as an abnormal trajectory of the mastoid segment of the facial nerve. After ossicular reconstruction (transcanal total ossicular replacement prosthesis) with cochleostomy, no surgical complications were recorded and hearing improvement was monitored by pre- and postoperative audiometry. *Conclusion*: Stapedial artery is a rare anatomical middle ear abnormality that can prevent proper surgical hearing restoration and can be associated with other simultaneous temporal bone malformations.

Keywords: persistent stapedial artery; cochleostomy; ossiculoplasty

1. Introduction

The persistent stapedial artery (PSA) is a rare vascular congenital abnormality originating from the second aortic arch, with a prevalence of 0.02–0.48% (5 out of 1045) as a temporal bone study shows [1]. Across embryonic development it connects the external and internal carotid arteries, only to involute during the 10th week of fetal development [2]. During this time, it shapes the stapes suprastructure as it passes along the promontory and then the obturator foramen, on its course from its origin in the external carotid artery to the middle cranial fossa, usually through a bony dehiscence of the facial canal wall just posterior from the cochleariform process; all the four subtypes of PSA described have in common that the PSA runs over the promontory and courses through the obturator foramen of the stapes to enter the facial canal. After exiting the facial canal just before the geniculate ganglion, the PSA travels anteriorly and cranially into the extradural space of the middle cranial fossa. If the stapedial artery persists into postnatal life, it supplies the middle meningeal artery.

PSA varies anatomically and among the known types there are described: the hyoido-stapedial artery, the pharyngo-stapedial artery, the stapedial artery with aberrant carotid artery and the pharyngo-hyo-stapedial artery, with the first type being the most described in literature. It is often an incidental discovery (discovered on CT scan images or intraoperatively during middle ear surgery), as it is mostly asymptomatic. It can also be associated with tinnitus, conductive hearing loss (by limiting the movement of the stapes, thereby mimicking otosclerosis), unilateral or bilateral pulsatile tinnitus or even dizziness or vertigo [3]. Sensorineural hearing loss has also been reported as a consequence of erosion of the otic capsule [4].

Given the anatomical variations of PSA and its trajectory through the middle ear, the surgeon must consider the risk of facial palsy, hearing loss, hemiplegia and account for the possibility of an aberrant internal carotid artery which can emerge in the hypotympanum without bone protection and can be easily injured during middle ear exploration [5]. Still, the utmost clinical significance is the hemorrhage as a consequence of accidental injury of the vessel. Other middle ear anomalies can be discovered in patients with PSA, from facial nerve anomalies [6,7], various blood vessel anomalies [8], to different stapes deformities [9–11].

The golden standard for diagnosing PSA is computed tomography (CT) scan which displays the absence of foramen spinosum and the abnormal widening of the anterior fallopian canal. Angiography, magnetic resonance angiography (MRA) or magnetic resonance imaging (MRI) scan are the only imaging tests which could specifically exhibit the artery and they might prove useful only in selected cases if one considers the variable diameter of this vessel (0.4–2 mm) [3].

We report a case of persistent stapedial artery associated with other rare middle ear malformations in a paediatric patient; informed written consent from the child's parents and approval from the Hospital's Ethics Committee were obtained (approval no. 45595/21 October 2022).

2. Case Presentation

We present the case of a 6-year-old male child who was first examined in our Department for bilateral hearing loss.

From history, the child was born by vaginal delivery, on term, and had no past medical problems. We also made the diagnosis of bilateral mixed hearing loss, with an air-bone gap (ABG) of 35 and 40 dB at 1000 Hz, respectively, and normal bilateral type A tympanogram (Figure 1). As such, the audiological investigations suggested an ossicular chain fixation.

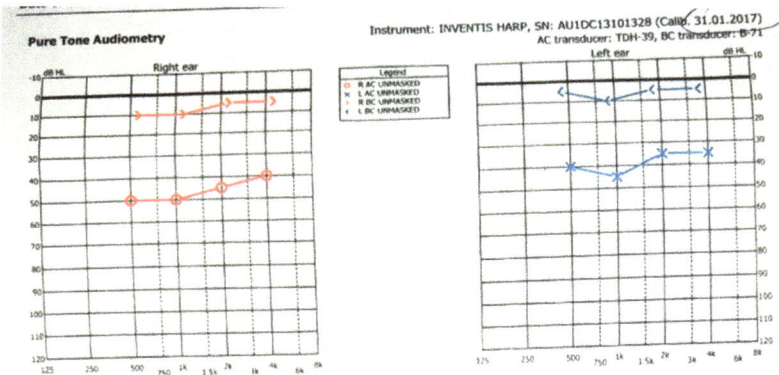

Figure 1. Audiogram from 31 January 2017 (Child age—6 years) showing bilateral conductive hearing loss with air-bone gap, suggesting bilateral middle ear affliction.

No family history of hearing problems could be elicited. A high resolution CT scan revealed bilateral middle ear anomalies. There were no images of the oval window and stapes suprastructure in his left ear, with abnormal facial nerve canal position and patent foramen spinosum (Figures 2 and 3). The stapes suprastructure and the oval window were also missing to the contralateral (right) ear with a wide facial nerve canal between the geniculate and the round window niche and an abnormal traject on its mastoid segment. No foramen spinosum was observable on the right side (Figures 4–6). Furthermore, surgery was carefully planned to investigate the middle ear.

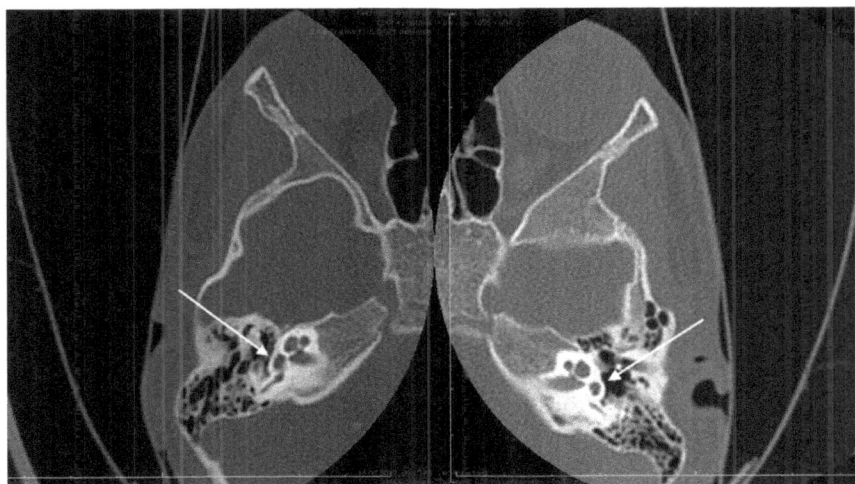

Figure 2. High resolution axial CT scan of left temporal bone showing a missing oval window and stapes suprastructure (arrow) on both sides.

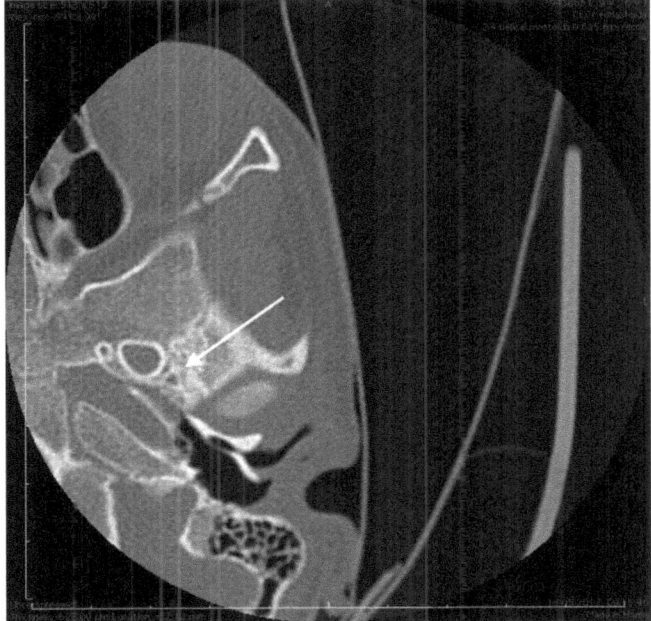

Figure 3. High resolution axial CT scan of left temporal bone exposing the patent foramen spinosum (arrow).

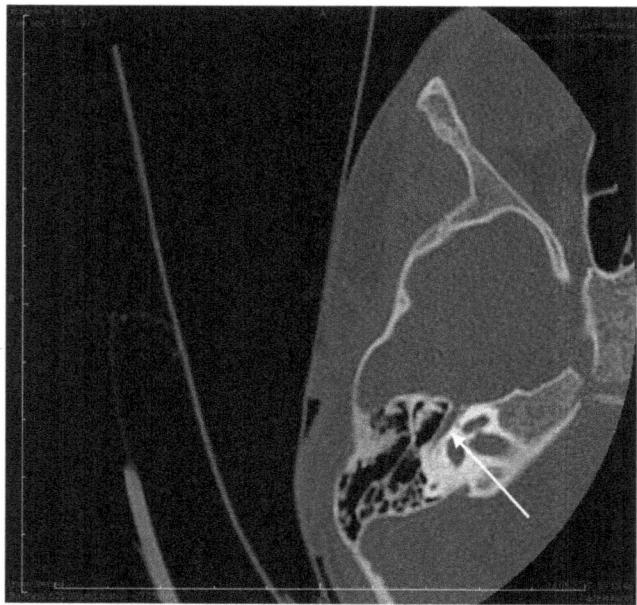

Figure 4. High resolution axial CT scan of right temporal bone exposing the unusual wide facial canal and the missing oval window on the right side (arrow).

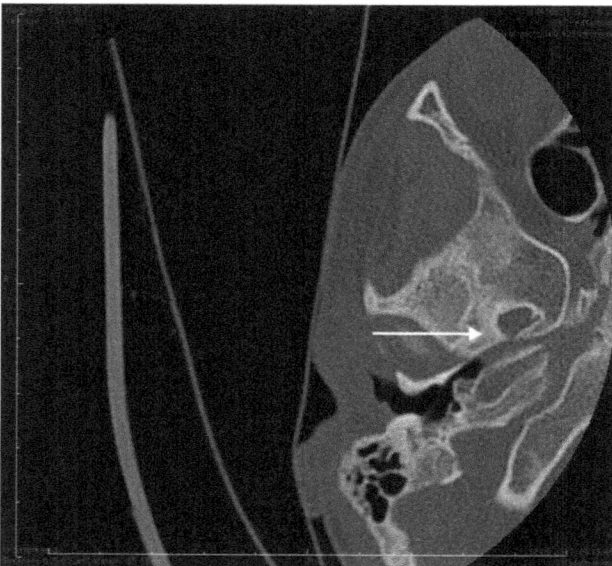

Figure 5. High resolution axial CT scan of right temporal bone exposing the missing foramen spinosum (arrow).

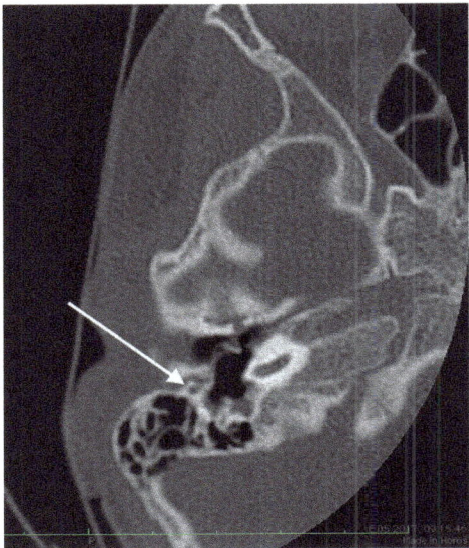 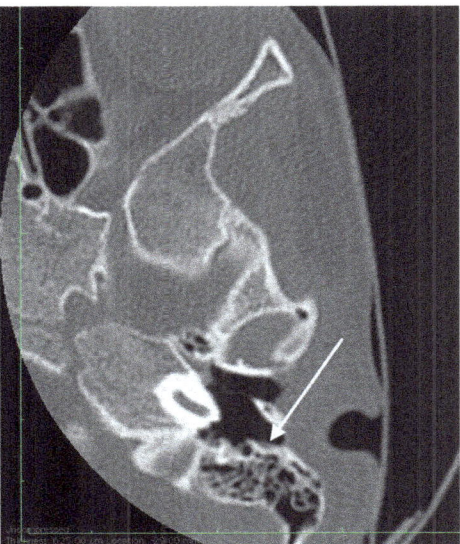

Figure 6. Abnormal position of the facial nerves in their mastoid segment, bilaterally (arrows).

The middle ear exploration of the right ear discovered a bright red pulsatile vessel across the promontory, in a cranial to caudal position, covering the round window and associating the absence of the stapes and the oval window. The diagnostic of persistent stapedial artery (PSA) was made, which resulted in postponing the right ear ossicular chain reconstruction.

During the following 3 years the child underwent surgical approaches for his left ear hearing loss. Stapes agenesis, but with oval window presence were recorded, with no associated PSA on that side. A stapedotomy and a Teflon wire piston attached to the incus were performed for reconstruction of the ossicular chain. This was followed by two other consecutive ossicular chain release surgeries, due to recurrent bony fixation of the incus and malleus to the middle ear walls, as observed intraoperatively. Hearing in the left ear had later degraded, as the monitoring audiograms showed, with minor improvement of the ABP persisting on long term follow-up (from 51.6 dB preoperatively to 41.6 dB after surgery).

Hearing loss in patient's right ear (with PSA) was addressed by performing an ossiculoplasty with a total ossicular replacement prosthesis (TORP). After a thorough preoperative planning based on prior surgical middle ear exploration and CT imaging, a transcanalar approach to the middle ear was used. A standard tympanomeatal flap was raised and the PSA was inspected. Large dimensions, complete coverage of the oval window site and crossing over the round window niche were again noted (Figure 7). The PSA went superiorly across the promontory and entered the facial nerve canal at the level where the normal oval window niche would have been located. Successful cochleostomy was carried out with a diamond burr posteriorly to the PSA and inferiorly to the facial nerve canal. Perichondrium was used to seal the cochlea opening and also served as a support for a total replacement ossicular prosthesis (Figure 8). The TORP was seated in place and covered with a mixed graft of cartilage and perichondrium with the tympanic membrane on top of it (Figures 9 and 10).

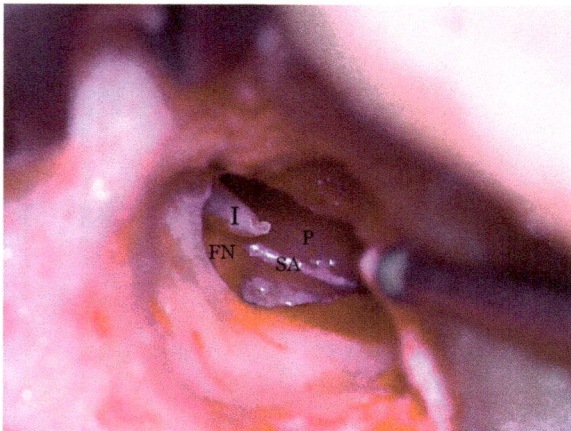

Figure 7. Transcanalar microscopic aspect of right middle ear: the Stapedial Artery (SA) can be seen runnning across the promontory (P) and joining with the facial nerve (FN) right under the incus (I) long process.

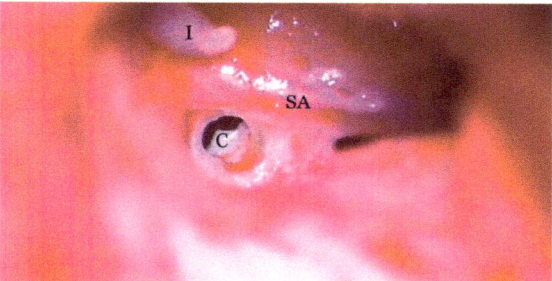

Figure 8. Transcanalar microscopic aspect of the right middle ear: the cochleostomy (C) orifice can be observed in the near vecinity of the stapedial artery (SA) and facial nerve (FN). The long process of the incus (I) can also be observed.

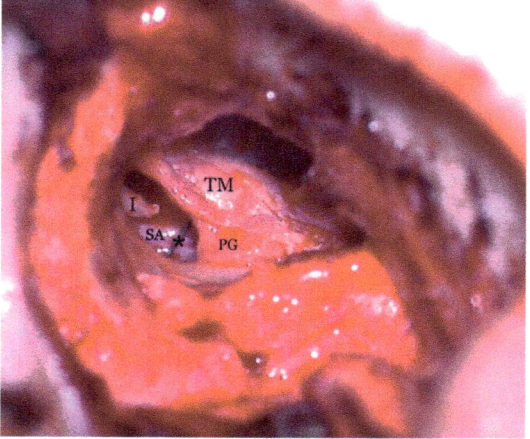

Figure 9. Transcanalar microscopic aspect of middle and external right ear: the handle of the TORP (*) can be observed lying in close contact with the stapedial artery (SA). The perichondrium graft (PG) stands between the plate of the TORP and the tympanomeatal flap (TM). (I) incus long process.

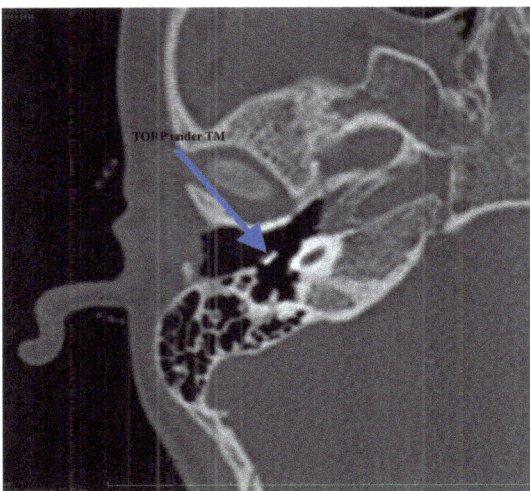

Figure 10. Final aspect of the right ear, with the perichondrium graft (PG) going under the tympanomeatal flap (TM) and sealing the middle ear space

The patient reported immediate postoperative good hearing but failed to present at our Department for performing an audiogram. His hearing was firstly evaluated at 2 months after right ear surgery demonstrating an air-bone gap of 41.6 dB (from 56.5 dB preoperatively). We could not explain at that moment the results but, at 9 months after surgery we were able to have another CT scan performed. The imaging showed good positioning of the ossicular prosthesis (Figures 10 and 11). Without surgical investigation of the middle ear is it impossible to know the precise reason why the hearing restoration is not as good as we expected. We can hypothesize about local healing changes but we cannot be sure.

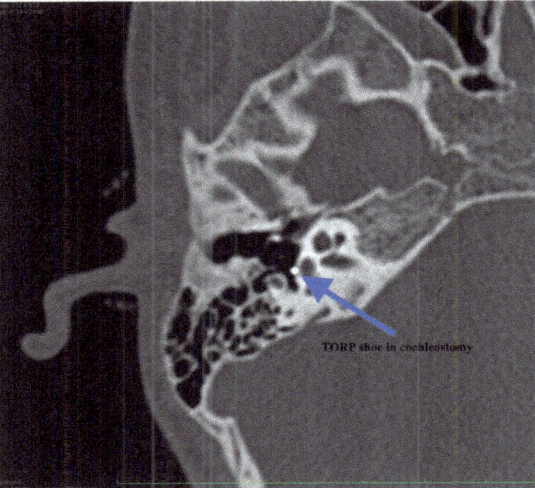

Figure 11. CT scan at 9 months after surgery, showing proper positioning of the prosthesis: TORP shoe in the cochleostomy.

Future surgical alternative approaches were contemplated in this case for hearing rehabilitation, considering the presented abnormalities, and the patient has been planned for osseointegrated implant surgery (OSIA).

3. Discussion

PSA is a rare condition of the middle ear, with an estimated incidence of 0.02–0.5%, discovered mostly incidentally, thus creating a great impact on surgeons who can be forced to discontinue interventions, such as Govaerts et al. show in their paper [12].

It evolves during embryologic stages from the hyoid artery, a branch of the external carotid artery which derives from the pharyngeal artery in the second aortic arch [13]. It runs across the promontory and shapes the stapes by passing between the crura. Above this point, it divides into an upper and a lower division, supplying the dura mater through the middle meningeal artery, the orbit, maxillary and mandibular structure through its other branches [14]. Its passage through the crus of the stapes limits the size of the artery, which can no longer supply the necessary blood to the final structures over a certain body size. This, and the later connection of the internal and external carotid artery through the anastomosis between the maxillomandibular division of the stapedial artery and the distal ventral pharyngeal artery, promote the involution of the stapedial artery in normal humans [15].

Understanding the embryological development of PSA can increase the confidence of handling it, either by cutting or coagulating it with CO_2 laser or simply avoiding it when possible. In our presented case, the large diameter of the vessel (possibly favored by stapes absence) prevented us from trying to coagulate or manipulate it, thus avoiding a high-risk bleeding that would have made the intervention impossible to be continued or extend it beyond its rehabilitation purposes. The absence of the stapes and the oval window, which would have oriented us towards a stapedotomy, forced us to perform a cochleostomy, while avoiding PSA trajectory.

The multitude of divisions of the stapedial artery pave the way for multiple anatomical variations of the PSA. Apart from this variety of anatomical disposals, literature review demonstrates that PSA is often associated with other middle ear structure deviations, like stapes footplate ankylosis [10,11], malformed stapes suprastructure [13], malpositioned facial nerve [7] or thickened middle ear mucosa that hides the PSA [9]. Particular to our case, we noted the PSA to be accompanied by bilateral congenital stapes agenesis, unilateral oval window atresia and bilateral abnormal facial nerve canal position. Since the first documentation of PSA existence (Hyrtl, 1836) we could only find few literature references about similar conditions, and only in one single reported case (Hoogland and Marres, 1977) PSA was associated with oval window atresia and aberrant stapes suprastructure.

Preoperative CT imaging of middle ear surgery patients is mandatory and careful interpretation of the results can sometimes prevent accidental injuries brought to a PSA. The usual findings are a small, abnormal, canaliculus leaving the carotid canal or the facial nerve, a straight line structure crossing over the promontory, an unusual widening of the fallopian canal or a different canal parallel to it between the geniculate and the oval window niche and absence of the foramen spinosum [16]. Our CT findings coincide with some of the aforementioned signs, as there can be seen no trace of the foramen spinosum in the affected ear (Figure 5), in contrast to the contralateral ear (Figure 3). There is also a widening of the facial nerve canal that can be observed in Figure 4. It came as no surprise that the stapes could not be described in the CT images, as the literature review acknowledges the possible stapes malformations that come along with PSA.

Even if there are many reports on CT findings and embryologic explanations on persistent stapedial artery, there are few literature data regarding the main surgical approaches to the persistent stapedial artery, as this can be an incidental CT or intraoperative finding complicating middle ear surgery or cochlear implantation, always a great dilemma to the surgeon, who must decide whether to abort or complete the procedure and how to manage the PSA. Successful surgical implantation in the presence of PSA has been described by some authors [17], also reconstruction of the ossicular chain (PORP, TPRP). stapes surgery without transaction of the PSA (stapedectomy with intact PSA—Baron 1963, House 1964, Pahor 1992; stapedotomy with intact PSA—Govaerts 1993, with profuse bleeding or floating footplate as complications, Pirodda 1994; maleostapedotomy with intact PSA—Sugimoto 2014) (reported in 9 ears) [18], stapes surgery combined with transaction of PSA (in 5 operated ears—PSA sectioned by Schweitzer 1984, Yamamoto 1988, Karosi 2008 with minor intraoperative bleeding; PSA transected by laser coagulation or cauterisation by Murphy 1995, Silbergleit 2000, Hitier, Goderie 2013, with intact stapes; clips on PSA by Fisch 1980, Araujo 2002, with intact stapes) have been described [18], sometimes with good hearing outcomes (hearing improvement and subsiding of the pulsatile tinnitus), manageable preoperative bleeding in four patients and no significant postoperative sequelae. Cited complications of surgery in cases of PSA are: profuse or minor intraoperative bleeding (controlled by pressure on the vessel, bipolar coagulation, Tabotamp application), floating footplate with consequent abortion of procedure [18].

Being sometimes asymptomatic, the act to manipulate the PSA or avoid it is a decision each surgeon has to take during intervention, based on the patients' needs and considering the significant risk of permanent hemiplegia, facial nerve paralysis, tabes dorsalis-like symptoms, and hearing loss, even if multiple papers describe successful discontinuations of the artery, as well. Carefully preparing of the surgery cannot rule out the possibility of misinterpreting the presence of the PSA but certain anatomical aspects of the CT imaging specific to the PSA can warn the surgeon of such possible malformation of the middle ear, thus making the approach more cautious.

Considering our case once again, we could try stapedial artery coagulation but with the risk of neurologic damage or impossibility to achieve useful hemostasis. That would have also incurred the presence of a normal oval window, in order to use it for TORP reconstruction. In our case, no such structure existed, leaving just the cochleostomy option as the only approach. We can also mention that the inferior traject of the stapedial artery partially covered the round window niche. Its presence and free movement is also important to consider when functional reconstruction is the target.

4. Conclusions

PSA is a rare disease, sometimes difficult to diagnose before surgery, even with imaging. Middle ear surgery in the presence of a PSA is possible without any major complications, but the surgeon alone must decide whether to manipulate the artery from its bed or to coagulate it. High resolution CT imaging is a good tool to assess the possibility of any middle ear associated abnormalities. Dimension of the artery is the main risk factor for final surgical outcome and intraoperative complications. Cochleostomy and ossicular chain reconstruction could represent an effective approach to managing hearing loss in cases with PSA. Different possible types of ossicular chain replacement prosthesis could eventually yield better results, in terms of hearing restoration.

Author Contributions: D.C.G.—writing—original draft, methodology, analysis, software; V.E., D.O.—data gathering, writing—review and editing; A.Z.-C.-A.—supervision and writing—review and editing. All authors have read and agreed to the published version of the manuscript.

Funding: This research received no external funding.

Institutional Review Board Statement: This study was conducted in accordance with the Declaration of Helsinki and approved by the Ethics Committee of M.S. Curie Hospital.

Informed Consent Statement: Written informed consent was obtained from the patient's parents both for diagnosis, surgery and inclusion in the study

Data Availability Statement: Data available on request to the corresponding author.

Conflicts of Interest: The authors declare no conflict of interest.

Abbreviations

PSA	persistent stapedial artery
TORP	total ossicular replacement prosthesis
CT	computed tomography
MRA	magnetic resonance angiography
MRI	magnetic resonance imaging
PG	perichondrium graft
TM	tympanomeatal flap
I	incus
SA	stapedial artery
FN	facial nerve
C	cochleostomy
P	promontory
ABG	air-bone gap

References

1. Moreano, E.H.; Paparella, M.M.; Zelterman, D.; Goycoolea, M.V. Prevalence of facial canal dehiscence and of persistent stapedial artery in the human middle ear: A report of 1000 temporal bones. *Laryngoscope* **1994**, *104 Pt 1*, 309–320. [CrossRef] [PubMed]
2. Hogg, I.D.; Stephens, C.B.; Arnold, G.E. Theoretical anomalies of the stapedial artery. *Ann. Otol. Rhinol. Laryngol.* **1972**, *81*, 860–870. [CrossRef] [PubMed]
3. Silbergleit, R.; Quint, D.J.; Mehta, B.A.; Patel, S.C.; Metes, J.J.; Noujaim, S.E. The persistent stapedial artery. *AJNR Am. J. Neuroradiol.* **2000**, *21*, 572–577. [PubMed]
4. Davies, D.G. Persistent stapedial artery: A temporal bone report. *J. Laryngol. Otol.* **1967**, *81*, 649–660. [CrossRef] [PubMed]
5. Celebi, I.; Oz, A.; Yildirim, H.; Bankeroglu, H.; Basak, M. A case of an aberrant internal carotid artery with a persistent stapedial artery: Association of hypoplasia of the A1 segment of the anterior cerebral artery. *Surg. Radiol. Anat.* **2012**, *34*, 665–670. [CrossRef] [PubMed]
6. Cureoglu, S.; Schachern, P.A.; Paparella, M.M. Persistent stapedial artery. *Otol. Neurotol.* **2003**, *24*, 833–834. [CrossRef] [PubMed]
7. Horn, K.L.; Visvanathan, A. Stapes surgery in the obscured oval window: Management of the ptotic facial nerve and the persistent stapedial artery. *Oper. Tech. Otolaryngol. Head Neck Surg.* **1998**, *9*, 58–63. [CrossRef]
8. Lau, C.C.; Oghalai, J.S.; Jackler, R.K. Combination of aberrant internal carotid artery and persistent stapedial artery. *Otol. Neurotol.* **2004**, *25*, 850–851. [CrossRef] [PubMed]
9. Karosi, T.; Szabo, L.Z.; Petko, M.; Sziklai, I. Otosclerotic stapes with three crura and persisting stapedial artery. *Otol. Neurotol.* **2008**, *29*, 1043–1044. [CrossRef] [PubMed]
10. Sugimoto, H.; Ito, M.; Hatano, M.; Yoshizaki, T. Persistent stapedial artery with stapes ankylosis. *Auris Nasus Larynx* **2014**, *41*, 582–585. [CrossRef] [PubMed]
11. Hill, F.C.; Teh, B.; Tykocinski, M. Persistent stapedial artery with ankylosis of the stapes footplate. *Ear Nose Throat J.* **2018**, *97*, 227–228. [CrossRef] [PubMed]
12. Govaerts, P.J.; Marquet, T.F.; Cremers, W.R.; Offeciers, F.E. Persistent stapedial artery: Does it prevent successful surgery? *Ann. Otol. Rhinol. Laryngol.* **1993**, *102*, 724–728. [CrossRef] [PubMed]
13. Marion, M.; Hinojosa, R.; Khan, A.A. Persistence of the stapedial artery: A histopathologic study. *Otolaryngol. Head Neck Surg.* **1985**, *93*, 298–312. [CrossRef] [PubMed]
14. Rodesch, G.; Choi, I.S.; Lasjaunias, P. Complete persistence of the hyoido-stapedial artery in man. Case report. Intra-petrous origin of the maxillary artery from ICA. *Surg. Radiol. Anat.* **1991**, *13*, 63–65. [CrossRef] [PubMed]
15. LoVerde, Z.J.; Shlapak, D.P.; Benson, J.C.; Carlson, M.L.; Lane, J.I. The Many Faces of Persistent Stapedial Artery: CT Findings and Embryologic Explanations. *AJNR Am. J. Neuroradiol.* **2021**, *42*, 160–166. [CrossRef] [PubMed]
16. Thiers, F.A.; Sakai, O.; Poe, D.S.; Curtin, H.D. Persistent stapedial artery: CT findings. *AJNR Am. J. Neuroradiol.* **2000**, *21*, 1551–1554. [PubMed]
17. Jones, H.; Hintze, J.; Gendre, A.; Wijaya, C.; Glynn, F.; Viani, L.; Walshe, P. Persistent Stapedial Artery Encountered during Cochlear Implantation. *Case Rep. Otolaryngol.* **2022**, *2022*, 8179062. [CrossRef] [PubMed]
18. Goderie, T.P.M.; Hussain, W.; Alkhateeb, F.; Smit, C.F.; Hensen, E.F. Surgical Management of a Persistent Stapedial Artery: A Review. *Otol. Neurotol.* **2017**, *38*, 788–791. [CrossRef] [PubMed]

Disclaimer/Publisher's Note: The statements, opinions and data contained in all publications are solely those of the individual author(s) and contributor(s) and not of MDPI and/or the editor(s). MDPI and/or the editor(s) disclaim responsibility for any injury to people or property resulting from any ideas, methods, instructions or products referred to in the content.

MDPI
St. Alban-Anlage 66
4052 Basel
Switzerland
www.mdpi.com

Medicina Editorial Office
E-mail: medicina@mdpi.com
www.mdpi.com/journal/medicina

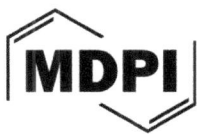

Disclaimer/Publisher's Note: The statements, opinions and data contained in all publications are solely those of the individual author(s) and contributor(s) and not of MDPI and/or the editor(s). MDPI and/or the editor(s) disclaim responsibility for any injury to people or property resulting from any ideas, methods, instructions or products referred to in the content.

www.ingramcontent.com/pod-product-compliance
Lightning Source LLC
LaVergne TN
LVHW070502100526
838202LV00014B/1773